A
BIOGRAPHICAL DICTIONARY
OF WOMEN HEALERS

A
BIOGRAPHICAL DICTIONARY
OF WOMEN HEALERS

Midwives, Nurses, and Physicians

Laurie Scrivener and J. Suzanne Barnes
with contributions by
Cecelia M. Brown and Dana Tuley-Williams

ORYX PRESS
Westport, Connecticut • London

The rare Arabian Oryx is believed to have inspired the myth of the unicorn. This desert antelope became virtually extinct in the early 1960s. At that time, several groups of international conservationists arranged to have nine animals sent to the Phoenix Zoo to be the nucleus of a captive breeding herd. Today, the Oryx population is over 1,000, and over 500 have been returned to the Middle East.

Library of Congress Cataloging-in-Publication Data

A biographical dictionary of women healers : midwives, nurses, and physicians / Laurie Scrivener . . . [et al.].
    p. cm.
   Includes bibliographical references and index.
   ISBN 1–57356–219–X (alk. paper)
   1. Women healers—Biography—Dictionaries. 2. Women in medicine—Biography—Dictionaries. 3. Women physicians—Biography—Dictionaries. I. Scrivener, Laurie.
   R692.B52 2002
   610'.82'0922—dc21   2001058031
   [B]

British Library Cataloguing in Publication Data is available.

Library of Congress Catalog Card Number: 2001058031
ISBN: 1–57356–219–X

First published in 2002

Oryx Press, 88 Post Road West, Westport, CT 06881
An imprint of Greenwood Publishing Group, Inc.
www.oryxpress.com

Printed in the United States of America

The paper used in this book complies with the Permanent Paper Standard issued by the National Information Standards Organization (Z39.48–1984).

10 9 8 7 6 5 4 3 2 1

Contents

Preface

Women have always been healers; they have helped each other through the birthing process, nursed the sick and wounded, and sought cures for illnesses and injuries. The names and biographical details of most of these women were never recorded or were not preserved; sometimes their work was taken for granted as part of women's traditional role as nurturers, sometimes it was overshadowed by the achievements of medical men, and sometimes it was forgotten through the accidents of history.

This book is meant to recognize and honor women healers; it summarizes the lives of 238 significant or representative women whose life stories were not lost. For the high school or college student, it serves as an introduction to the lives of these healers; some students may be inspired to do further research on them or to become healers themselves. For women's studies scholars, biographers, and historians of science, medicine, or nursing, we hope that they find the biographies useful starting points for more in-depth research. Each biography provides references for further reading and study.

Although women healers have worked, and are working, in many different occupations, this book is limited to those engaged in the "core" professions of midwifery, nursing, and medicine (exclusive of psychiatry) and whose careers were/are primarily spent in the United States and Canada, from colonial times to the present. A number of those who initially practiced one of the healing arts but who later became administrators, researchers, teachers, or leaders in professional organizations are also included. We have made a particular effort to include biographies of women who either devoted their careers and lives to caring for women or were advocates for women's entering and succeeding in the healing professions. Some of the women included here were notable firsts in their fields, such as Dr. Elizabeth Blackwell, or women who made significant achievements in their professions, such as nurse Adelaide Nutting; others, such as midwife Pearlie Burton and physician Florence Huson, are representative of the countless unknown women who quietly went about their craft and were forgotten by history.

With few exceptions, the women in this book are labeled as midwives (43), nurses (82), or physicians (113). Past figures are emphasized over present ones, except in the case of midwives. We have adopted broad interpretations of these three professional categories, making allowances for historical changes in the professions and changes in the circumstances of women's employment in them. Thus, the category of "physician" here includes women who were denied admittance to medical schools but who sought training through informal methods, as well as women with traditional training in medical schools. Elizabeth Blackwell, for example, the first woman to earn an M.D., was admitted to the all-male Geneva Medical College in western New York and graduated in 1849. Most women who sought to become physicians in the nineteenth century, however, were denied entrance into medical schools and were denied practical clinical experience as well; they had to seek training through preceptorships or self-study and had to establish their own medical schools and hospitals. The first women's medical school was the Female (later, Woman's) Medical College of Pennsylvania in Philadelphia, established in 1850. "Sectarian" medical schools (homeopathic, botanic, hydropathic, or other nonconventional schools) were quicker to admit women than conventional institutions; hence, many early women physicians sought training at these institutions, and a number of these women are listed here. (Present-day physicians practicing what is now considered to be alternative or complementary medicine, however, have not been included.) Medicine was the second most popular profession for women in the nineteenth century, behind teaching; by 1910, there were more than 9,000 women physicians in the United States. However, as medicine became more professionalized and scientific, and as the women's medical colleges began to close their doors, the number of women in medicine declined; it did not rise again until the 1970s.

Apart from a few notable exceptions (such as significant Civil War nurses), the category of "nurse" here includes only women who received formal nurse's training. As is the case with medicine, the training available to nurses has changed dramatically over the years. Until the mid-nineteenth century, women who worked as hospital nurses had little or no training and were considered to be of the lowest moral character. But, as

hospitals evolved from institutions for the poor into complex medical facilities, trained nurses were needed to staff them. Emulating the nursing and hospital reforms of English nurse Florence Nightingale, socially prominent American women established training schools for nurses in hospitals; the first schools were established in New York City; New Haven, Connecticut; and Boston in 1873. These schools were an integral part of hospitals, and nursing students became their primary nursing staff. The education and training that early hospital schools provided were more often on-the-job experience than classroom instruction. As the profession grew, nursing leaders sought to transfer education of nurses from the hospital to the university environment; nevertheless, as late as 1971, hospital diploma schools graduated more nurses than university or college programs combined.

"Midwife" is interpreted in a very broad sense to include lay midwives with little or no formal training, as well as trained midwives and modern-day nurse-midwives. In colonial and early American times, childbirth was regarded as a natural, woman-centered event, with the midwife as the primary attendant and caregiver. Although the midwife was a highly regarded member of the community, her role was often not regarded as worthy of particular note; there was little formal training or certification involved in the practice of midwifery. At least partially for this reason, there is little documentation of the lives and practices of midwives of this time period, and few eyewitness accounts or diaries are extant. In the late eighteenth century, male physicians began to displace midwives as the primary attendants and caregivers at childbirth. By the late nineteenth century, childbirth had become almost fully "medicalized" for the middle and upper classes, a "disease" requiring the attendance of a physician. Midwives continued to be in use among women at the lower end of the socioeconomic scale, however. By the early twentieth century, certification programs for midwives began to be instituted, but certified midwives continued to exist side by side with uncertified lay midwives. The 1970s saw a resurgence of interest in midwifery as a result of a number of social and medical trends. In this book, midwives are labeled as "midwife" "nurse-midwife" "nurse, midwife"; or "midwife, nurse" according to their certification, self-designation, or primary practice.

Work was begun on this book in mid-1997 and continued through mid-2001. The first step was to compile a list of potential candidates for inclusion in the book. An invaluable reference tool for beginning this list was *Women in Particular: An Index to American Women* (Oryx Press, 1984), which lists women in all fields of activity together with their accomplishments. Among the works that we consulted in pursuing our research into the women on this preliminary list were Vern Bullough's three-volume set *American Nursing: A Biographical Dictionary* (Garland, 1988 and 1992; Springer, 2000) and Martin Kaufman's *Dictionary of American Nursing Biography* (Greenwood, 1988), the two editions (Edward T. James et al., and Barbara Sicherman, and Carol Hurd Green) of *Notable American Women* (Belknap Press of Harvard University Press, 1971, 1980), Sandra Chaff's *Women in Medicine: A Bibliography of the Literature on Women Physicians* (Scarecrow Press, 1977), and other reference works. In addition, we searched the periodical literature of medicine, nursing, history, and women's studies, and read the standard monographic histories of the fields (see the Bibliography), such as Regina Markell Morantz-Sanchez's *Sympathy and Science: Women Physicians in American Medicine* (Oxford University Press, 1985), Susan Reverby's *Ordered to Care: The Dilemma of American Nursing, 1850–1945* (Cambridge University Press, 1987), and Judy Barrett Litoff's *American Midwives: 1860 to the Present* (Greenwood Press, 1978). In the course of this research, we found that some of the women on our preliminary list did not meet our criteria for inclusion; at the same time, we discovered the names of other women who did meet them.

Because there is not a great deal of pub-lished biographical information on modern-day midwives, we contacted Internet discussion groups that focus on midwifery to solicit the names of possible candidates for inclusion in our book. Our inquiries resulted in many responses, but relatively few bore fruit. Many practicing midwives could not, or would not, furnish us with biographical information about themselves. Undoubtedly, many women are not included who should be recognized.

Sources used to write the biographical essays include the reference books mentioned earlier, periodical articles, archival materials, Internet Web sites, and interviews. In each biography, we include the following information about each woman, if it is available: name; date of birth (and death, if the woman is deceased); birthplace; parents' names; family information (number of siblings and place of residence while growing up; if she married or had children, those facts are mentioned in the body of the essay); education (formal or informal); motivation to become a woman healer; professional accomplishments; obstacles encountered; and major awards, publications, and other achievements. The book is organized alphabetically, and each essay has two or more references for further reading. There are cross-references to women mentioned in other entries, so the reader may understand how the lives and influences of these women interlaced. At the end of the book are appendices, the first listing all women by occupation and the second chronologically listing notable events, a bibliography of works on women and health, and a general index.

The authors would like to thank Deborah L. Thompson for contributing the essay on Maude Callen and assisting with the compilation of the bibliography; Calvin S. Byre for his advice and guidance; the Inter-Library Loan Departments from the University of Oklahoma Libraries, Santa Monica Public Library, and Oklahoma City Community College; the librarians at Oklahoma City Community College, particularly Rachel Butler; archivists Joanne Grossman and Barbara Williams of MCP

Hahnemann University; Sabrina Cuddy, owner of the Midwife Internet discussion group; midwives Alicia Huntley and Raven Lang; and our editor at Oryx, Henry Rasof.

Finally, we would especially like to thank Joseph Soliz, Scott McCaulley, Lennit Williams, and Lee Krumholz for their support and patience.

A

Abbott, Maude Elizabeth Seymour (1869–1940)
Physician

Maude Abbott was a Canadian pathologist famous for her research on heart disease. She was born on March 18, 1869, at St. Andrews East, Quebec, the second daughter of Reverend Jeremiah Babin and Elizabeth Frances (Seymour) Abbott. Her father left home before she was born, and her mother died shortly afterward. Consequently, Abbott and her older sister, Alice, were adopted by their maternal grandparents. Abbott's early education was with governesses, but in 1884 she attended the Misses Symmers and Smith private school in Montreal.

Upon graduation from Symmers and Smith in 1885, Abbott won a scholarship to the Donalda Department for the Arts Education of Women at McGill University in Montreal. She graduated with a B.A. in 1890 as class valedictorian and wished to continue at McGill to study medicine; however, the university did not admit women into its medical program. Hearing that Abbott wanted to study medicine at McGill, a group of local women formed the Association for the Professional Education of Women and pledged to raise the money necessary to accommodate women's medical study at McGill. Nonetheless, Abbott's request for admission to the Department of Medicine's 1889–1890 session was denied, and McGill did not admit women medical students until 1917. Abbott therefore studied medicine at the less prestigious University of Bishops College of Montreal, graduating in 1894 with the Senior Anatomy Prize and the Chancellor's Prize for the best final examinations.

After graduation, Abbott spent three years studying in Europe and Britain. There she became intrigued by pathology and returned to Montreal in 1897 with a microscope and a collection of specimen slides. Although she would have preferred a teaching or research position at McGill, she opened a private practice for women and children. A chance meeting with Dr. Charles Martin, a McGill medical school faculty member, led to an invitation to work with him on heart murmur research. The significance of this research resulted in Abbott's election into the Medico-Chirurgical Society, its first woman member. Concurrently, Abbott was conducting research on her slide collection with John Adami, also from McGill. Although the paper from this research was presented by a man, it was the first paper authored by a woman to be presented at the Pathological Society of London, England.

In 1898 Abbott became the first woman

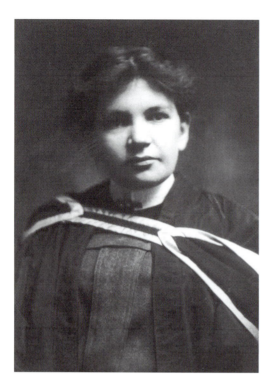

Maude Elizabeth Seymour Abbott. National Library of Medicine.

on staff at the McGill Medical School when she was appointed as assistant curator of the Medical Museum. She was promoted to the position of curator in 1899. As curator, she established a classification method for a previously unorganized collection of thousands of medical specimens, including a large number of diseased hearts. Her system of classification became the basis by which congenital heart diseases are understood. She remained at McGill except for a two-year term (1923–1925) as a professor of pathology and bacteriology and director of clinical laboratories at the Woman's Medical College of Pennsyl-

vania in Philadelphia. When she returned to McGill, she was appointed assistant professor of medical research at the McGill University Clinic in the Royal Victoria Hospital, becoming the first female professor of medicine. She retired in 1936.

After suffering a cerebral hemorrhage in July 1940, Abbott died on September 2, 1940.

Selected Additional Achievements

In 1907, Abbott organized the International Association of Medical Museums. McGill awarded Abbott three honorary degrees, M.D. (1910), C.M. (Master in Surgery, 1910), and LL.D. (Doctor of Laws, 1936). She authored numerous books, including *Historical Sketch of the Medical Faculty of McGill University* (1902), *Women in Medicine* (1911), *Florence Nightingale as Seen in Her Portraits with a Sketch of Her Life* (1916), *History of Medicine in the Province of Quebec* (1931), *Atlas of Congenital Cardiac Diseases* (1931), and *Classified and Annotated Biography of Sir William Osler's Publications* (1939). Two scholarships were established in her name for women medical students at McGill; one was given anonymously and the other by the Federation of Medical Women of Canada.

References

Abbott, Maude Elizabeth Seymour. 1959. "Autobiographical Sketch." *McGill Medical Journal* 28:127–152.

Hacker, Carlotta. 1974. *The Indomitable Lady Doctors.* Toronto: Clarke, Irwin.

MacDermot, H. E. 1941. *Maude Abbott, a Memoir.* Toronto: Macmillan.

Peitzman, Steven J. 1984. "Abbott, Maude." In *Dictionary of American Medical Biography*, edited by M. Kaufman, S. Galishoff, and T. L. Savitt. Westport, Conn.: Greenwood Press.

CMB

Aikens, Charlotte Albina (ca. 1868–1949)
Nurse

Charlotte Aikens was the author of several nursing texts and editor of *Trained Nurse and Hospital Review*. She was born around 1868, in Mitchell, Ontario, Canada and at-

tended Alma College in St. Thomas, Ontario. In 1897 she graduated from the Stratford Hospital School of Nursing in Stratford, Ontario, and then received additional education in ward administration at the New York Polyclinic Hospital.

During the Spanish-American War, Aikens volunteered as a nurse. Next, she was director of Sibley Memorial Hospital in Washington, D.C. While there, she came to recognize the contradictory missions of the hospital and the hospital nurse-training school. At the time, hospitals used student nurses to provide most nursing care. The result for the student was often a limited range of experience and limited exposure to nursing theory. Aikens strongly believed that nursing administrators should develop a standard curriculum that allowed students to learn theory and gain a variety of nursing experiences. She promoted her ideas at meetings of the American Society of Superintendents of Training Schools for Nurses and wrote of them in the *Trained Nurse and Hospital Review* and in the *National Hospital Record*.

Aikens was named associate editor of the *National Hospital Record* in 1902. Not long after, she was superintendent of nurses at Methodist Hospital in Des Moines, Iowa, and then at Columbia Hospital in Pittsburgh. In both positions, she collected data for a report, "The Relation of the Training School to Hospital Efficiency," which she gave at the American Hospital Association's (AHA) 1908 convention. After this presentation, she was invited to join the staff of *Trained Nurse and Hospital Review*. In 1911 she retired from hospital work to become full-time associate editor of the journal at its headquarters in Detroit; she became editor four years later. In 1912, she was named chair of the AHA's Committee on the Grading of Nurses. The committee studied hospital service to determine which services could be provided by trained nurses and which could be done by attendants. The 1916 report of the committee introduced the controversial idea of different levels of nursing, based on education and type of nursing.

Aikens wrote several nursing texts; the most influential was *Studies in Ethics for Nurses* (1st ed. 1916). The book was written to "emphasize the importance of ethical training of nurses, and to aid teachers and students in the study of conduct and duty as it relates to nurses and nursing life" (Aikens, p. 10). The text was translated into 14 languages. In 1920, Aikens went to South America to survey hospital administration for the Methodist Church Mission Board. She resigned her editorship at *Trained Nurse and Hospital Review* in 1922.

At the age of 55, Aikens adopted two children. She died on October 20, 1949, in Detroit.

Selected Additional Achievements

Hospital Housekeeping (1st ed., 1906); *Hospital Training-School Methods and the Head Nurse* (1907); *Clinical Studies for Nurses: A Text-Book for Second and Third Year Pupil Nurses and a Hand-Book for All Who Are Engaged in Caring for the Sick* (1st ed., 1909); *Primary Studies for Nurses: A Text-Book for First Year Pupil Nurses* (1st ed., 1909); *Hospital Management: A Handbook for Hospital Trustees, Superintendents, Training-School Principals, Physicians, and All Who Are Actively Engaged in Promoting Hospital Work* (1911); *The Home Nurse's Handbook of Practical Nursing* (1st ed., 1912); *Lessons from the Life of Florence Nightingale* (1915); *Training School Methods for Institutional Nurses* (1919). Organized Detroit Nursing Home Association (1913). Vice president, American Hospital Association.

References

Aikens, Charlotte A. 1937. *Studies in Ethics for Nurses.* 4th ed. Philadelphia: W. B. Saunders.

"Charlotte A. Aikens—One of TN's Own Editors." 1949. *Trained Nurse and Hospital Review* 123 (December):279.

Fulton, Janice, and Vern L. Bullough. 1988. "Charlotte Albina Aikens." In *American Nursing: A Biographical Dictionary*, edited by V.L. Bullough, O.M. Church, and A.P. Stein. New York: Garland.

"Mrs. Aikens Dead at 82." 1949. *Detroit News* (October 22):2.

LS

Alexander, Virginia M. (1900–1949)
Physician

Virginia Alexander was one of the first African American women physicians. She was born in Philadelphia on February 4, 1900, the fourth of five children of Hilliard and Virginia (Pace) Alexander. She graduated from William Penn High School and then entered the University of Pennsylvania. There she met Sadie Tanner Mossell, who had been awarded a medical school scholarship. Mossell, who would eventually become Alexander's sister-in-law, did not wish to study medicine, and the donor agreed to transfer the scholarship to Alexander. Alexander matriculated at the Woman's Medical College of Pennsylvania (now MCP Hahnemann University) after her graduation from Pennsylvania in 1921.

After graduating from Woman's Medical in 1925, Alexander completed an internship at Wheatly Provident Hospital in Kansas City, Missouri, and spent the following year as the first woman staff member of Kansas City General Hospital. She returned to Philadelphia to establish an obstetrics and gynecological practice in an overcrowded black neighborhood in north Philadelphia. In an effort to reduce the high infant mortality rate among African American babies, she opened the Aspiranto Health Home (1931) in her own house to teach infant care to new mothers. She later opened a Well Baby Clinic.

In 1938 Alexander graduated from the Public Health Department at Yale University and the same year traveled to Norway, Denmark, and Sweden to study public health problems in those countries. After her return to the United States, she was appointed as physician in charge of women students at Howard University in Washington, D.C. Concurrently, she maintained a private practice and was associated with Freedman's Hospital in D.C.

At the outbreak of World War I, Alexander volunteered at the U.S. Department of Health as a public health physician at Schlossfield Hospital in Birmingham, Alabama. Her patients were primarily coal and iron miners. She also worked with the miners' families on child health and birth control issues. In 1946, she returned to private practice in Philadelphia and was on staff at the Woman's Medical College. She died from lupus on July 24, 1949. The Doctor Virginia M. Alexander Scholarship Foundation was created in her memory four years later.

References

Alexander, Virginia M. Deceased Alumnae Files, Special Collections on Women in Medicine, Archives and Special Collections, MCP Hahnemann University, Philadelphia.

Galloway-Wright, Brenda. 1993. "Alexander, Virginia M." In *Black Women in America: An Historical Encyclopedia*, edited by D.C. Hine, E. Barkley, and R. Terborg-Penn. Brooklyn, N.Y.: Carlson.

JSB

Angwin, Maria L. (1849–1898)
Physician

Maria Angwin was the first woman licensed to practice medicine in Halifax, Nova Scotia, Canada. She was born on September 21, 1849, in Newfoundland, the ninth of 10 children of Thomas and Louisa Emma (Gill) Angwin. The family moved to Dartmouth, Nova Scotia, in 1865, and in 1866, Angwin entered the liberal arts program at Wesleyan Ladies' Academy at Mount Allison College in New Brunswick. She graduated in 1869, the only woman in the class. Although she successfully completed her studies, her mistress of liberal arts was awarded as a diploma rather than a degree because no universities in the British Empire awarded degrees to women at that time.

Returning home to Dartmouth, Angwin originally intended to pursue a legal career. She was inspired to become a physician, however, after reading *Eminent Women of the Age* (1868) by James Parton, which included several biographies of female physicians of the day, including Elizabeth and Emily Blackwell. In order to earn money for medical school, she decided to become a schoolteacher and enrolled in the Provincial Normal School at Truro, Nova Scotia. She obtained a teaching license and returned to Dartmouth (1874), where she spent five years teaching. Angwin was forced to pursue her medical training in the United States because no schools were open to women in Canada. She had saved enough by 1879 to register at the Woman's Medical College of the New York Infirmary, founded by Elizabeth Blackwell in 1868. She graduated in 1882 and undertook a year of postgraduate work at the New England Hospital for Women and Children in Boston, founded by Marie Zakrzewska in 1862 and run entirely by a female staff dedicated to the care of women and children.

In 1883, while in Dartmouth for the summer, Angwin became the subject of much notoriety when the local paper, the *Morning Herald*, ran a sensational front-page story on her medical career. The antagonistic reporter attempted to provoke her anger with such questions as whether she felt that all her training would be lost once she married and by proposing that she would be boycotted by the local male doctors. In response, Angwin said that the motto that would hang in her office would be "If God be for us, who can be against us?" and that she saw no reason "why a married woman shouldn't practice medicine as well as bending over the washtub, or dragging out a miserable existence with a drunken husband."

In 1884, Angwin traveled abroad and spent two months attending at the Rotunda Hospital in Dublin, Ireland. She returned to Canada in September 1884 and opened a medical practice, becoming the first woman in the Medical Register of Nova Scotia and therefore the first woman physician licensed to practice in that province. She chose to work in Halifax because she believed that Halifax needed a woman doctor who would strive to improve the health of mothers and young women through the promotion of health education and good personal hygiene. She became a local personality who protected herself with a hatpin, wore her hair short, and took a strong stand against drinking and cigarettes. In 1889, she became the superintendent for scientific temperance instruction for the Woman's Christian Temperance Union, and in 1890 she served as the organization's superintendent for hygiene and heredity.

In April 1898, Angwin moved to New York City to conduct postgraduate research at the New York Infirmary for Women and Children. On route to New York, however, she stopped at Ashland, Massachusetts, and underwent minor surgery, from which she developed a fatal infection. She died on April 25, 1898.

See also Blackwell, Elizabeth; Blackwell, Emily; Zakrzewska, Marie Elizabeth

References

"Dartmouth's Lady Doctor." 1883. *Morning Herald* (August 13):1.

Hacker, Carlotta. 1974. *The Indomitable Lady Doctors.* Toronto: Clarke, Irwin.

Kernaghan, Lois K. 1991. "Someone Wants the Doctor: Maria L. Angwin, M.D. (1849–1898)." *The Collections of the Royal Nova Scotia Historical Society* 43:33–48.

The Maritime Medical News. 1898. 10 (May): 175.

Nichols, R. Bond. 1950. "Early Woman Doctors of Nova Scotia." *Nova Scotia Medical Bulletin* 29:14–21.

CMB

Apgar, Virginia (1909–1974)
Physician

Virginia Apgar was an anesthesiologist noted for her innovations in obstetrics and birth defects prevention. In particular, her Apgar score is a system used worldwide to gauge quickly an infant's health and development at birth. She was born on June 7, 1909, in Westfield, New Jersey, the youngest of two surviving children of Charles Emory and Helen May (Clarke) Apgar.

In 1929, Apgar graduated from Mount Holyoke College, where she studied zoology, chemistry, and physiology. With the intention of becoming a surgeon, she entered Columbia University's College of Physicians and Surgeons. She graduated in 1933 and became the fifth woman to earn the prestigious surgical internship at Presbyterian Medical Center in New York City. After interning for two years and performing over 200 operations, the department chair convinced her that a woman could not support herself as a surgeon. She reluctantly gave up surgery and turned to anesthesiology, a new field that she reasoned would provide more opportunities for women. She began her training at Columbia University and then completed residencies at the University of Wisconsin and at Bellevue Hospital in New York.

In 1936, Apgar was appointed instructor of anesthesiology at Columbia University. Two years later, she became assistant professor and director of the anesthesiology division at Columbia-Presbyterian Medical Center and was the first woman to head a medical division at Columbia. She advanced to associate professor in 1942. When the division became a department in 1949, she hoped to be named chair but was passed over by a male colleague. She was, however, appointed to full professor and became the country's first full professor of anesthesiology and the first woman to hold a full professorship at Columbia. She remained at Columbia until 1959, directing one of the most highly regarded anesthesiology departments in the country.

In 1952, Apgar presented a paper to the International Anesthesia Research Society proposing the use of Newborn Scoring System, a method of evaluating the condition of newborn babies within one minute of birth. The system, now commonly called the Apgar score, consists of rating five aspects of the newborn's condition: heart rate, respiratory effort, reflex irritability, muscle tone, and color. Now standard practice in hospitals worldwide, the Apgar score alerts physicians to the need for emergency treatment as soon as possible.

In 1959, Apgar earned a master's degree from Johns Hopkins University School of Hygiene and Public Health in Baltimore. The same year, she was appointed by the Na-

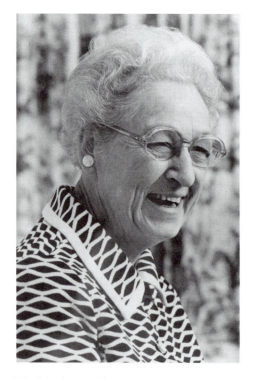

Virginia Apgar. Photo © Bettmann/COR-BIS.

tional Foundation-March of Dimes to head its congenital malformations division. She subsequently held the positions of director of the basic research department (1967–1974), vice president for medical affairs (1968–1973), and senior vice president (to 1974). She traveled the world on behalf of the foundation, educating the public on the importance of research and prevention in the area of birth defects. Her work is credited with bringing the study of birth defects into a place of prominence in the medical field. Concurrently, she held the first birth defects faculty position (1965–1971) at Cornell University Medical College and was appointed lecturer of genetics at Johns Hopkins School of Public Health (1973).

Apgar was once asked if discrimination against women exists in medicine; she replied, "Heavens, no. Never! You just had to be twice as smart as the men" ("For Healthier Babies," vertical file). She died on August 7, 1974, from cirrhosis of the liver.

Selected Additional Achievements

Awards include the Elizabeth Blackwell Citation, New York Infirmary (1960); Distinguished Service Award, American Society of Anesthesiologists (1961); honorary doctor of science degree, Woman's Medical College of Pennsylvania (1965);

first woman recipient, Gold Medal for Distinguished Achievement in Medicine, Alumni Association of the Columbia Medical College of Physicians and Surgeons (1967); Ralph M. Waters Award, American Society of Anesthesiology (1967). Publications include *Is My Baby All Right? A Guide to Birth Defects* (1972) and several articles in scientific and popular journals.

References

Apgar, Virginia. 1953. "A Proposal for a New Method of Evaluation of the Newborn Infant." *Current Researches in Anesthesia and Analgesia* (July–August):260–267.

Duffin, Jacalyn. 1999. "Apgar, Virginia." In *American National Biography*, edited by J.A. Garraty and M.C. Carnes. New York: Oxford University Press.

"For Healthier Babies." 1968. *Medical World News* (November 15). Vertical file. Special Collections on Women in Medicine, Archives and Special Collections, MCP Hahnemann University, Philadelphia.

The National Cyclopaedia of American Biography. 1960. Current volume 1. New York: James T. White.

Waldinger, Robert J. 1980. "Apgar, Virginia." In *Notable American Women: The Modern Period: A Biographical Dictionary*, edited by B. Sicherman and C.H. Green. Cambridge: Belknap Press of Harvard University Press.

JSB

Aragon, Jesusita (ca. 1908–   )
Midwife

Jesusita Aragon is one of the last representatives of the long tradition of Hispanic midwifery in the culturally and geographically unique area of northern New Mexico. Her career is one of the longest and best-documented within that tradition, and she is one of its most revered figures. She has attended many thousands of births, and although some infants did not survive, she has not lost any of the mothers whom she assisted. She was born around 1908 in Trujillo, northern New Mexico; she was the first of her mother's eight pregnancies to survive.

Her mother later had two more girls who also lived.

By 1918, Aragon's family was living in Las Vegas, New Mexico, where her father worked as a laborer. The same year, her mother, pregnant and ill with the flu, died, and the family returned to its ranch in Trujillo. There Aragon "was raised out like a boy" (quoted in Buss, p. 120). She tended animals, sheared sheep, and worked the fields, but she also helped with the more traditional female chores of cooking and cleaning. Through trial and error and experience assisting her midwife grandmother, she became the local expert who was called upon to help the animals that were having a difficult time giving birth.

Because her family considered an eighth grade education sufficient, Aragon was unable to continue her schooling and fulfill her lifelong desire to become a nurse. Instead, she decided to become a midwife. The decision was a natural one since her grandmother was a midwife, as had been her great-grandmother. Her grandmother began passing on her knowledge of midwifery to Aragon at a very young age. She taught Aragon to maintain a positive attitude, to keep her "mouth shut," and not to "get scared" (quoted in Chester, p. 38) during a delivery; she also showed her how to use olive oil and a gentle touch to reduce a mother's discomfort. The first time that Aragon delivered an infant alone, her grandmother was 40 miles away attending another birth. The favorable outcome began Aragon's eight-decade career as a midwife, the success of which she attributes to the God-given ability of her hands to "feel everything" (quoted in Chester, p. 39). The only formal instruction that she received was 15 days of midwifery training from the state of New Mexico, which culminated in the receipt of a home nursing pin.

When Aragon was in her early 20s and still living with her father, she had two out-of-wedlock children. The births were not well received by her family, so she moved her young family to a home on the Trujillo ranch that she built with her own hands. While her children were young, she ran a small farm in addition to practicing midwifery. In 1952, when her eldest was ready to start high school, she moved to Las Vegas, New Mexico, and hand-built another home. In Las Vegas, she continued to serve as a midwife. For additional income, she took in laundry and worked in a parachute factory, where the manager allowed her to leave work to attend births.

Aragon still lives in Las Vegas and continues to deliver infants, employing her traditional methods. In 1989, Aragon was awarded the Sage Femme Award by the Midwives' Alliance of North America in recognition of her years of dedicated midwifery.

References

Buss, Fran Leeper. 1980. *La Partera: Story of a Midwife.* Ann Arbor: University of Michigan Press.

Chester, Penfield. 1997. *Sisters on a Journey: Portraits of American Midwives.* New Brunswick, N.J.: Rutgers University Press.

CMB

Armstrong, Penny Bradbury (1946–   )
Nurse-midwife

Penny Armstrong is a nurse-midwife who spent many years in Lancaster County, Pennsylvania, delivering babies for Amish families. She surmounted many objections to her practice from local physicians in order to provide midwifery care for Amish women. She was born on January 23, 1946, in Aroostook County, Maine, one of three children of Gerald A. and Arlene (Howard) Bradbury. Her great-grandmother, Gertrude Bradbury, was a lay midwife. During her youth, Armstrong had the opportunity to assist a veterinarian delivering lambs. The veterinarian allowed her to turn a stuck lamb, which created in her a great interest in the birthing process. She spent her early life in Maine, but her father's profession as an airline pilot forced the family to move frequently. She graduated from Myers Park High School in Charlotte, North Carolina, in 1964.

After attending Northeastern University in Boston, Armstrong moved to Coral Gables, Florida, to attend the University of Miami. She received a bachelor's degree in psychology in 1969. During the early 1970s, she worked as a regional health planner in Portland, Maine, directing a drug abuse education council. In 1976, she received a bachelor's degree in nursing from Saint Louis University in Missouri. The following year, she began attending Glasgow College of Midwifery in Scotland, receiving a certificate in midwifery in 1978. Upon her return to the United States, she moved to Philadelphia to attend the foreign-trained midwives program at Booth Maternity Center. Here she became aware of the opportunities for attending births in the nearby Amish communities.

In 1979, Armstrong became director of the Dry Hill Clinic in Gordonville, Pennsylvania. As part of her job, she attended approximately 1,400 births, mostly in the Amish and Mennonite communities around Lancaster County, Pennsylvania. While the Amish were not opposed to using doctors or hospitals for their births, they preferred simple home births attended by midwives. Armstrong's experiences working with the Amish are recounted in her book *A Midwife's Story* (1986). An incident that she described in the book demonstrates the prejudice that midwives often face. In 1980, she was granted privileges at a small hospital in Lancaster County, which she prefers not to name. The following day, five physicians, the entire senior medical staff, resigned in protest. Additionally, the volunteers who ran the hospital's snack bar closed it and threatened to cancel their charity ball. Nonetheless, local doctors eventually started referring patients to her, and she was accepted by most as a legitimate health care provider. After a few years, her home birth practice had grown so much that she left the hospital to concentrate on home births.

Armstrong returned to Maine in 1989 and worked as a family planning practitioner in Houlton. In 1990, she moved to Cooperstown, New York, to serve as a staff nurse-midwife in a group practice of seven certified nurse-midwives and four obstetricians at Bassett Hospital. She earned a master's degree in nursing from Case Western Reserve University in Cleveland, Ohio, in 1993. She has begun focusing on education for midwives, having held positions with the Community-Based Nurse-Midwifery Education Program at the Frontier School of Midwifery and Family Nursing, a program that offers continuing education for practicing nurse-midwives and on-line courses for students. Currently, she is the project director of the Behavioral Science and Community Health Curriculum Project at the University of New England College of Osteopathic Medicine in Biddeford, Maine. She lives in Cape Elizabeth, Maine, with her husband, Dick.

Selected Additional Achievements

A Wise Birth: Bringing Together the Best of Natural Childbirth with Modern Medicine (with Sheryl Feldman, 1990); several articles in childbirth, midwifery, and other publications. Armstrong has held teaching positions at a number of institutions, including the University of New England College of Osteopathic Medicine, Case Western Reserve University, and the University of Pennsylvania.

References

Armstrong, Penny. May 18, 30, 2001. Interview with author via E-mail.
Armstrong, Penny Bradbury. 2001. Résumé.
Armstrong, Penny, and Sheryl Feldman. 1986. *A Midwife's Story.* New York: Arbor House.
Chester, Penfield. 1997. *Sisters on a Journey: Portraits of American Midwives.* New Brunswick, N.J.: Rutgers University Press.

DTW

Arnstein, Margaret Gene (1904–1972)
Nurse

Margaret Arnstein was a leader in public health nursing whose career included 20 years with the U.S. Public Health Service. She was born on October 27, 1904, in New York City, the second of four children of Leo and Elsie (Nathan) Arnstein. Her father was a businessman who sat on the Board of Directors of nurse Lillian Wald's Henry Street

Settlement, and her mother was involved with the settlement's social work. Arnstein was influenced by Wald's efforts and decided at a young age to become a nurse. After graduating from the Ethical Culture School in 1921, she entered Smith College in Northampton, Massachusetts and studied the biological sciences. She graduated in 1925 with an A.B. and three years later earned a diploma in nursing from New York Presbyterian Hospital School of Nursing.

After graduating, Arnstein took a job at the Westchester County Hospital in White Plains, New York, and also earned a master's degree in public health nursing at Teachers College, Columbia University (1929). In 1934, she earned a master's degree in public health from Johns Hopkins University and became a consultant nurse in the communicable disease division of the New York State Department of Health. She taught public health nursing at the University of Minnesota for two years (1938–1940) before returning to the New York Health Department. She believed that nurses must systematically study how to be most effective in the health care system and began to research the issue in her position with the New York Health Department.

Arnstein took a leave of absence from the department from 1943 to 1945 to work with the United Nations Relief and Rehabilitation Administration in the Balkan countries. In 1946, she began a long association with the U.S. Public Health Service (USPHS) when she accepted a position as assistant to the chief nurse, Lucile Petry Leone. In 1949 Arnstein was promoted to chief of the division of nursing resources and rose through the ranks to become chief of the division of nursing in 1960. Within the USPHS, she traveled widely to survey conditions in her jurisdiction and directed studies analyzing patient problems and nursing methods. One such study of the head nurse's daily routine showed that nurses were frequently running errands and performing clerical duties for physicians; as a result of this research, some hospitals began to hire clerical staff and messenger services to perform those tasks. She also studied international issues in public health and wrote *A Guide for National Studies of Nursing Resources* (1953) for the World Health Organization. Additionally, she directed the first International Conference on Nursing Studies in Sèvres, France, in 1956. In 1958, she took a leave of absence from the USPHS to become the first holder of the Annie W. Goodrich Chair of Nursing at the Yale University School of Nursing.

In 1964 Arnstein moved from the USPHS nursing division to its international health office, where she worked with physicians to study public health needs in developing countries. She strongly believed in adapting nursing practices to meet the needs of developing nations. In 1966, she left the USPHS to become a professor and head of the public health nursing program at the University of Michigan but was soon called on by Yale University to become the dean of its School of Nursing. She remained at Yale until her retirement in 1972.

She died of cancer on October 8, 1972, in New Haven, Connecticut.

See also Goodrich, Annie Warburton; Leone, Lucile Petry; Wald, Lillian D.

Selected Additional Achievements

Numerous articles in the nursing literature; *Communicable Disease Control* (with Gaylord Anderson, 1941). Several honorary degrees; Lasker Award (1955); first woman awarded the $10,000 Rockefeller Public Service Award (1965); American Public Health Association Sedgwick Memorial Award (1971).

References

Fondiller, Shirley H. 1988. "Margaret Gene Arnstein." In *American Nursing: A Biographical Dictionary*, edited by V.L. Bullough, O.M. Church, and A.P. Stein. New York: Garland.

Milio, Nancy. 1980. "Arnstein, Margaret Gene." In *Notable American Women: The Modern Period: A Biographical Dictionary*, edited by B. Sicherman and C.H. Green. Cambridge: Belknap Press of Harvard University Press.

"Yale Nursing School Alumnae Meet New Visiting Professor." 1958. *New Haven Evening Register* (February 23): 17.

LS

B

Bagshaw, Elizabeth (1881–1982)
Physician

Elizabeth Bagshaw served as medical director for the first birth control clinic in Canada. She was born in rural Ontario, Canada, on October 19, 1881, the youngest of four daughters of farmers John and Eliza (Beatty) Bagshaw. Her early education was in local schools. In high school her interest in medicine was peaked by a friend's accounts of her female physician cousin, who practiced in Rochester, New York. Bagshaw had not been aware that women could practice medicine. Her desire to become a doctor increased as she read about the pioneering Canadian women physicians of the time, including Emily Stowe, Augusta Stowe Gullen, and Maude Abbott.

Although Bagshaw's mother was opposed to the idea, her father was determined to lend support to his adventurous and independent daughter. Consequently, Bagshaw set out for Toronto in September 1901 to study medicine. Although she took most of her classes at the Ontario Medical College for Women, she also enrolled at the University of Toronto as an "occasional" student, so that her degree would be granted from the more prestigious institution.

Eight women and 140 men graduated with Bagshaw in 1905. To be licensed to practice medicine by the College of Physicians and Surgeons of Ontario, new graduates were required to complete a year of work in either a recognized hospital or under a doctor's supervision in a private practice and then take an examination. At the time, very few hospital internships were available to women. Bagshaw, therefore, chose to work in a private practice under Emma Leila Skinner, an 1896 graduate of the University of Toronto whose specialty was obstetrics. The year was successful; Bagshaw passed the required examination and became licensed to practice medicine in Ontario.

In the summer of 1906, Bagshaw acted as a substitute for a woman physician in Hamilton, Ontario, and in the fall began her own practice there. Initially, the majority of her patients were maternity cases from the large European immigrant population in Hamilton. These women readily accepted her, as they had been accustomed to obtaining their obstetrical care from female midwives in Europe. Victorian modesty still prevailed during Bagshaw's early years of practice, so nonimmigrant women also turned to her because they were more comfortable being examined by a female physician.

In 1932, Mary Chambers Hawkins approached Bagshaw and asked her to become the medical director of the Birth Control Society of Hamilton, Canada's first birth control clinic. Hawkins founded the clinic in early 1932 to prevent undesired pregnancies. Although the clinic was technically operating illegally, Bagshaw accepted the position. The work appealed to her sense of social responsibility for the prevention of unwanted childbirths, especially for economically disadvantaged women.

Since Bagshaw had not received instruction in contraception in medical school, she traveled to Margaret Sanger's New York clinic to learn birth control techniques. Then, from the spring of 1932 until 1966, she worked at the clinic almost every Friday afternoon, fitting diaphragms and providing instruction in their use. The Criminal Code of Ontario made the provision of, and instruction in, birth control illegal; however, a caveat in the code exempting those who could prove they were acting for the public good prevented her from prosecution.

The Criminal Code was not amended until 1969, three years after Bagshaw retired as medical director of the clinic, which had become part of the Planned Parenthood Society. After retirement from the clinic, she continued her medical practice, serving primarily as a support for elderly patients until 1976. She never married, but in 1926, she adopted a son, John, who became a physician, and a daughter, Voureen. Bagshaw died on January 5, 1982.

See also Abbott, Maude Elizabeth Seymour; Gullen, Augusta Stowe; Sanger, Margaret Louise Higgins; Stowe, Emily Jennings

Selected Additional Achievements

Life member, Ontario Medical Association (1954); senior member, Canadian Medical Association (1969); Citizen of the Year (Hamilton, 1970); Elizabeth Bagshaw Elementary School in Hamilton named in her honor (1971); Order of Canada Medal (1973); honorary doctor of laws degree from McMaster University (Hamilton, 1974); life member, College of Family Physicians of Canada, (1978); guest lectureship established in her name by the Hamilton Academy of Medicine (1981).

References

Arnup, Katherine, Andrée Lévesque, and Ruth Roach Pierson. 1990. *Delivering Motherhood: Maternal Ideologies and Practices in the 19th and 20th Centuries.* London: Routledge.
Hacker, Carlotta. 1974. *The Indomitable Lady Doctors.* Toronto: Clarke, Irwin.
Hellstedt, Leone McGregor. 1978. *Women Physicians of the World: Autobiographies of Medical Pioneers.* Washington, D.C.: Hemisphere.
"Obituary." 1982. *Macleans* 95:4.
Wild, Marjorie. 1984. *Elizabeth Bagshaw.* Markham, Ont.: Fitzhenry and Whiteside.

CMB

Baker, S. [Sara] Josephine (1873–1945)
Physician

S. Josephine Baker was a physician whose public health work for mothers and children in New York City in the early twentieth century was a model for the nation and the world. She was born on November 15, 1873, in Poughkeepsie, New York, the third of four children of Orlando Daniel Mosher Baker and Jenny Harwood Brown Baker. Her early education was at the Misses Thomas' school in Poughkeepsie. When Baker was 16, her father and brother died, leaving the family with limited financial resources. Realizing that she might eventually have to support them, Baker decided to go to medical school, using part of the family savings.

After studying privately for a year, in 1894 Baker entered the Woman's Medical College of the New York Infirmary, founded 26 years earlier by Dr. Elizabeth Blackwell. Baker graduated second in her class in 1898 and then took an internship at the New England Hospital for Women and Children in Boston, founded by Dr. Marie Zakrzewska in 1862. She also worked in a clinic in the slums of

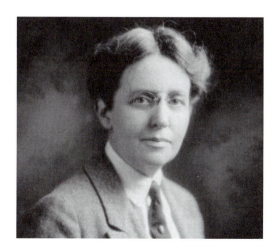

Josephine S. [Sara] Baker. National Library of Medicine.

Boston. In 1899, she and another female physician established a private practice in New York City, which she maintained until 1914. Making only $185 the first year, she sought additional income as an insurance company medical examiner and took a part-time job as a medical inspector for the city of New York in 1901. Her duties for the city included inspecting schoolchildren for signs of illness and, in the summer of 1902, seeking out sick babies among the Irish immigrant and African American families on New York's West Side. In her autobiography, *Fighting for Life* (1939), she described it as "an appalling summer, . . . with an average of fifteen hundred babies dying each week" (1980 reprint, p. 58).

In 1907, Baker became assistant to the health commissioner and helped to vaccinate the population against smallpox and to apprehend the notorious typhoid carrier Mary Mallon. In her work, Baker saw a great deal of death and disease, particularly in babies and young children, and she was determined to do something to fight them. She realized that the way to lower the death rate was through preventive action. Accordingly, in the summer of 1908, she designed an experiment in which 30 trained nurses would teach child care, breast-feeding, bathing, ventilation, and proper clothing to a portion of New York's population. Their efforts re-

sulted in 1,200 fewer infant deaths from the previous year and to the creation of the Bureau of Child Hygiene within the city health department. Baker was appointed director of the bureau and held the position for 15 years.

Under Baker's leadership, the bureau began tackling New York City's public health problems. Among her first actions was regulating the city's midwives. Unlike many physicians, however, she supported the midwife, saying that "a well-trained midwife deserves all possible respect as a practical specialist" (Baker, p. 114). Her innovations included placing orphaned babies with poor foster mothers to give the babies the affection that they were lacking in institutions, establishing baby health stations where mothers were able to buy clean milk, and founding Little Mothers' Leagues to educate young girls who had to take care of their younger siblings. Her actions were so successful that she often provoked the ire of the city's physicians, who found themselves with fewer sick children to treat.

From 1915 to 1930 Baker lectured on public health at New York University-Bellevue Hospital Medical School. She agreed to do so on the condition that she could enter the institution's public health doctoral program. At first, school administrators refused her as a student, and she refused to teach. After being unable to find an alternative qualified teacher, the administrators relented, and she was admitted. She earned a doctorate of public health in 1917, the first woman to do so.

By the time Baker retired from the bureau in 1923, New York City's infant death rate was less than half of what it was when she started, and her programs had been copied by city and state governments in the United States and around the world. She remained active in many medical societies and was a consultant to the federal Children's Bureau and Public Health Service and to the New York State Department of Health. She lived the last years of her life with the novelist and writer Ida Wylie and physician Louise Pearce in Bellemead, New Jersey. She died of cancer on February 22, 1945, in New York City.

See also Blackwell, Elizabeth; Zakrzewska, Marie Elizabeth

Selected Additional Achievements

Baker wrote *Healthy Babies* (1920); *Healthy Mothers* (1920); *Healthy Children* (1920); *The Growing Child* (1923); and *Child Hygiene* (1925). She also contributed about 200 articles to the popular press and more than 50 to the medical literature. Founder (1909) and president (1917–1918), American Child Hygiene (later, Health) Association; representative of the United States to the Health Committee of the League of Nations (1922–1924); president, American Medical Women's Association (1935–1936); College Women's Equal Suffrage League; Heterodoxy Club (a discussion group).

References

Baker, S. Josephine. 1980. *Fighting for Life*. Reprint ed. Huntington, N.Y.: Robert E. Krieger. Original edition, New York: Macmillan, 1939.

Baumgartner, Leona. 1971. "Baker, Sara Josephine." In *Notable American Women, 1607–1950: A Biographical Dictionary*, edited by E.T. James, J.W. James and P.S. Boyer. Cambridge: Belknap Press of Harvard University Press.

Morantz-Sanchez, Regina. 1999. "Baker, Sara Josephine." In *American National Biography*, edited by J.A. Garraty and M.C. Carnes. New York: Oxford University Press.

"One of the World's Great Citizens: S. Josephine Baker, M.D., D.P.H." 1922. *Medical Woman's Journal* 29 (8):180–182.

LS

Ballard, Martha Moore (1735–1812)
Midwife

Martha Ballard was a successful midwife in Maine in the late eighteenth and early nineteenth centuries. Her name, like the names of most early American midwives, would have disappeared from history if not for the meticulous diary that she kept for 27 years. She was born on February 20, 1735, in Oxford, Massachusetts, the daughter of Elijah and Dorothy (Learned) Moore. In 1754, she married Ephraim Ballard, a miller and surveyor, and the couple eventually had nine children, three of whom died during a diphtheria epidemic in 1769.

In 1775, Ephraim moved to Hallowell, Maine, where he leased sawmills and gristmills. Martha Ballard and the children joined him in October 1777. She was already practicing midwifery when she began writing in her diary on January 1, 1785, but left no record of where or how she learned to be a midwife. She probably apprenticed with an older woman while still in Oxford. Although it was becoming increasingly common for physicians to attend births at the time that Ballard practiced midwifery, women were the primary assistants and caregivers during the birthing process. When a woman went into labor, she called the local midwife as well as female relatives and neighbors to her side and often gave birth resting in the arms or on the laps of these women assistants. Ballard required at least two women aides during a birth. Following the birth, an afternurse attended to the woman, who was considered recovered from childbirth when she could make her own bed and get back into the kitchen.

From 1785 to 1812, Ballard recorded 816 births in her diary; she had attended more than 200 before that, bringing her total number of deliveries to over 1,000. Until 1800, she performed two-thirds of Hallowell's deliveries, and her services were used by all levels of the town's society. Her practice reached its peak, an average of about 50 deliveries per year, after 1790, when her daughters were old enough to take care of the household. She charged six shillings for a birth, which was equivalent to what her husband made for a day spent appraising an estate. Her fee could be paid in cash, in credit, or in kind, and she frequently accepted textiles, food, and household goods instead of cash. She was nearly always paid, although not always at the time of delivery. She recorded an "XX" in her diary when an account was settled.

For each birth, Ballard also recorded the father's surname, the sex of the child, the location of the birth, the number of hours that the woman was in labor, the hour of her summons and departure, and the condition of the mother and baby. She usually wrote that she left a woman "cleverly" or that she had "safe delivered" the woman of a baby, indicating that the birth had proceeded with few complications. Most births were normal, but she did encounter breech and multiple births, obstructions, and fainting mothers. She handled such complications capably on her own, calling for a physician's assistance only twice in her long career. None of the women whom she attended died during a delivery, although five died a few days later, and she had only 19 babies born dead or die shortly after birth.

In addition to being a midwife, Ballard knew how to treat illnesses and injuries with herbs in preparations such as teas, syrups, pills, poultices, ointments, and salves, with common garden plants like onions and green beans, and with household items such as vinegar, soap, and flour. A frequent complaint of nursing mothers was breast abscess, which she treated with poultices of sorrel, yellow lily roots, or even lancing. Her remedies were not unlike physicians' treatments, except that she did not set bones, administer opiates, or let blood. She also assisted in laying out the dead of the community and attended four autopsies during her career.

In 1802, Ballard delivered only 11 babies; her practice declined because of ill health, advancing age, and the fact that she had moved to a house in a more isolated area. When another local midwife died in 1809, Ballard's business increased, but she attended her last birth only three years later, on April 26, 1812. She returned from the birth feeling unwell and never recovered. Her final diary entry was written May 7, and she died about May 19, 1812. Her diary was passed down to her great-great-granddaughter, physician Mary Hobart, who donated it to Maine State Library in 1930. A digitized version and a transcribed version of the diary are available on the Internet through Harvard University's Film Study Center at http://www.dohistory.org.

References

Ulrich, Laurel Thatcher. 1990. *A Midwife's Tale: The Life of Martha Ballard, Based on Her Diary, 1785–1812.* New York: Alfred A. Knopf.

Ulrich, Laurel Thatcher. 1999. "Ballard, Martha Moore." In *American National Biography*, edited by J.A. Garraty and M.C. Carnes. New York: Oxford University Press.

LS

Barringer, Emily Dunning (1876–1961)
Physician

Emily Dunning Barringer was the first woman intern and first woman staff member at a New York City municipal hospital. She was born in Scarsdale, New York, on September 27, 1876, the second of six children of Edwin James and Frances Gore (Lange) Dunning. She decided to pursue a medical career the night her mother gave birth to her youngest child. The birth was difficult, and an obstetrician was called to the house. She later wrote in her autobiography, *Bowery to*

Bellevue (1950), that "it was at this time that the great desire was born in me to help the sick and suffering" (p. 28).

In 1897, Barringer graduated from Cornell University and enrolled at the Woman's Medical College of the New York Infirmary for Women and Children, established by physicians Elizabeth and Emily Blackwell in 1868. In 1899, Emily transferred the students to Cornell's new coeducational medical school, where Barringer earned her M.D. in

1901. After graduation, she was refused internships at New York's Mount Sinai and Gouverneur Hospitals because of her sex, despite earning the highest score on the examinations for both positions.

With no internship, Barringer worked under L. Emmet Holt, a prominent pediatrician, and was assistant to pioneering female physician Mary Putnam Jacobi. She did not give up on finding a place in a general hospital, convinced that "women must be willing to go up, to be knocked down again and again, before the general hospitals will be opened" (Barringer, p. 74). She wrote a letter to Mayor Seth Low, urging him to allow women physicians appointments in city hospitals. The mayor agreed, and on January 1, 1903, she was accepted for an internship at Gouverneur, becoming the first woman intern at a New York City general hospital. She met with strong opposition by the male staff members of the hospital, who protested her appointment on the grounds that it would begin a precedent of hiring female staff members who would eventually be promoted into supervisory positions over men. At Gouverneur, she was required to make ambulance calls, making her the first female ambulance surgeon in the city. During her one-year internship, she earned two promotions.

In 1905, Barringer established a private medical practice and was assistant gynecologist at New York Polyclinic Hospital, becoming the first woman regular staff member at a New York City general hospital. She was also attending surgeon at the New York Infirmary for Women and Children (1905–1916). After 1916, she was the infirmary's consultant in gynecology and obstetrics and was lecturer in gynecology at the Woman's Medical College of Pennsylvania in Philadelphia. Around this time, she was also director of gynecology at Brooklyn's Kingston Hospital. During the war years, she headed an unsuccessful committee for the American Medical Women's Association (AMWA) to secure military commissions for female physicians. However, during World War II, with Barringer as president of the AMWA (1941–1942), the campaign was successful, and women physicians entered World War II with commissioned status. From 1937 to 1940, she was director of the venereal disease department for the New York City Department of Health. As a result of this work, she played an important role in the passage of legislation in New York state designed to curb the spread of syphilis and gonorrhea.

She was married to Benjamin Stockwell Barringer, with whom she had two children. She died in New Milford, Connecticut, on April 8, 1961.

See also Blackwell, Elizabeth; Blackwell, Emily; Jacobi, Mary Corinna Putnam

Selected Additional Achievements

Barringer wrote several articles and book chapters on gynecological and venereal subjects. Delegate, International Congress of Women Physicians (1937); member, house of delegates, American Medical Association and Medical Society of the State of New York; member, general advisory board, American Social Hygiene Association; president, Women's Medical Society of New York State (1918) and Women's Medical Association of New York City (1914, 1939–1942); fellow, American College of Surgeons, New York Academy of Medicine and the American Neiserian Society; member, Medical Women's National Association.

References

Barringer, Emily Dunning. 1950. *Bowery to Bellevue: The Story of New York's First Woman Ambulance Surgeon*. New York: W. W. Norton.

German, Lisa Broehl. 1999. "Barringer, Emily Dunning." In *American National Biography*, edited by J.A. Garraty and M.C. Carnes. New York: Oxford University Press.

Marks, Geoffrey, and William K. Beatty. 1972. *Women in White*. New York: Charles Scribner's Sons.

JSB

Barry, James Miranda Stuart (ca. 1795–1865)
Physician

James Barry was possibly the first woman to practice medicine in Canada. Her birthplace was London, England, but her parentage and date of birth (between 1790 and 1795) are not well established. Her parents died shortly after her birth, leaving her to be raised by persons of unknown identity. At some point in her youth, she decided to portray herself as a man; therefore, when she enrolled as a literary and medical student at the University of Edinburgh in Scotland, she did so as a man. She completed her M.D. in 1812 and in 1813, after passing the British Army Medical Board examination, became a hospital assistant for the Army Medical Department. She quickly rose through the ranks of the army, serving in Canada, India, Jamaica, and South Africa.

In 1857, Barry was assigned the post of inspector general of hospitals in Montreal. Her inspection of the Canadian military facilities revealed monotonous, nutritionally poor diets and barracks without adequate sewage and drainage systems. She also discovered the lack of separate sleeping quarters for married soldiers; wives shared their husbands' beds in the same barracks that housed the single men. Consequently, she instituted a larger variation in diet, improved the sanitation of the lodgings, and established separate facilities for married couples. She also made reforms in the overcrowded Montreal hospitals that had been inadequately equipped with straw bedding. In 1859, she became ill with influenza and was deemed unfit for service by the Army Medical Board. She was thus forced into retirement, a ruling that she bitterly and unsuccessfully contested.

Barry concealed her sex until her death on July 25, 1865. As her body was being prepared for burial, her long-held secret was revealed. An inquest following the discovery corroborated the suspicion that she was female; however, no official statement was ever made, and her personal records have disappeared.

References

Brunton, Lauder. 1992. "Some Women in Medicine." *Canadian Medical Association Journal* 146 (6):955–961.

Hacker, Carlotta. 1974. *The Indomitable Lady Doctors.* Toronto: Clarke, Irwin.

Kirby, Percival. 1970. "Dr. James Barry, Controversial South African Medical Figure: A Recent Evaluation of His Life and Sex." *South African Medical Journal* 44 (April):506–516.

McSherry, James. 1992. "Some Women in Medicine." *Canadian Medical Association Journal* 147 (3):291–293.

Rae, Isobel. 1958. *The Strange Story of Dr. James Barry.* London: Longmans, Green.

CMB

Barton, Clarissa Harlowe [Clara] (1821–1912)
Nurse

Clara Barton is most notable for her work as a volunteer Civil War nurse and as the founder of the American Red Cross. She was born on Christmas Day 1821, in North Oxford, Massachusetts, the last child of Stephen and Sarah (Stone) Barton. Named Clarissa Harlowe, she soon adopted her lifelong nickname, Clara. Her first experience caring for the sick came at age 11 when she nursed her brother, David, through a two-year illness. From that point on, she derived her greatest sense of usefulness alleviating the pain of others.

Although later known for her great courage, Barton was an insecure and self-effacing child. In an effort to cure Barton of her shyness, her mother turned to phrenologist Lorenzo Fowler (husband of pioneering

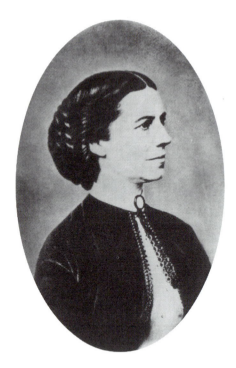

Clarissa Harlowe [Clara] Barton. National Library of Medicine.

woman physician Lydia Folger Fowler). Fowler examined Barton and determined somewhat prophetically that while Barton would always be shy, she would be fearless on the behalf of others. Fowler suggested that Barton begin a teaching career, which she did at the age of 18. For the next 10 years, Barton taught in and around North Oxford. She interrupted her teaching career in 1850 to attend the Liberal Institute in Clinton, New York. After leaving Clinton, she returned to teaching in Bordentown, New Jersey, where she was responsible for establishing one of the state's first public schools.

In 1854 Barton left New Jersey for Washington, D.C., to clerk in the U.S. Patent Office. In 1857 an administrative change led to the firing of all female clerks in the office. She was called back to her position in 1860, just before the outbreak of the Civil War. On April 19, 1861, she learned that wounded soldiers from the Sixth Massachusetts Regiment had arrived in Washington. The next day, she arrived at the soldiers' quarters with

food and clothing. As more troops camped in Washington, she was there to provide relief to soldiers who were often sick and hungry. Afterward, she began a public solicitation for more supplies that was so successful she was required to rent storage space.

As more and more local women followed Barton's example, she decided to use her skills on the battlefield. She comforted soldiers and assisted surgeons after the Battles of Cedar Mountain, Second Bull Run, Chantilly, South Mountain, Antietam, and Fredericksburg. Barton biographer Elizabeth Pryor provides this image of Barton at work: "With her skirt pinned up around her waist and a face blue from gunpowder, she served gruel, extracted bullets and held the hands of the dying . . . she assisted at surgery, dressing wounds with green corn leaves when the bandages were exhausted" (1999, p. 290). Her work blunted criticism that women were of no use on the battlefield. She was the best-known of the female Civil War nurses but was quick to recognize the work of lesser-known women, such as Mary Bickerdyke, Dorothea Dix, and Mary Safford.

Barton was commissioned with the army for a short time in 1864 as acting head nurse for the Army of the James. By 1863, however, her role in the field had diminished as formal relief organizations gained experience and recognition. In 1865, Barton received permission from President Lincoln to open an office in Annapolis, Maryland, for the purpose of compiling a record of the names of missing Civil War casualties. This turned into a massive, four-year project in which she compiled the names of tens of thousands of soldiers. From 1866 to 1868, Barton toured the United States, lecturing on her nursing experiences.

Total exhaustion sent Barton to Europe for rest in 1869, but this goal would not be realized. In Switzerland, she learned of the existence of the International Red Cross. This organization, founded in 1863 to provide relief to war victims, was ratified by 11 governments during the Geneva Treaty of 1864. Disturbed to learn that the United States was not among the 11 countries, she campaigned for U.S. ratification. Her plans were postponed in 1870, while she volunteered in France with the International Red Cross during the Franco-Prussian War. Another case of exhaustion sent her to a sanatorium in Dansville, New York, in 1873. However, the outbreak of the Russo-Turkish War in 1877 revived her interest in the International Red Cross. She spent the next five years engaged in a public campaign to convince the U.S. government to sign the Geneva Treaty. It was not until 1882 that President Arthur and Secretary of State Blaine signed the treaty. During her campaign, Barton stressed that the Red Cross could also be of assistance after domestic disasters. This vision became a reality in 1884, when the Geneva Convention added the American Amendment to the treaty, sanctioning Red Cross activities during peacetime disasters.

By 1881, Barton had already formed the American Association of the Red Cross, a national organization in name only. The Red Cross did not become a federally recognized organization until June 6, 1900, when President McKinley signed a bill issuing its federal charter. From 1881 to 1904, Barton's energies were totally concentrated on the Red Cross. The only interruption was for six months in 1883, when the governor of Massachusetts asked her to be superintendent of the Woman's Reformatory Prison in Sherborn, after the resignation of physician Eliza Mosher. During her tenure with the Red Cross, Barton was in the field during natural disasters at home and abroad and also provided relief during the Spanish-American War (1898). One of her later actions was to persuade Dr. Anita McGee, founder of the United States Army Nurse Corps, to require that the head of that organization be a graduate nurse.

Always efficient with time and money, Barton chose to assist only where help was most needed and did not stay longer than necessary. She refused to organize disaster relief from behind a desk; she went to the field herself, working side by side with the strongest victims to help the weakest. However, as the Red Cross grew in size and importance, her own board challenged her administrative skills. Although the public continued to admire her good works, there was a general lack of confidence in her ability to run the growing organization. Constant criticisms from the board forced her resignation in 1904. Leadership of the Red Cross was handed to Mabel Thorp Boardman, Barton's most staunch detractor. Barton's last important act was the formation of the Red Cross' National First Aid Society, which today provides instruction to thousands in the use of emergency first aid.

Barton spent her retirement years in Glen Echo, Maryland. Throughout her life, she was a strong supporter of woman's rights. She died on April 12, 1912.

See also Bickerdyke, Mary Ann Ball; Dix, Dorothea Lynde; Fowler, Lydia Folger; McGee, Anita Newcomb; Mosher, Eliza Maria; Safford, Mary Jane

Selected Additional Achievements

The Red Cross: A History of This Remarkable International Movement in the Interest of Humanity (1898); *The Red Cross in Peace and War* (1899); *The Story of My Childhood* (1907); and *A Story of the Red Cross* (1918). Barton received medals of honor from Germany, Russia, Turkey, and Siberia.

References

Barton, William E. 1922. *The Life of Clara Barton: Founder of the American Red Cross.* 2 vols. Boston: Houghton Mifflin.

Curti, Merle. 1971. "Barton, Clara." In *Notable American Women, 1607–1950: A Biographical Dictionary,* edited by E.T. James, J.W. James, and P.S. Boyer. Cambridge: Belknap Press of Harvard University Press.

Hawkins, Joellen Watson. 1988. "Barton, Clarissa Harlowe." In *Dictionary of American Nursing Biography,* edited by M. Kaufman. New York: Greenwood Press.

Pryor, Elizabeth Brown. 1987. *Clara Barton: Professional Angel.* Philadelphia: University of Philadelphia Press.

Pryor, Elizabeth B. 1999. "Barton, Clara." In *American National Biography,* edited by J.A. Garraty and M.C. Carnes. New York: Oxford University Press.

JSB

Bass, [Mary] Elizabeth (1876–1956)
Physician

Elizabeth Bass was one of the first women physicians appointed to the faculty of a medical school in the American South, cofounder of a hospital for women and children, and a historian of women in medicine. She was born on April 5, 1876, in Marion County, Mississippi, the second of eight children of Isaac Esau and Mary Eliza (Wilkes) Bass. Bass' early education was in local schools; she graduated from Columbia High School (Mississippi) in 1893 and earned teaching certificates in 1892 and 1896. She then taught in public schools in Mississippi and Texas.

Bass' brother, Dr. Charles C. Bass, encouraged Elizabeth and her sister Cora to study medicine. Because women were not permitted in southern medical schools, in 1900 Bass and her sister went north to attend the Woman's Medical College of Pennsylvania in Philadelphia (now MCP Hahnemann University). Bass graduated from the school in 1904 and then interned at the Woman's Hospital of Philadelphia (1904–1905). After her internship, she moved to New Orleans and opened a private practice. At the time, women were not allowed to practice in the city's hospitals. In response, Bass, Dr. Sara Mayo, and five other women physicians (including her sister, Cora Bass) established the New Orleans Hospital and Dispensary for Women and Children in June 1905. The hospital was the only one in the South governed entirely by women.

In December 1911, Bass and another woman doctor became the first women to be appointed to the faculty at Tulane University's School of Medicine. Within two years of her appointment to the nonsalaried position of assistant demonstrator of surgical pathology, Bass advanced to the position of instructor in the Clinical Medicine Laboratory. She remained at Tulane until 1941, when she retired from her positions of professor of laboratory diagnosis in the Graduate School of Medicine and associate professor of medicine in the School of Medicine. During

World War II, she returned to private practice due to a shortage of doctors. She was also house physician at the Jung Hotel, which was her place of residence. In 1949, she quit the practice of medicine to care for her aging mother.

Bass was very interested in the history of women in medicine; in a speech she once said that the subject was "very dear to [her] heart and one of boundless scope and fascination" (Bass, Deceased Alumnae Files). After leaving Tulane, she devoted much of her time to assembling what would become a vast collection of newspaper clippings, pictures, photographs, glass magic lantern slides, books, and medical school catalogs on women in medicine. She used these materials as the basis for her "These Were the First" columns on outstanding women physicians in the *Journal of the American Medical Women's Association* (1946–1956). She gave her collection to the Rudolph Matas Library of Tu-

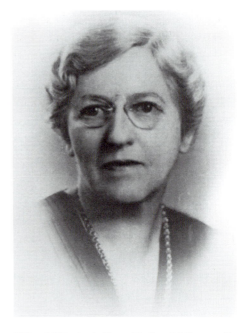

[Mary] Elizabeth Bass. National Library of Medicine.

lane University's School of Medicine after she retired from teaching.

Bass died in New Orleans on January 26, 1956, of cancer.

See also Mayo, Sara Tew

Selected Additional Achievements

In addition to her regular columns in the *Journal of the American Medical Women's Association*, Bass wrote many articles on the history of women in medicine. Member, Equal Rights Association of New Orleans; first woman elected to active membership (1913), secretary (1921–1922), vice president (1923), Orleans Parish Medical Society; vice president (1919), president (1925–1927), Women Physicians of the Southern Medical Association; member and president (1921–1922), Medical Women's National Association. Alumnae Achievement Award, Woman's Medical College of Pennsylvania (1952); Elizabeth Blackwell Centennial Medal (1953). After her death, the Elizabeth Bass Memorial Student Loan Fund was established at Tulane.

References

Bass, Elizabeth. Deceased Alumnae Files, Special Collections on Women in Medicine, Archives and Special Collections, MCP Hahnemann University, Philadelphia.

Burns, Chester, and Melinda Nelson. 1980. "Bass, Mary Elizabeth." In *Notable American Women: The Modern Period: A Biographical Dictionary*, edited by B. Sicherman and C.H. Green. Cambridge: Belknap Press of Harvard University Press.

Elizabeth Bass Collection on Women in Medicine. Online. http://www.tulane.edu/~matas/bass .html. 16 February 1999.

"In Memoriam: Elizabeth Bass 1876–1956." 1956. *Bulletin of the Orleans Parish Medical Society* 27 (4):6, 8.

LS

Bates, Mary Elizabeth (1861–1954)
Physician

Mary Elizabeth Bates was the first woman to be awarded an internship at Chicago's Cook County Hospital in 1881. She was born in Manitowoc, Wisconsin, on February 25, 1861, one of two children of William Wallace and Marie (Cole) Bates, a graduate of the New York Hydropathic Medical College. She became interested in medicine after attending a graduation ceremony at the Woman's Medical School in Chicago (now part of Northwestern University). In 1881, she earned a medical degree from the same institution.

After graduation, Bates and six male doctors took a competitive civil service examination for an internship at Cook County Hospital in Chicago. As a result of her scores, she was awarded the internship, along with the distinction of becoming the first woman to intern at the hospital. She was the only graduate in her class of 26 women to take the examination. At that time, internships were not required to practice medicine, and few women graduates chose to complete them. Bates, however, feared that "the doors might close on internship for women if some didn't take the examination" (quoted in Minney, p. 31). After completing the internship, she returned to her alma mater to serve as lecturer in minor surgery and demonstrator of anatomy. Afterward, she spent a year at the General Hospital in Vienna studying anatomy, dissection, and obstetrics. She returned to the United States in 1885 to open a private practice in Chicago, where she was also professor of anatomy at the Woman's Medical College and on the staff of the Chicago Hospital for Women and Children. In 1891, she settled permanently in Denver, where she maintained a large practice specializing in diseases of women and children.

In addition to her regular medical duties, Bates served as secretary of the Colorado Medical Women's War Service League. She was also surgical editor of the *Medical Woman's Journal* and founder of the Denver

School for Practical Nurses. She introduced and conducted the Baby Health Contest in Colorado and Utah and published the Model Baby Health Score Card. In 1894, she established the *Woman Voter*, the first woman suffrage circular in the West, and was instrumental in founding the Woman's Protective League. She successfully lobbied for a law protecting children from lewd advances (1905), an age of consent law (1907), and a "white slavery law" (1911). She was also instrumental in the passage of a law requiring physical examinations of schoolchildren (1909) and chaired the School Health Committee of the National Education Association.

Bates died in 1954.

Selected Additional Achievements

Founder, White Star Society; secretary, Denver Dumb Friends League; president, Humane Education Society (animal rights organizations); vice president, Colorado State Bureau of Child and Animal Protection; founder, Clean City Club.

References

Minney, Doris. 1948. "Mary Elizabeth Bates, M.D." *Medical Woman's Journal* 55 (7):30–31.

The National Cyclopaedia of American Biography. 1922. Vol. 18. New York: James T. White.

Who Was Who in America with World Notables: Vol. IV, 1961–1968. 1968. Chicago: Marquis-Who's Who.

JSB

Batterham, Mary Rose (ca. 1870–1927)
Nurse

Mary Batterham, a North Carolina nursing leader, was the second American woman to become a registered nurse. She was born in England around 1870 to William and Mary Rose Batterham and came to New York at about age 20. After graduating from the Brooklyn City Hospital nursing program in 1893, she began postgraduate work at City Hospital. Before earning a degree, she went to North Carolina, where she held positions in public health and private nursing, was head nurse at the Oakland Heights Sanitarium, and was a Metropolitan Life nurse.

In 1902 North Carolina became the first state to require the registration of nurses, and on June 5, 1903, Batterham registered in Buncombe County, becoming the country's second registered nurse. While she is often considered to be the first, research shows that this distinction actually goes to Josephine Burton, who registered in Craven County one day before Batterham (Wyche, p. 52). Nonetheless, Batterham remains one of nursing's pioneers. She was a charter member of the North Carolina State Nurses' Association and in 1902, became its first vice president. In 1916, she and 11 other nurses organized the association's public health section, to

which she was elected chair the following year.

Throughout her career, Batterham spoke out on behalf of nurses and their patients. She advocated shorter hours and better working conditions for her colleagues and supported a broad nursing school curriculum to strengthen nurses' cultural backgrounds. She urged nurses to take opportunities to care for those who could not afford such care and to study the relationship between social problems and health. In addition to writing for many nursing journals, she was a member of the North Carolina State Red Cross Nursing Committee and a charter member of her alumnae association (1895).

Batterham died on April 4, 1927, of acute appendicitis and acute chronic myocarditis.

References

Hawkins, Joellen Watson. 1988. "Batterham, Mary Rose." In *Dictionary of American Nursing Biography*, edited by M. Kaufman. New York: Greenwood Press.

"Obituary." 1927. *American Journal of Nursing* 27 (5):410.

Stein, Alice P. 1992. "Mary Rose Batterham." In *American Nursing: A Biographical Dictionary,* edited by V.L. Bullough, L. Sentz, and A.P. Stein. New York: Garland.

Wyche, Mary Lewis. 1938. *History of Nursing in North Carolina*. Chapel Hill: University of North Carolina Press.

JSB

Beard, Mary (1876–1946)
Nurse

Mary Beard was a leading figure in public health nursing, notable particularly for her work in raising the standards of public health nursing education. She was born in Dover, New Hampshire, on November 14, 1876. She was the fourth of five children of Ithamar Warren and Marcy (Foster) Beard. As a child, she contracted diphtheria, and a nurse was hired to care for her. Impressed by the nurse, the young Beard was inspired to pursue the same occupation. After completing her early education at Dover public schools, she entered the New York Hospital School of Nursing (1899). She graduated in 1903 and then served as staff nurse and director of the Waterbury Visiting Nurse Association in Connecticut (1904–1909). From 1910 to 1912, she was engaged in cancer research at the Laboratory of Surgical Pathology at Columbia University in New York.

Beard felt a calling to return to nursing, however, and in 1912 she accepted the directorship of the Boston Instructive District Nursing Association (BIDNA), an organization devoted to providing nursing care to Boston's low-income residents. In 1922, the BIDNA became known as the Community Health Association (CHA) after Beard facilitated its merger with the Baby Hygiene Association. With Beard as its head, the CHA continued its original work and also persuaded the city of Boston to establish more infant health programs. The year before Beard came to the organization, the staff had made 112,000 visits to 11,000 patients. By the time she resigned in 1924, the number of visits increased to 440,000 for over 52,000 patients, making the BIDNA the largest visiting nurse association in the country.

Concurrently, Beard accepted a committee appointment (1918) with the Rockefeller Foundation to study the education of public health nurses. In 1923, the committee published the Winslow-Goldmark report, *Nursing and Nursing Education in the United States*, the first extensive study of nursing education and practice. The report advocated high standards in nursing education and resulted in the closing of schools that could not meet those standards.

In 1924, Beard left Boston for New York to begin a career with the Rockefeller Foundation. After a short assignment studying maternal health programs in England, she continued the original work that she had begun on the Goldmark committee, pursuing higher standards for public health nursing. As special assistant to the director of the division of studies (1925–1927), she oversaw the allocation of $4 million to help nursing schools establish the committee's proposed standards. Afterward, she was assistant to the director of the division of medical education (1927–1930). In this position she was in charge of encouraging more college-educated women to enter nursing. From 1930 to 1938, she served as associate director of the foundation's international health division, in which she studied nursing practices in Europe and Asia. She was responsible for establishing schools of nursing in many of these countries and arranged for over 400 nurses from 38 countries to come to the United States for training.

Beard left the foundation in 1938, after her appointment as director of nursing services for the American Red Cross. In this capacity, she was in charge of directing the wartime recruitment of military nurses without depleting nursing resources for civilian needs. She was also responsible for the creation of nurse's aide educational and home nursing programs. One of her most important programs was the Camp Community Emergency Nursing Service, which provided maternal and child care for families of servicemen. Beard was the first chairperson of the Subcommittee on Nursing of the Health and Medical Committee of the Office of Defense Health and Welfare Services. She also chaired the Council of National Defense's Subcommittee on Public Health Nursing and served on the National Nursing Council. By the time she left the Red Cross in 1944, 50,000 nurses had been recruited for the war effort at home and abroad.

Beard considered public health programs to be the greatest achievement of our age. She died on December 4, 1946, in New York.

Selected Additional Achievements

Board of Directors (1912–1946), vice president (1915–1916), and president (1916–1919), National Organization for Public Health Nursing; member, nursing committee, Henry Street Nursing Service; member, advisory committee on nursing, New York City Department of Health;

honorary membership, Grand Council of the International Council of Nurses, the Association of Collegiate Schools of Nursing, and the Old Internationals Association; honorary doctoral degree, University of New Hampshire (1934) and Smith College (1945). In addition to her many professional journal articles, Beard published *The Nurse in Public Health* (1929).

References

Beard, Mary. 1936. "Creative Nursing." *American Journal of Nursing* 36 (1):69–78.

Buhler-Wilkerson, Karen. 1988. "Mary Beard." In *American Nursing: A Biographical Dictionary*, edited by V.L. Bullough, O.M. Church, and A.P. Stein. New York: Garland.

Carey, Charles W. 1999. "Beard, Mary." In *American National Biography*, edited by J.A. Garraty and M.C. Carnes. New York: Oxford University Press.

Gifford, Alice J. 1974. "Beard, Mary." In *The Dictionary of American Biography: Supplement 4, 1946–1950*, edited by J.A. Garraty and E.T. James. New York: Charles Scribner's Sons.

Higgins, Loretta P. 1988. "Beard, Mary." In *Dictionary of American Nursing Biography*, edited by M. Kaufman. New York: Greenwood Press.

JSB

Beeman, Ruth Coates (1925–   )
Nurse-midwife

Ruth Beeman was a leading figure in the development of some of the first accredited nurse-midwifery training programs in the United States and abroad. She was born on January 10, 1925, in Harriston, Virginia, and received her nursing education at West Baltimore General Hospital. During her last six months as a student, she obtained practical experience as a cadet nurse in an army paraplegic and amputee hospital. She became a registered nurse in 1946 and then served as a public health nurse with the Instructive Visiting Nurse Association in Baltimore until 1947.

In 1950, Beeman earned both a bachelor's degree in public health nursing from the University of Pennsylvania and certification from the Maternity Center Association (MCA) School of Nurse-Midwifery in New

York. After completing an internship at MCA's Berwind Clinic, she was a nurse-midwife for the MCA home birth service (1950–1952). Around this time she was instrumental in the formation of the American College of Nurse-Midwifery. As chair of the College's Committee on Approval, she led the development of the first standards of accreditation for nurse-midwifery programs.

Around 1952, Beeman went to the Belgian Congo in West Africa with the United Christian Missionary Society. She spent about three years in Africa training midwives, delivering babies, and caring for patients with tropical diseases. She also earned a diploma from the Institute of Tropical Medicine in Antwerp, Belgium (1953).

After returning to the United States in 1956, Beeman earned a master's of public health degree from Columbia University (1957) and then instituted a graduate program in maternity nursing at Indiana University. She served as assistant professor of the program until 1959, when she rejoined the MCA as assistant professor of its Downtown Campus of the State University of New York in Brooklyn. Concurrently, she taught students from Johns Hopkins, Columbia, and Yale Universities.

In 1962, Beeman began an appointment as professor and chairman of the department of maternity nursing and nurse-midwifery at the Graduate School of Nursing of New York Medical College. She instituted a maternity program, an advanced clinical program in maternity nursing and nurse-midwifery, and a postgraduate training program. She and other faculty established the first nurse-midwifery service at Metropolitan Hospital and developed a series of short-term training programs for family-planning nurses.

Beeman married in 1970 and the same year began working for the New York Bureau of Family Planning as a family-planning nurse consultant. For the next six years, she led the development of family-planning programs in all but two New York counties. In 1976, she relocated to Arizona, where she was associate professor at Arizona State University (ASU) College of Nurse-Midwifery. After one year, she went to work for the Arizona Bureau of Maternal and Child Health, where she directed the midwifery licensing program and implemented prenatal services in rural counties. She continued to collaborate with ASU faculty, however, carrying out and publishing surveys on the outcome of cases overseen by licensed midwives.

In 1983, Beeman became director of Kentucky's Frontier School of Midwifery and Family Nursing. She created a program allowing nursing students from Case Western Reserve University to earn graduate credits toward midwifery certification. She also led the creation of the Community-Based Nurse-Midwifery Education Program (CNEP). In 1985, when the Frontier School endowed the Mary Breckinridge chair of nurse-midwifery, she was the first to occupy that position.

Throughout her career, Beeman continued the international work that she had begun in the 1950s. In 1957, she was a member of the U.S. delegation to the International Confederation of Midwifery in Stockholm. She developed and codirected a school of nurse-midwifery in Ponce, Puerto Rico, and has been an American Public Health Association consultant for midwifery and family planning in the Virgin Islands, Benin, Togo, and The Gambia.

Beeman retired from the Frontier School in 1988 and from the CNEP in 1994. She is currently an honored fellow of the American College of Nurse-Midwives.

See also Breckinridge, Mary

References

Biographical Directory of the American Public Health Association, 1979. 1979. New York: R.R. Bowker.
U.S. Department of Health and Human Services. 1985. "First Nurse-Midwifery Chair in U.S. Endowed." *Public Health Report* 100 (March/April):247.
"Who's Who among Newly Inducted ACNM Fellows." 1996. *Journal of Nurse-Midwifery* 41 (4):298–304.

JSB

Bennett, Alice (1851–1925)
Physician

One of the first women to hold an administrative position at a mental hospital in the United States, Alice Bennett is known for her courageous and innovative ideas and practices in the treatment of the mentally ill. She was born on January 31, 1851, in Wrentham, Massachusetts, the youngest of six children of Isaac Francis and Lydia (Hayden) Bennett.

Her early education was at the Day's Academy in Wrentham. She earned money for her medical education by teaching at local schools (1868–1872). In 1872, she entered the Woman's Medical College of Pennsylvania in Philadelphia and graduated four years later.

Bennett then worked at a dispensary in Philadelphia for seven months. In October 1876, she was appointed demonstrator of anatomy at her alma mater, a position that she held for the next four years. At the same time, she maintained a private practice and worked toward her doctorate in anatomy at the University of Pennsylvania. In 1880, she became the first woman to earn a Ph.D. from the university.

In July 1880, Bennett was appointed superintendent of the women's section at the State Hospital for the Insane at Norristown, Pennsylvania. Under her direction, the institution became one of the first mental hospitals in the United States where women patients were entirely under the care of women physicians. She espoused a philosophy of nonrestraint and abolished straitjackets, chains, and cells. She also challenged the use of sedating drugs and initiated occupational therapy for her patients in the form of handicrafts, music, and painting. Bennett gave all her patients gynecological exams, which eventually led her to question the assumed connection between a woman's reproductive system and her vulnerability to mental illness. She believed that her responsibility to patients did not end when they were discharged and followed up with such patients through letters and visitations. Her innovative practices in the care of the mentally ill were noticed and adopted by other hospitals.

Despite all her positive innovations, Bennett was forced to defend her professional judgment in 1892, when she was accused of allowing ovariotomies to be performed on nonconsenting patients. Six operations were performed (though not by Bennett), but they had been done with the consent of the patients' nearest relatives and with pathological conditions present. Bennett was eventu-ally cleared of any wrongdoing, but when questions about the operations arose again in 1895, she resigned the following year, weary of defending herself.

Afterward, Bennett served as a private-duty physician, caring for a mentally ill woman (1896–1898), and then she returned to private practice in her hometown. In 1910, she began working at the New York Infirmary for Women and Children, which had been founded by pioneering women physicians Elizabeth and Emily Blackwell and Marie Zakrzewska in 1857. Bennett worked at the infirmary for the remainder of her life, without compensation. While there, she assisted in the delivery of 2,000 babies.

Bennett died on May 31, 1925, at the New York Infirmary for Women and Children.

See also Blackwell, Elizabeth; Blackwell, Emily; Zakrzewska, Marie Elizabeth

Selected Additional Achievements

Bennett wrote several articles, primarily on mental illness and its treatment. Member, American Medical Association, American Psychiatric Association, National Association for the Protection and Prevention of Insanity, Pennsylvania State Medical Society, Philadelphia Neurological Society, and Philadelphia Medical Jurisprudence Society; member and first woman president, (1890) Montgomery County Medical Society.

References

Kutler, Stanley I. 1971. "Bennett, Alice." In *Notable American Women, 1607–1950: A Biographical Dictionary*, edited by E.T. James, J.W. James, and P.S. Boyer. Cambridge: Belknap Press of Harvard University Press.

McGovern, Constance M. 1984. "Doctors or Ladies? Women Physicians in Psychiatric Institutions, 1872–1900." In *Women and Health in America: Historical Readings*, edited by J.W. Leavitt. Madison: University of Wisconsin Press. Reprinted from *Bulletin of the History of Medicine* 55 (1981):88–107.

McGovern, Constance M. 1999. "Bennett, Alice." In *American National Biography*, edited by J.A. Garraty and M.C. Carnes. New York: Oxford University Press.

Willard, Frances E., and Mary A. Livermore. 1967. *A Woman of the Century: Fourteen Hundred-*

Seventy Biographical Sketches Accompanied by Portraits of Leading American Women in All Walks of Life. Reprint ed. Detroit: Gale Re-search. Original edition, Buffalo, N.Y.: Charles Wells Moulton, 1893.

LS

Berryhill, Elizabeth (1923–   )
Nurse-midwife

Elizabeth Berryhill is a Canadian-born nurse-midwife. Throughout her career, she has been instrumental in establishing maternal and child health programs in South America, Africa, and the United States. She was born in 1923 in London, Ontario, Canada, the only child of Gordon and Lillian Marguerita Berryhill. After completing high school, she earned a nursing diploma from the Victoria Hospital School of Nursing in London, Ontario (1946), and a bachelor's degree in public health nursing administration at the University of Western Ontario (1947). Between 1948 and 1951 she held public health positions with the Victorian Order of Nurses and at the Community Health Nursing Program in Collingwood, Ontario.

In 1951, Berryhill entered the nurse-midwifery course at the Maternity Center Association (MCA) in New York City. In addition to daytime classes at the MCA, she was on call for home deliveries four to five nights a week. After earning her certificate of nurse-midwifery, she returned to Victoria Hospital, where she was the lead labor and delivery nurse.

In 1953, Berryhill began a career as a Presbyterian missionary. Her first assignment was as supervisor of obstetrical and gynecological outpatient services at the Clinica Colombo-Americano in Barranquilla, Colombia (1953–1954). The hospital closed within a year, and she continued her missionary work with the Indians of Tabacundo, Ecuador (1954–1958) and at a clinic in Bucaramanga, Colombia (1959–1964).

Berryhill returned to Canada, where she earned a bachelor's degree in nursing in 1967 from the University of Western Ontario. She then moved to North Carolina and received a master's degree in public health from the University of North Carolina in Chapel Hill in 1968. Afterward, Berryhill served as the eastern project coordinator for the North Carolina State Migrant Health Project and was a regional health education consultant for the North Carolina Department of Human Resources (1968–1972). She was then assistant professor for the Obstetrics and Gynecology Graduate Nursing Program at the University of North Carolina, where she helped establish prenatal, family planning, well-woman gynecology, and postpartum clinics for the nursing students (1972–1975). During this period, she was also the nurse-midwife and project consultant for African Health Training Institutions through the U.S. Agency for International Development. In this role, she traveled to many African countries training nurse-midwife and medical school administrators.

In 1975, Berryhill was appointed as regional child health consultant for the North Carolina Department of Human Resources. In this position she was responsible for developing maternal–child health services for migrant workers in public health departments and clinics in 33 counties. Concurrently, she held two consecutive terms on the North Carolina Board of Nursing (1984–1989). During her tenure on the board, she was instrumental in the creation of the nurse-midwifery program at East Carolina University in Greenville.

Berryhill retired from the Department of Human Resources in 1992. However, she continues volunteer public health work in South America and Africa. Today she is listed on the American College of Nurse-Midwives Roster of Honored Fellows.

Selected Additional Achievements

Founding member, American College of Nurse-Midwifery (1955) and the North Carolina Chapter, American College of Nurse-Midwives (1981).

References

American College of Nurse-Midwives. *Roster of ACNM Fellows.* Online. http://www.acnm.

org/about/FROSTER.HTM. 29 October 2000.

Bergstrom, Linda, Marie E. Pokorny, Margaret B. Davis, and Terrell O. Wootten. 1999. "Full Circle: The Nurse-Midwifery Careers of Elizabeth Berryhill and Gabriela Olivera." *Nursing History Review* 7:29–45.

"Who's Who among Newly Inducted ACNM Fellows." 1996. *Journal of Nurse-Midwifery* 41 (4):298–304.

JSB

Bickerdyke, Mary Ann Ball (1817–1901)
Nurse

Mary Bickerdyke was a U.S. Civil War nurse. Although well known during her lifetime, her work is now overshadowed by that of other Civil War nurses, such as Clara Barton. Bickerdyke was born on July 19, 1817, in Knox County, Ohio, the daughter of Hiram and Annie (Rodgers) Ball. After her mother died in December 1818, she and her siblings were raised by relatives in Ohio. Details of her education are uncertain. She may have attended Oberlin College in 1833. Her medical studies consisted of either a course for nurses (1837) under Dr. Reuben Mussey or classes at the Physio-Botanic Medical College in Cincinnati, run by a Dr. Hussey. She may have provided nursing assistance during the Cincinnati cholera epidemic of 1849.

In 1847, she married Robert Bickerdyke, and the couple had two surviving children, James and Hiram. The family moved to Galeston, Illinois, in 1856, where Robert died three years later. Bickerdyke's notable work was inspired by an 1861 sermon by the Reverend Edward Beecher on the fate of Civil War soldiers camped in Cairo, Illinois. In June that year, she went to Cairo to oversee the distribution of food and medical supplies collected by Beecher's congregation. There, she found hungry, wounded, and sick soldiers lying in filthy, ill-equipped hospital tents. Without seeking permission, she bathed and fed the soldiers, cleaned the tents, and laundered clothes and bedsheets.

In November, General Ulysses S. Grant appointed her as matron of the Cairo military hospital, despite opposition from the male surgeon in charge.

Bickerdyke continued her work for the duration of the war, even though regulations barring women from the battlefield generated resentment from some male officers. A surgeon once asked Bickerdyke under whose authority she worked; she replied, "I have received my authority from the Lord God Almighty. Have you anything that ranks higher than that?" (quoted in Baker, p. 101). General Grant, however, valued her services and issued an order stating, "All . . . military authorities will pass and re-pass Mrs. Mary A. Bickerdyke from any point within the lines, and all military railroads and chartered steamboats will grant her free transportation" (quoted in Erlandson, p. 630). This freedom of movement facilitated her ability to secure food and medical supplies.

In February 1862, Bickerdyke and Mary Safford, another volunteer nurse, made several trips on the *City of Memphis* hospital ship to care for soldiers during the Battle of Fort Donelson. On one occasion, Bickerdyke wandered the battlefield in the middle of the night looking for any sign of life among the dead. Stories of this midnight search were told in many civilian newspapers. Her experience at Fort Donelson convinced her that need was greatest at the front, and she decided to join Grant's troops at the Battle of Shiloh, where she again nursed the troops without any official sanction. In April 1862, she was appointed as agent in the field by the Northwestern Sanitary Commission, thus allowing her to draw on supplies that the commission collected for the troops. Later the same year the commission sent her on a fund-raising tour.

Early in 1863, General Grant sent Bickerdyke to work at a Memphis, Tennessee, hospital. The medical director at Memphis was opposed to a woman's working at his hospital, so he appointed her to Fort Pickering, the site of a smallpox hospital. Administering the hospital had proved difficult as military personnel feared contracting the disease and refused to enter the hospital. Bickerdyke, however, accepted the challenge and began her usual work of cleaning the hospital, feeding the soldiers, and laundering their clothes. Many recovered, and those who did not at least died in relative comfort.

Satisfied with her work at Fort Pickering, Bickerdyke returned to Memphis as matron of the Gayoso military hospital. She found the hospital diet inadequate and traveled to Illinois to collect contributions of chickens and cows as a source of milk and eggs for the soldiers. Successful in this task, she again joined Grant's army in July 1863 at the Battle of Vicksburg. Later General William Sherman assigned her to his army. She joined Sherman, caring for his soldiers until the end of the war in April 1865. The following month, Bickerdyke was seated next to the general during a victory parade. After assisting in the demobilization of soldiers, she resigned her position as spokesperson for the Sanitary Commission.

Bickerdyke's postwar career consisted of one year as assistant superintendent of Chicago's Home for the Friendless and as co-ordinator of a project to provide farmwork for unemployed veterans. In 1870, she was a missionary for New York City's Protestant Board of City Missions. In 1874, she moved to Great Bend, Kansas (where her sons lived), and raised relief funds after locusts plagued that state. Two years later, she moved to San Francisco to work for the Salvation Army and to clerk at the San Francisco Mint. She also organized the California branch of the Woman's Relief Corps. Her concern for Civil War veterans never ceased; she often went to Washington, D.C., in support of veterans' pension claims. In 1886, she herself was given a pension of $25 a month. She returned to Kansas in 1887, where, on July 19, 1897, the state celebrated Mother Bickerdyke Day. She died in Bunker Hill, Kansas, on November 8, 1901. She is buried in the Linwood Cemetery in Galesburg, Illinois. There, a statue of her stands, which reads, " 'She outranks me' General Sherman."

See also Barton, Clarissa Harlowe; Safford, Mary Jane

References

Adams, George W. 1971. "Bickerdyke, Mary Ann Ball." In *Notable American Women, 1607–1950: A Biographical Dictionary*, edited by E.T. James, J.W. James, and P.S. Boyer. Cambridge: Belknap Press of Harvard University Press.

Baker, Nina Brown. 1952. *Cyclone in Calico: The Story of Mary Ann Bickerdyke.* Boston: Little, Brown.

Erlandson, E.V. 1920. "The Story of Mother Bickerdyke." *American Journal of Nursing* 20 (8):628–631.

Gordon, Sarah H. 1999. "Bickerdyke, Mary Ann Ball." In *American National Biography*, edited by J.A. Garraty and M.C. Carnes. New York: Oxford University Press.

Webster's American Military Biographies. 1978. Springfield, Mass.: G. and C. Merriam.

JSB

Birtles, Mary Ellen (1859–1943)
Nurse

Mary Ellen Birtles was one of the first trained nurses in the Canadian west. She was born in 1859 in Hepworth, a village near Yorkshire, England. In 1883, her family emigrated to Brandon, Manitoba, Canada, where Birtles taught school with her father. In July 1886, she began working at Winnipeg General Hospital. When a nurse training school opened at the hospital, she enrolled. Training was two years, and she graduated with the first class in May 1889.

Birtles worked at a small hospital in North Dakota for a short time and then became an assistant nurse at the Medicine Hat General Hospital (1890) in the province of Alberta. Birtles was one of only two nurses there, who also did the work of orderlies and cooks. Typhoid was prevalent in Medicine Hat, and Birtles contracted the disease while caring for a patient. In October 1892 she returned to Manitoba and became the head nurse at a hospital in Brandon, where she remained for two years.

In 1894, Birtles was named matron of Calgary General Hospital. While a new hospital building was under construction, she worked at the old cottage hospital. It was meant to hold only eight patients but often served many more. At first, her only help was an orderly and an assistant, who quit after refusing to properly bathe a typhoid patient. Because the hospital was utilizing the expensive services of a local drugstore to procure prescriptions, Birtles asked for, and received permission to purchase, the raw materials to mix the drugs herself. In 1895 Birtles moved to the new hospital facilities and, with the acceptance of a student nurse, created the Calgary General Hospital Training School. In 1898, she returned to Brandon and became matron of the General Hospital, remaining there until her retirement on August 31, 1919.

Birtles died on June 22, 1943.

Selected Additional Achievements

Charter member, Manitoba Association of Graduate Nurses (1913); Order of the British Empire (1935).

References

Birtles, William. 1995. "A Pioneer Nurse." *Alberta History* (Winter):2–6.

Richardson, Sharon. 2000. "Mary Ellen Birtles." In *American Nursing: A Biographical Dictionary*, edited by V. L. Bullough and L. Sentz. New York: Springer.

Slattery, Anne. 1929. *Pioneers of Nursing in Canada*. Montreal: Gazette Printing.

LS

Black, Elinor Frances Elizabeth (1905–1982)
Physician

Elinor Black was the first female Canadian physician to head a major medical department. For 13 years she was the head of obstetrics and gynecology at the University of Manitoba and at Winnipeg General Hospital. She was born in Nelson, British Columbia, on September 9, 1905, one of five surviving children of Francis Mollison and Margaret Elizabeth (McIntosh) Black. After living in Calgary, Alberta, Canada, and Edinburgh, Scotland, the family settled in Winnipeg, Manitoba, Canada, in 1918.

Black decided to pursue medicine, although her parents and brother, a physician, firmly opposed her career choice. Undaunted, she matriculated at the University of Manitoba Medical School and graduated cum laude in 1930. During her postgraduate internship at Winnipeg General Hospital, she decided to specialize in obstetrics and gynecology. After a three-month residency at Children's Hospital, she studied at the Annie McCall Maternity Hospital in London. She learned most of the techniques of childbirth at the hospital and came to relish the challenge of delivering breech babies safely. She also worked at Chelsea Hospital for Women and attended lectures at London hospitals.

Black returned to Winnipeg in 1931 and established a private obstetrics and gynecology practice. Two years later she was appointed assistant in obstetrics and gynecology at the Winnipeg General Hospital and assistant demonstrator in obstetrics and gynecology at the University of Manitoba. In 1936, she was promoted to the rank of lecturer at the university. The following year, she returned to England to study for the membership examination of the Royal College of Obstetricians and Gynaecologists. As part of her membership requirements, she completed a six-month residency in gynecology at the South London Hospital for Women. In 1938 Black passed the examination and earned the distinction of being the first female Canadian member of the Royal College. After earning her certification, she returned to her positions at Winnipeg General and at the university. She also resumed her private practice and taught at St. John Ambulance. In 1948, she furthered her education during a tour of American and European hospitals and clinics.

Black returned to Winnipeg in 1949 and that year became the first woman elected fellow of the Royal College of Obstetricians and Gynaecologists. In 1951, she was appointed chair and full professor of obstetrics and gynecology at the University of Manitoba. Her new position came with an auto-

matic appointment as head of the Department of Obstetrics and Gynaecology at Winnipeg General. In addition to running a university department and a hospital department, Black continued her private practice.

In 1961, Black became the first woman president of the Society of Obstetricians and Gynaecologists of Canada. Three years later she retired from the university and Winnipeg General. In 1969, she took a temporary professorship of obstetrics and gynecology at the University of the West Indies in Jamaica. In her later years, she suffered a variety of health problems, including a stroke and a broken pelvis and arm. Black died in 1982. Today the Elinor Black room of the University of Manitoba's Department of Obstetrics, Gynecology and Reproductive Sciences exists in her honor.

Selected Additional Achievements

Several medical articles in the *Manitoba Medical Review*, the *University of Manitoba Medical Journal*, and the *Canadian Medical Association Journal*. Member, Winnipeg Medical Society, Manitoba Medical Association, Canadian Medical Association; fellow, International College of Surgeons (1955). Honorary LL.D (Winnipeg, 1970).

References

Hacker, Carlotta. 1974. *The Indomitable Lady Doctors*. Toronto: Clarke, Irwin.
Simpson, Kieran, ed. 1980. *Canadian Who's Who: A Biographical Dictionary of Notable Living Men and Women*. Vol. 15. Toronto: University of Toronto Press.
Vandervoort, Julie. 1992. *Tell the Driver: A Biography of Elinor F. E. Black, M.D.* Winnipeg: University of Manitoba Press.

JSB

Blackwell, Elizabeth (1821–1910)
Physician

Elizabeth Blackwell was the first woman to earn a medical degree in the United States and the first formally recognized female physician in England. She also founded a medical

school devoted to the care of women and to providing women with a quality medical education. She described her struggles and successes as America's earliest woman physician

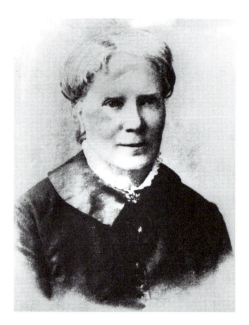

Elizabeth Blackwell. National Library of Medicine.

in her autobiography, *Pioneer Work in Opening the Medical Profession to Women* (1895).

Blackwell was born on February 3, 1821, in Counterslip, England, one of nine surviving children of Samuel Blackwell, a sugar refiner, and Hannah (Lane) Blackwell. She was influenced by her father, who championed women's rights, temperance, and the abolition of slavery. Samuel's daughters received the same education as his sons, an uncommon practice for the time.

The family emigrated to the United States in 1832, first to New York, then to New Jersey in 1835. In 1838, the Blackwells settled in Cincinnati, Ohio; Samuel died later the same year. To support the family, Blackwell, her mother, and sisters ran a boarding school until 1842. In 1844, Blackwell was offered a position as the head of a girls' school in Henderson, Kentucky. Blackwell accepted but soon became bored with teaching, and life among the Kentucky slaveholders outraged her sense of justice. She resigned her position later the same year.

After her return to Cincinnati Blackwell decided to become a physician. She was inspired by a woman friend, dying of cancer, who believed examination by a physician of the same sex would have lessened her suffering. Friends and family enthusiastically supported Blackwell's decision. However, many male doctors advised her that while her goal was admirable, it was impossible for a woman to obtain a medical education. Yet, with every discouragement, her desire "gradually assumed the aspect of a great moral struggle" (Blackwell, p. 29).

Between 1845 and 1847, Blackwell studied medicine privately with sympathetic physicians, first with Dr. John Dickson in Asheville, North Carolina, and then with his brother, Samuel, in Charleston, South Carolina. Her ambition was to become the first American woman surgeon, so she moved to Philadelphia, then considered the seat of medical learning in the United States, and began applying to the best colleges. However, she was rejected by every medical school in Philadelphia and New York and by Harvard, Yale, and Bowdoin, despite recommendations of her physician friends. One professor of surgery said that he would allow her to attend his lectures under the condition that she disguise herself as a man. Instead, she continued private study in Philadelphia with Dr. Joseph Allen and began applying to smaller rural colleges.

In 1847, Blackwell was admitted to Geneva Medical College in western New York. The faculty was opposed to accepting a woman but left the decision to a vote by the students. While the students first met the situation with laughter, they voted unanimously in her favor. She arrived in Geneva in November 1847 to finally begin her formal training. The students and professors, who met the first woman medical student with curiosity, soon developed an admiration for her. Life outside school proved more difficult. The Geneva townspeople considered her either insane or evil and would gather in groups to stare at her. To avoid the unfriendly glares, she walked swiftly to the college, where she could "shut out all unkindly criticism" (Blackwell, p. 70).

During her first summer break, Blackwell was accepted for clinical study at Blockley, a

Philadelphia almshouse. The medical staff did not support her admittance and often left the room when she appeared. They ceased to write diagnoses and treatments on patient cards kept at the head of each bed, leaving her to her own resources for her clinical education. She worked in the women's syphilis department, where she developed the conviction that women must be educated about their own bodies and the spread of disease. In 1848, an outbreak of typhus at Blockley further convinced her of the need for sanitation and personal hygiene. She wrote her graduation thesis, "Ship Fever: An Inaugural Thesis," on her observations of this outbreak.

In 1849, Blackwell received her medical degree along with the distinction of earning the highest scores on final examinations. She then traveled to Paris for training as a student midwife at La Maternité. There, she treated an infant with purulent ophthalmia, a contagious eye disease. Blackwell contracted the disease, lost sight in one eye, and was left with limited vision in the other. Thus, she abandoned her dream of becoming the first woman surgeon. After recovering, she went to London for further study at St. Bartholomew's hospital under Dr. James Paget. She noted in her autobiography the irony that she was allowed into most of the hospital wards *except for the department for female diseases!* (p. 164).

In 1851, Blackwell returned to New York to begin her medical career. As a woman, she was unable to find employment in any clinics or hospitals, was ignored by colleagues, and was even attacked in anonymous letters. Building owners were reluctant to rent office space to a "lady physician," a term that referred to female abortionists. Patients came slowly, and she spent her time preparing lectures on the principles of good hygiene. These lectures were published in 1852 as *The Laws of Life, with Special Reference to the Physical Education of Girls.* During this lonely time, she adopted Katharine Barry, a seven-year-old orphan.

In 1853, Blackwell opened a one-room dispensary in New York. In 1857, with the help of her sister, Dr. Emily Blackwell, and

Dr. Marie Zakrzewska, the dispensary was expanded into the New York Infirmary for Women and Children, the first U.S. hospital conducted entirely by women. The infirmary gave women the opportunity to consult physicians of the same sex and provided clinical experience to female medical students. In 1867, Blackwell appointed Dr. Rebecca Cole as "sanitary visitor," whose job was to visit patients' homes to give simple, practical advice on proper hygienic practices. This was the first form of social medicine in the United States.

In 1858, Blackwell went to England to deliver a series of lectures on the value of medical study for women. She was proud of the progress made in the United States and hoped to advance medical opportunities for women in England. The following year, she became the first woman to be entered onto the Medical Register of the United Kingdom. In 1859, she returned from abroad to add a women's medical school to the New York Infirmary. These plans were interrupted by the outbreak of the Civil War. The war inspired the leaders of the infirmary to form the National Sanitary Aid Association and the Ladies' Sanitary Aid Association, both designed to organize the training and selection of nurses to be dispatched to the battlefield.

After the war, Blackwell refocused her energies on building the women's medical school, an addition that she felt was necessary, as there were few other avenues available for aspiring women physicians. In 1868, the New York Infirmary was expanded into the Woman's Medical College of the New York Infirmary. Entrance examinations were required for admission, before the state required such exams. The college also offered longer terms than other schools, opportunities for clinical experience, and an examining board made up of the most prestigious physicians in the state; no medical college of that day had adopted such rigid academic standards. Blackwell held the Chair of Hygiene, and the college was the first to require a course in hygiene, now known as preventive medicine. The college functioned until 1899, when Cornell University Medical School opened its doors to women.

In 1869, Blackwell left the operation of the college and infirmary to Emily and returned to England to lecture on the importance of women in medicine. She argued that women should play an integral part in improving overall human health; as physicians, women were simply extending their natural role as the family caretaker. Blackwell established a successful practice in London and in 1871, formed the National Health Society, whose motto was "Prevention is better than cure" (Blackwell, p. 247). In 1875, she accepted the Chair of Gynecology at New Hospital and London School of Medicine for Women. Declining health led to her retirement from the New Hospital after only one year. After a headlong fall down a staircase in 1907, Blackwell never fully regained her strength. She died on May 31, 1910, in Argyllshire, Scotland.

See also Blackwell, Emily; Cole, Rebecca J.; Zakrzewska, Marie Elizabeth

Selected Additional Achievements

In *Counsel to Parents on the Moral Education of Their Children* (1878), Blackwell proposed the sexual education of children. Other writings include *The Religion of Health* (1871); *Wrong and Right Methods of Dealing with Social Evil* (1883);

The Human Element in Sex (1884); *The Purchase of Women: The Great Economic Blunder* (1887); *The Influence of Women in the Profession of Medicine* (1889); and *Essays in Medical Sociology* (1892).

References

Blackwell, Elizabeth. 1895. *Pioneer Work in Opening the Medical Profession to Women*. London: Longmans, Green.

Fulton, John F. 1927. "Blackwell, Elizabeth." In *The Dictionary of American Biography*, edited by A. Johnson. New York: Charles Scribner's Sons.

Morantz-Sanchez, Regina Markell. 1985. *Sympathy and Science: Women Physicians in American Medicine*. New York: Oxford University Press.

Morantz-Sanchez, Regina. 1999. "Blackwell Elizabeth." In *American National Biography*, edited by J.A. Garraty and M.C. Carnes. New York: Oxford University Press.

The National Cyclopaedia of American Biography. 1899. Vol. 9. New York: James T. White.

Thomson, Elizabeth H. 1971. "Blackwell, Elizabeth." In *Notable American Women, 1607–1950: A Biographical Dictionary*, edited by E.T. James, J.W. James, and P.S. Boyer. Cambridge: Belknap Press of Harvard University Press.

Wilson, Dorothy Clarke. 1970. *Lone Woman: The Story of Elizabeth Blackwell, the First Woman Doctor*. Boston: Little, Brown.

JSB

Blackwell, Emily (1826–1910)
Physician

Emily Blackwell was one of the first women in the United States to earn a medical degree. With her sister, Elizabeth, she formed the country's first hospital run by women. This hospital played a critical role in opening the doors of medicine to women by providing a place for women physicians to work.

Emily Blackwell was born on October 8, 1826, in Bristol, England, one of nine surviving children of Samuel and Hannah (Lane) Blackwell. She was the younger sister of Elizabeth Blackwell, the first woman to receive a medical degree in the United States. Like Elizabeth, Emily lived in a stimulating

and enlightened family atmosphere. The family emigrated to the United States in 1832, first to New York and then to New Jersey. The family moved to Cincinnati, Ohio, in 1838, a few months before her father died.

In 1848, Blackwell decided to follow in her sister's footsteps and begin a medical career. Elizabeth supported her sister's goal but cautioned her that society was largely still opposed to the woman physician. She wrote to Emily: "I really have no *medical friend*; all the gentlemen I meet seem separated by an invincible, invisible barrier. . . . It will not al-

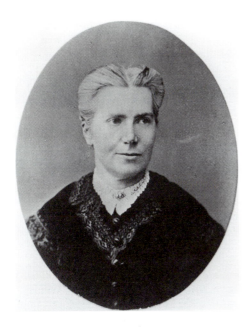

Emily Blackwell. Sophia Smith Collection, Smith College.

ways be so; when the novelty of the innovation is past, men and women will be valuable friends in medicine, but for a time that cannot be" (Blackwell, p. 172). Blackwell studied medicine privately with Dr. John Davis, an anatomy professor at the Medical College of Cincinnati. To earn money for medical school, she took teaching positions, first in Henderson, Kentucky, and then in Cincinnati. She did not find satisfaction in teaching and was eager to begin a formal medical education.

Blackwell was rejected by 11 schools, including Geneva Medical College, which had earlier graduated Elizabeth. She attended clinical lectures at New York's Bellevue Hospital in the summer of 1852 and later that year was finally accepted into Rush Medical College in Chicago. She studied only one year because the Medical Society of Illinois censured the school for admitting a woman. The following summer, Blackwell worked with Elizabeth at her dispensary for women in New York. The next fall, she was accepted into the medical college at Western Reserve University in Cleveland and graduated with honors in 1854. Marie Zakrzewska was also accepted into Western Reserve. There, she would earn her medical degree and later join Elizabeth and Emily in their pioneering work.

After graduation, Blackwell pursued clinical education in Europe. She traveled to Edinburgh, where she studied with Dr. James Young Simpson. Simpson helped Blackwell gain entrance into clinics in London, Paris, Berlin, and Dresden. In 1856, she returned to New York to work in her sister's dispensary, which, with the help of Dr. Zakrzewska, became the New York Infirmary for Women and Children in 1857. The infirmary was the first to give women the opportunity to seek medical attention from physicians of their own sex and to provide clinical experience to women physicians. Both Elizabeth and Emily believed that women should study medicine alongside men. But, as most schools and hospitals would not accept women, the infirmary provided an otherwise unavailable opportunity.

Blackwell's administrative skills were invaluable in converting the sisters' rented house into a 16-bed hospital. She took the major responsibility for the management of the infirmary, overseeing surgery, nursing, and bookkeeping. In 1859, she made a successful trip to Albany to urge the state legislature to place the infirmary on the list of institutions receiving state support. Blackwell so ably managed the hospital that they twice moved to larger quarters, once in 1860 and again in 1874. The hospital treated 3,680 patients in 1860 and 7,549 patients in 1876. In 1868, Woman's Medical College was established at the infirmary.

When Elizabeth moved to England in 1869, the full responsibility of the infirmary and the college was left to Emily. For 30 years she served as dean and professor of obstetrics and diseases of women. The opportunities for clinical training and education at the college were among the best in the United States. By 1876, a three-year graded course was obligatory, a length of training that was required by few other medical schools. The next year, the school term was lengthened to eight months, up to three months longer than at many medical schools. In 1893, the full course was expanded to four years. When Cornell University Medical College began accepting women in 1899, Blackwell closed Woman's Medical College and arranged to have her students transferred to Cornell. At the time of its closing, the college had graduated 364 women physicians. She continued to work with the infirmary until her retirement in 1900.

While Elizabeth is the better known of the Blackwell sisters, it was Emily's "quiet, efficient leadership that placed New York Infirmary . . . in the front rank of medical institutions in this country" (L'Esperance, p. 258). Blackwell spent her retirement years in a house in York Cliffs, Maine, with her adopted daughter, Anna, and Dr. Elizabeth Cushier. She died of enterocolitis on September 7, 1910, only three months after her sister died.

See also Blackwell, Elizabeth; Cushier, Elizabeth; Zakrzewska, Marie Elizabeth

Selected Additional Achievements

Blackwell's publications include "Medicine as a Profession for Women" (1860); "Address on the Medical Education of Women" (1864); "The Industrial Position of Women," *Popular Science Monthly* (1883); "Need of Combination among Women for Self-Protection," *The Philanthropist Series*, no. 14; "Regulation Fallacies: It Will Exist While the World Lasts," *The Philanthropist Series*, no. 22.

References

Blackwell, Elizabeth. 1895. *Pioneer Work in Opening the Medical Profession to Women*. London: Longmans, Green.

L'Esperance, Elise S. 1949. "Influence of the New York Infirmary on Women in Medicine." *Journal of the American Medical Women's Association* 4 (6):255–261.

Morantz-Sanchez, Regina. 1999. "Blackwell, Emily." In *American National Biography*, edited by J.A. Garraty and M.C. Carnes. New York: Oxford University Press.

The National Cyclopaedia of American Biography. 1899. Vol. 9. New York: James T. White.

Thomson, Elizabeth H. 1971. "Blackwell, Emily." In *Notable American Women, 1607–1950: A Biographical Dictionary*, edited by E.T. James, J.W. James, and P.S. Boyer. Cambridge: Belknap Press of Harvard University Press.

Withington, Alfreda B. 1978. "Blackwell, Emily." In *Dictionary of American Medical Biography: Lives of Eminent Physicians of the United States and Canada, from the Earliest Times*, edited by H.A. Kelly and W.L. Burrage. West Newfield, Maine: Longwood Press. Original ed. New York: Appleton, 1928.

JSB

Blanchfield, Florence Aby (1884–1971)
Nurse

Florence Blanchfield was superintendent of the Army Nurse Corps during World War II and the first woman to hold a permanent commission in the United States Army. She was born on April 1, 1884, in Shepherdstown, West Virginia, the fourth of eight children of Mary Louvenia (Anderson), a practical nurse, and Joseph Plunkett Blanchfield, a stonemason and cutter. Blanchfield attended public schools in Walnut Springs, Virginia, and the private Oranda Institute in Virginia.

In August 1902, Blanchfield entered the South Side Hospital Training School for Nurses in Pittsburgh. She graduated in 1906 and then worked as a private-duty nurse in Baltimore, where she also did postgraduate work at Dr. Howard Kelly's Sanatorium and at Johns Hopkins Hospital. She then held supervisory positions at hospitals in Pennsylvania, (1906–1913), worked as a surgical nurse and anesthetist at Ancon Hospital in the Panama Canal Zone (1913), and was the emergency surgical nurse at U.S. Steel Corporation in Bessemer, Pennsylvania (1914–1915). In August 1917, in the midst of World War I, she joined the Army Nurse Corps (ANC), which was established in 1901 largely through the efforts of Dr. Anita McGee.

Blanchfield sailed for France in September 1917 and served at Angers and Camp Co-etquidan as a surgical nurse and acting chief nurse. In June 1920 an Army Reorganization Act authorized relative rank for army nurses, and she was appointed to the relative rank of first lieutenant. Relative rank permitted nurses to wear the insignia of their grade and was an improvement in status. Nurses were not afforded the full rights, privileges, and basic pay of male officers of comparable rank, however.

From 1920 to 1935, Blanchfield served in several states and also overseas. Beginning in 1935, she worked in the Office of the Su-perintendent of the ANC, becoming super-intendent in June 1943. Upon accepting her assignment, she assured skeptical reporters that army nurses were prepared for assign-ment in theaters of war, saying that "they are hardened, I assure you" (quoted in "New Nurse," p. 22).

Blanchfield was an effective administrator of the corps. She oversaw the dramatic and successful increase of nurses from a prewar level of 700 to a high of 57,000 during World War II. She established basic training centers for new nurses to learn military cus-toms and regulations and assigned nurses to hospitals close to the front lines to maximize care. She also obtained permission for nurses to wear battle fatigues in war zones, rather than impractical, traditional white nursing uniforms.

Throughout her career, Blanchfield's ma-jor concern was eliminating the bias in mili-tary status of army nurses. She fought to have nurses recognized as Regular Army person-nel. With Congresswoman Frances Payne Bolton, her goal was partially achieved in 1944, when nurses were given full military rank for the duration of the war plus six months. Finally, after passage of the Army-Navy Nurse Act of 1947, nurses were given permanent commissioned officer status. To recognize the role that Blanchfield played in this achievement, on June 19, 1947, she was the first nurse, as well as the first woman, commissioned in the Regular Army, receiv-ing the rank of lieutenant colonel. She retired from the army a few months later, in Septem-ber 1947.

Blanchfield died on May 12, 1971, in Washington, D.C., of heart disease. She was buried in Arlington National Cemetery with full military honors.

See also McGee, Anita Newcomb

Selected Additional Achievements

Blanchfield wrote numerous articles on military nursing. Honors include the Distinguished Service Medal of the United States Army (1945); the Florence Nightingale Medal of the International Red Cross (1951); and induction into the Amer-ican Nurses Association Hall of Fame (1996). The United States Army hospital at Ft. Campbell, Ken-tucky, was named the Colonel Florence A. Blanch-field Army Community Hospital in her honor (1982).

References

Bombard, Charles F., Wynona M. Bice-Stephens, and Karen L. Ferguson. 1988. "The Soldiers' Nurse: Colonel Florence A. Blanchfield." *Mi-nerva: Quarterly Report on Women and the Military* 6 (4):43–49.

Henry, Linda J. 1980. "Blanchfield, Florence Aby." In *Notable American Women: The Mod-ern Period: A Biographical Dictionary*, edited by B. Sicherman and C.H. Green. Cambridge: Belknap Press of Harvard University Press.

"New Nurse Chief Takes Oath in Presence of Army Officials." 1943. *New York Times* (June 2):22.

Reeves, Connie L. 1999. "Blanchfield, Florence Aby." In *American National Biography*, edited by J.A. Garraty and M.C. Carnes. New York: Oxford University Press.

LS

Breckinridge, Mary (1881–1965)
Nurse-midwife

Mary Breckinridge introduced nurse-midwifery to the United States through her establishment of the Frontier Nursing Service (FNS) in the rural Kentucky mountains. The FNS brought the region modern health care and midwifery service. She was born on February 17, 1881, in Memphis, Tennessee, to Katherine (Carson) and Clifton Rodes Breckinridge, a congressman and diplomat. In her childhood, she lived in Washington, D.C., and in St. Petersburg, Russia. In addition to her education by governesses, she attended schools in Switzerland and Connecticut.

Her parents disapproved of women attending college, so Breckinridge spent her young adulthood with family and relatives, waiting to marry. She found the lifestyle repressive, writing later in her autobiography, *Wide Neighborhoods* (1952), "As the seasons of my aimless girlhood passed, I tried to effect a

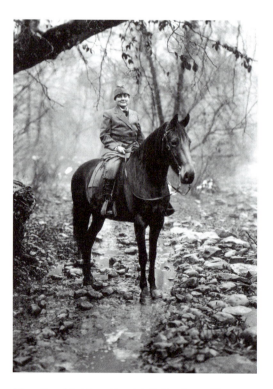

Mary Breckinridge. Special Collections: Photographic Archives, University of Louisville.

reconciliation between the life I longed to live and the life allowed me" (1981 reprint, p. 46). In 1904, she married Henry Ruffner Morrison. When he died just two years later, she felt unfit to do anything useful. Then, while tending a child sick with typhoid, she realized that she could be of great service to children if she studied nursing. In 1907, she entered St. Luke's Hospital School of Nursing in New York City and graduated in 1910. She then spent a year at her parents' home in Arkansas at the request of her ailing mother.

On October 8, 1912, Breckinridge married Richard Ryan Thompson, president of Crescent College and Conservatory for Young Women in Eureka Springs, Arkansas. She taught French and hygiene at the school. In 1914, a son was born to the couple. Breckinridge delighted in caring for her son, but her marriage and life in Eureka Springs were otherwise unfulfilling. In 1916, she had a daughter, who died shortly after birth. Then, in January 1918, her son fell ill and died suddenly. Soon thereafter, she left her husband (divorcing him in 1920) and turned again to nursing as an outlet for her grief.

Breckinridge decided to volunteer her services to the American Red Cross in war-devastated France. While awaiting assignment, she spent time at the Boston Instructive District Nursing Association, where she received training in public health nursing. She also worked in Washington, D.C., for three months with the Children's Bureau. Before she could be assigned to Europe, the war ended, so she volunteered for the American Committee for Devastated France. She was assigned to Vic-sur-Aisne, where she provided disaster relief and initiated a special program of medical and nutritional care for children and pregnant women.

Breckinridge considered her time in France as important preparation for the FNS. In France and in visits to England, she encountered British nurse-midwives who impressed her greatly. Inspired by the nurse-midwives and her relief work in France, she decided to initiate a nursing service in the rural United States. She left France in 1921 and studied public health nursing at Teachers College, Columbia University in New York. She chose Leslie County in Eastern Kentucky, one of the poorest regions in Appalachia, as the site for her nursing experiment. She spent the summer of 1923 surveying the health needs of women and children in the area and that fall sent her report and a proposal for a maternal and child health service to the American Child Health Association. The association denied her funding, however.

In the fall of 1923, Breckinridge received midwifery training at London's British Hospital for Mothers and Babies and attended lectures at the Royal College of Surgeons, the Midwives Institute, and the York Road General Lying-In Hospital in London. To increase her knowledge of what would be needed in a rural nursing service, she went to Scotland in August 1924 to study the methods of the Highlands and Islands Medical and Nursing Service.

Upon returning to the United States in 1925, Breckinridge established the Kentucky Committee for Mothers and Babies, which was renamed the Frontier Nursing Service in 1928. She served as director of the service until her death. Without public funding, the FNS relied on the support of private donors and an inheritance from Breckinridge's mother. The FNS eventually consisted of six outpost nursing centers, approximately 10 miles apart, centered on her home in Hyden, Kentucky. On Christmas Day in 1925, Breckinridge dedicated her home, Wendover, and the nursing service to the people of the region. Wendover served as a small hospital as well as Breckinridge's home before the FNS opened Hyden Hospital in 1928.

FNS nurses provided care to people in a 700-square-mile area. The nurse-midwives, many of whom were British, rode horseback to get to their patients and carried all their supplies in saddlebags. They provided general preventive care as well as midwifery serv-

ice and stressed prenatal care. Ninety percent of births took place in patients' homes, and once a woman was in labor, the nurses never left her. The excellent care provided by FNS nurses resulted in a reduced mortality and morbidity rate for mothers and babies in the region. By 1951, nurse-midwives of the FNS had delivered 8,596 patients, with only 10 maternal deaths.

In 1939, when many British nurses returned home during World War II, Breckinridge established the Frontier Graduate School of Midwifery to teach American nurses midwifery skills. Classes began on November 1, 1939, with just two students. The school eventually flourished and exists today as the Frontier School of Midwifery and Family Nursing. After taking two year's leave to write *Wide Neighborhoods*, Breckinridge never resumed the level of daily contact that she had had with FNS operations. She died in Hyden, Kentucky, on May 16, 1965, of leukemia and a stroke. Ten years after her death, a new hospital, named in her honor, opened in Hyden. The Frontier Nursing Service continues today.

Selected Additional Achievements

Breckinridge established the *Frontier Nursing Service Quarterly Bulletin* in 1925 to provide progress reports of the organization. She edited the journal and contributed many signed and unsigned articles to it. Among the awards that she received are the Médaille Reconnaissance Française and the Mary Adelaide Nutting Award of the National League for Nursing. She was inducted into the American Nurses Association Hall of Fame in 1982, and on November 9, 1998, the U.S. Postal Service honored Breckinridge with a 77-cent stamp of her likeness.

References

Breckinridge, Mary. 1927. "The Nurse-Midwife—A Pioneer." *American Journal of Public Health* 17 (11):1147–1151.

Breckinridge, Mary. 1981. *Wide Neighborhoods: A Story of the Frontier Nursing Service*. Reprint ed., Lexington: University Press of Kentucky. Original ed., New York: Harper and Brothers, 1952.

Bullough, Vern L. 1988. "Mary Breckinridge." In *American Nursing: A Biographical Dictionary*, edited by V.L. Bullough, O.M. Church, and A.P. Stein. New York: Garland.

Dye, Nancy Schrom. 1984. "Mary Breckinridge, the Frontier Nursing Service, and the Introduction of Nurse-Midwifery in the United States." In *Women and Health in America: Historical Readings*, edited by J.W. Leavitt. Madison: University of Wisconsin Press. Reprinted from *Bulletin of the History of Medicine* 57 (1983): 485–507.

Faust, Drew Gilpin. 1980. "Breckinridge, Mary." In *Notable American Women: The Modern Period: A Biographical Dictionary*, edited by B. Sicherman and C.H. Green. Cambridge: Belknap Press of Harvard University Press.

LS

Broomall, Anna Elizabeth (1847–1931)
Physician

Anna Broomall was an innovative professor of obstetrics at Woman's Medical College of Pennsylvania in Philadelphia. She was born on March 4, 1847, in Upper Chichester Township, Pennsylvania, the younger of two children of John Martin and Elizabeth (Booth) Broomall. Her mother died when Broomall was one year old, and relatives raised her until her father remarried in 1853.

After graduating from Bristol Boarding School in 1866, Broomall matriculated at Woman's Medical College of Pennsylvania (now MCP Hahnemann University). In 1869, she and her classmates were among the first female medical students to receive permission to attend clinical lectures at Pennsylvania Hospital, an event that sparked protests by male medical students opposed to coeducational medical education. After earning her medical degree in 1871, Broomall interned for one year at the College's Woman's Hospital and then traveled to Vienna to study diseases of the skin, nose, and throat. While in Vienna, she learned that Emeline Cleveland, chair of obstetrics at Woman's Medical, had been diagnosed with cancer and wanted Broomall to succeed her after Cleveland's death. Broomall thus altered her course of study to obstetrics under prominent physicians in Vienna and Paris.

After returning to Philadelphia in 1875, Broomall was appointed as chief resident physician at Woman's Hospital and as instructor of obstetrics at Woman's Medical.

She succeeded Cleveland as chair in 1879 and was also professor of obstetrics (1880–1903). Seeking to improve the students' obstetrical education, she established the Out-Practice Maternity Department in an impoverished Philadelphia neighborhood (1888), one of the first institutions of its kind in the country. The obstetrical students received clinical experience while providing the highest-quality obstetrical care to poor women. In 1896, the department expanded to include inpatient care at Maternity Hospital of Woman's Medical College. An innovator in the use of obstetrical surgical techniques, Broomall read German, Italian, and French medical literature to keep her students abreast of European obstetrical advancements. The extremely low mortality rate at Maternity Hospital is a testament to her skills and teaching methods.

During her career, Broomall also maintained a private practice and was gynecologist at the Friends' Asylum for the Insane in Philadelphia. In 1890, she traveled to Asia and India to lecture and visit medical missionaries who were former students. In 1903, she resigned from the chair of obstetrics at Woman's Medical College and moved to Chester, Pennsylvania. In her later years she pursued an interest in historical preservation and was museum curator of the Delaware County Historical Society. She died from a septic bladder on April 4, 1931.

See also Cleveland, Emeline Horton

Selected Additional Achievements

Broomall was one of the first female members of the Philadelphia Obstetrical Society and the first woman physician to publish in its *Transactions.* Writings include "The Operation of Episiotomy as a Prevention of Perineal Ruptures during Labor," *American Journal of Obstetrics and Diseases of Women and Children* (1878); "Three Cases of Symphysiotomy, with One Death from Sepsis," *American Journal of Obstetrics and Diseases of Women and Children* (1893); member, Delaware County Institute of Science; member, Delaware County Botanical Society. The Broomall Maternity ward of Woman's Medical College and the Anna E. Broomall Medical Club were formed in her honor.

References

Broomall, Anna E. Deceased Alumnae Files, Special Collections on Women in Medicine, Archives and Special Collections, MCP Hahnemann University, Philadelphia.
"Broomall, Dr. Anna E." 1931. *Medical Woman's Journal* 38 (5):130.
Griscom, Mary W. 1931. "A Beloved Physician." *Medical Woman's Journal* 38 (7):183–185.
Ward, Patricia Spain. 1971. "Broomall, Anna Elizabeth." In *Notable American Women, 1607–1950: A Biographical Dictionary*, edited by E.T. James, J.W. James, and P.S. Boyer. Cambridge: Belknap Press of Harvard University Press.

JSB

Brown, Charlotte Amanda Blake (1846–1904)
Physician

Charlotte Brown was an early woman physician in California who helped found a women's and children's hospital in San Francisco. She was born on December 22, 1846, in Philadelphia, the second of five children of Charles Morris Blake, a teacher and Presbyterian minister, and Charlotte A. (Farrington) Blake. She graduated from Bangor High School in Maine in 1861 and from Elmira College in Elmira, New York in 1866. After college, she moved to Arizona, where her father was chaplain to an army regiment.

In 1867, she married Henry Adams Brown of Riverside, Maine, and the next year the couple's first child, Adelaide, was born. In 1869, they had their second child, Philip, and the Browns and Charlotte's parents moved to Napa, California. In California, she began to study medicine with a family doctor. Medicine was something of a tradition in her family, as her father had begun a medical education in Philadelphia in the 1840s, and her older brother was a physician. In 1872, after her third child, Harriet, was born, Brown left her home in Napa and went to Woman's Medical College of Pennsylvania in Philadelphia to study medicine. She graduated from the college in 1874.

After graduation, Brown and her family moved to San Francisco, where she opened a private practice. Brown had spent her senior year at Woman's Medical as a hospital intern, and as a result, she was a great believer in such practical training. Accordingly, in 1875 she and several other women joined together to form a dispensary for women and children that would provide women physicians clinical experience, as well as allow women to receive medical care from their own sex. The Pacific Dispensary for Women and Children opened in 1875 with Brown as one of the first two attending physicians. During its first 10 months, 267 patients were treated at the dispensary; most ailments were related to malnutrition. In 1878, the dispensary was reorganized as a hospital, and in 1880 the hospital added the first nurse training program west of the Rockies. By 1885, the hospital emphasized children's care, and it was renamed San Francisco Hospital for Children and Training School for Nurses (also called Children's Hospital). Brown was a staff physician at the hospital from 1885 to 1895.

Brown was an innovator; in 1878 she was the first woman on the Pacific Coast to perform an ovariotomy. In 1887, she advocated

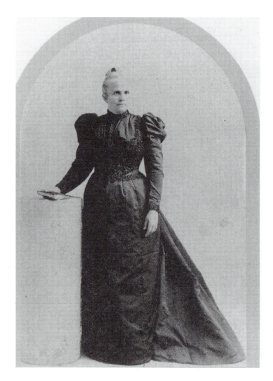

Charlotte Amanda Blake Brown. Archives & Special Collections on Women in Medicine, MCP Hahnemann University.

a tumor registry, and in 1889, she designed and introduced a milk sterilizer. She was also an advocate for better training for nurses and doctors and a supporter of social responsibility and public hygiene. Among the causes that she supported were treating children with contagious diseases at public expense and the sterilization of milk. In an 1896 article, Brown also supported "the establish-ment . . . of out of door gymnastic fields, especially for women" (p. 197).

In 1895, Brown resigned from Children's Hospital. She and two of her children who had also become physicians, Adelaide and Philip, opened a small private practice, and she worked with them until her death. Brown died in San Francisco of intestinal paralysis on April 19, 1904.

Selected Additional Achievements

Brown published 18 articles in medical journals. Member, California Medical Society (1876), San Francisco Medical Society (1878), standing committee on training schools for nurses for the National Conference of Charities and Corrections.

References

Brock, Lois. 1950. "The Hospital for Children and Training School for Nurses." *Journal of the American Medical Women's Association* 5 (1): 28–30.

Brown, Adelaide. 1926. "The History of the Development of Women in Medicine in California." *Medical Woman's Journal* 33 (1):17–20. Reprinted from *California and Western Medicine* (May 1925).

Brown, Charlotte B. 1896. "The Health of Our Girls." *Transactions. California State Medical Society* 26:193–202.

Jensen, Joan M. 1971. "Brown, Charlotte Amanda Blake." In *Notable American Women, 1607–1950: A Biographical Dictionary*, edited by E.T. James, J.W. James, and P.S. Boyer. Cambridge: Belknap Press of Harvard University Press.

LS

Brown, Dorothy Lavinia (1919–   )
Physician

Dorothy Brown is one of the first African American women surgeons to practice in the South and one of the first to be admitted to the American College of Surgeons. She was born in Philadelphia on January 7, 1919. Her mother, Edna Brown, was unwed at the time and placed her baby in a Troy, New York, orphanage when Brown was five months old. At age 15, Brown enrolled in Troy High School and lived with foster parents.

In 1937, Brown entered Bennett College in Greensboro, North Carolina. She decided to be a physician at the age of five, when her tonsils were removed. She took science courses in preparation for her future career and graduated second in her class in 1941. In 1944, she entered the Meharry Medical College in Nashville, Tennessee. While Meharry lacked prestige, it was affordable, and Brown reasoned, "You could go to any small place, because you're going to learn as much as you want anyhow" (*They Have Overcome*, p. 8). She earned her M.D. in 1948 and completed a one-year internship at Harlem Hospital. This was followed by a five-year surgical residency at Meharry, despite opposition to her appointment by male doctors.

She began her career at Meharry's George W. Hubbard Hospital as assistant professor of surgery and director of Student Health Services. Beginning in 1959, she also served as chief of surgery at Nashville's Riverside Hospital. Brown was general surgeon and clinical professor of surgery at Meharry Medical College before her retirement in January 2000.

Selected Additional Achievements

Fellow, American College of Medicine, Nashville Academy of Medicine, R.F. Boyd Medical Society, and National Medical Association; Award for Outstanding Achievement, Delta Sigma Theta Sorority (1963); honorary degrees from Russell Sage College, Bennett College, and Cumberland University. First woman to hold a seat in the Tennessee state legislature and the first single woman in Tennessee to legally adopt a child. The women's building at Meharry Medical College is named after her.

References

Dunn, Lois L. 1992. "Dorothy Brown." In *Notable Black American Women*, edited by J.C. Smith. Detroit: Gale.

Lunardini, Christine A. 1993. "Brown, Dorothy Lavinia." In *Black Women in America: An Historical Encyclopedia*, edited by D.C. Hine, E. Barkley, and R. Terborg-Penn. Brooklyn, N.Y.: Carlson.

"Our Lady Asclepiads." 1968. *Journal of the National Medical Association* 60 (2):136–137, 163.

They Have Overcome: Dr. Dorothy Brown. 1967. Pleasantville, N.Y.: Warren Schloat Productions. Transcript of filmstrip.

JSB

Browne, Helen Edith (1911–1987)
Nurse-midwife

Helen Browne was a prominent nurse-midwife, educator, and administrator who devoted much of her career to the Frontier Nursing Service of rural Kentucky, which became a model for nurse-midwifery in the United States. She was born on February 3, 1911, in Bury St. Edmonds, England, to Phil and Agnes (Rice-Capon) Browne. Her early education was with governesses and at Ipswich High School in Suffolk, England. She always wanted to be a nurse, particularly after meeting the nurses and midwives who cared for her mother when her younger sister was born. From 1931 to 1934 Browne studied at the St. Bartholomew's Hospital School of Nursing in London, England. She then took a one-year course in midwifery (1934–1935) at British Hospital for Mothers and Babies in London and became a certified midwife.

While studying at British Hospital, Browne was nurse-in-charge at St. Bartholomew's. From 1935 to 1938, she also worked in private practice as a nurse-midwife, and in 1937, she was midwifery supervisor for British Hospital for Mothers and Babies. In 1938, a nursing school teacher told Browne of an opportunity to go to the United States and work for the Frontier Nursing Service (FNS), founded by Mary Breckinridge in 1925. Working in a rural area that required riding horses to reach patients appealed to Browne, and she arrived in Leslie County, Kentucky, in July 1938.

Browne worked for the FNS for the next 38 years, beginning as a district midwife at the Red Bird-Flat Creek Clinic. She started at the FNS at a time when many other British nurse-midwives were returning home to aid their country in the war effort. She stayed in the United States and steadily took on more responsibility for the administration of the FNS. She joined the faculty of the FNS' training school, Frontier Graduate School of Midwifery, in 1940. Browne believed strongly in the value of nursing in keeping people well and often said to incoming classes, "Now, remember, you're a nurse and always remember that nursing cares and medicine cures" (Browne, p. 38). During World War II, she became supervisor of the FNS hospital, Hyden Hospital, and was later made assistant director of the FNS (1947).

In 1965, after the death of Mary Breckinridge, Browne was unanimously elected the new FNS director. She led the organization through a period of great change in health care delivery and administration, helping the FNS adjust to the advent of Medicare and Medicaid. She also saw the need for a new hospital in the area and was a major fundraiser and force behind the building of Mary Breckinridge Hospital. Additionally, she helped visitors from foreign countries learn and adapt the practices of the FNS for their own locales. She was also instrumental in merging the FNS-based American Association of Nurse-Midwives with American College of Nurse-Midwifery to form American College of Nurse-Midwives because she believed that midwives should speak with one voice. In 1970, she combined the family nursing and nurse-midwife elements of Frontier Graduate School of Midwifery into one educational curriculum, and the school was renamed Frontier School of Midwifery and Family Nursing.

Although Browne retired in 1975, she continued to raise funds and speak on behalf of the FNS. She died on January 20, 1987, at her home in Milford, Pennsylvania, after suffering a heart attack. Both the Frontier Nursing Service and its Frontier School of Midwifery and Family Nursing continue today.

See also Breckinridge, Mary

Selected Additional Achievements

Member, American Nurses Association, Royal College of Nurse Midwives, National League for Nursing; member and director (1954–1958), Kentucky Nurses Association; Distinguished Service Award, Berea College (1976); American Nurses Association Honorary Recognition Award (1976); honorary doctorate in nursing from Eastern Kentucky University (1976); officer of Most Excellent Order of the British Empire (1964); and Commander of the Most Excellent Order of the British Empire (1976).

References

Browne, Helen. 1979. Interviews by Carol Crowe-Carraco and by Dale Deaton. Tape Recordings, March 26, 27. Frontier Nursing Service Oral History Project, Division of Special Collections and Archives, University of Kentucky Libraries, Lexington.

Calley, Linda M. 1992. "Helen Edith Browne." In *American Nursing: A Biographical Dictionary*, edited by V.L. Bullough, L. Sentz, and A.P. Stein. New York: Garland.

Hawkins, Joellen Watson. 1988. "Browne, Helen E." In *Dictionary of American Nursing Biography*, edited by M. Kaufman. New York: Greenwood Press.

"A Life of Service: Miss Helen E. Browne, C.B.E." 1987. *Frontier Nursing Service Quarterly Bulletin* 62 (3):1–3.

LS

Buckel, C. [Cloe] Annette (1833–1912)
Physician, Civil War nurse

C. Annette Buckel was one of the earlier women physicians in the United States. In addition to practicing medicine in several cities, she used her medical skills to serve as a nurse during the Civil War. She was born on August 25, 1833, in Warsaw, New York, to Thomas Buckel and his wife, known only by her maiden name of Bartlett. Both died before Buckel reached her first birthday, so she was taken in by her paternal grandparents. They died when she was about four, and she was left in the care of two teenage aunts. She attended a local district school, as well as a more advanced school in a nearby town. By age 14, Buckel was teaching in elementary schools in New York state and in Canada, and by age 15, she knew that she wanted to be a doctor.

To earn money for her medical education, Buckel worked in a Connecticut burnishing factory and borrowed against a life insurance policy. In 1856, she entered Female (later, Woman's) Medical College of Pennsylvania in Philadelphia. She graduated in 1858, writing her thesis on insanity. After graduation, she spent one year doing postgraduate work at the Blackwell sisters' and Marie Zakrzewska's New York Infirmary for Women and Children. Buckel began her medical career in Chicago in December 1859 by founding a dispensary there for women and children.

In 1863, with the Civil War raging, Buckel felt compelled to volunteer her services. As women physicians were not recognized by the military, she served as a nurse. The United States Army's acting surgeon general authorized her to select and appoint female nurses, and by the fall of 1864, she was the chief of female nurses at Jefferson General Hospital in Jeffersonville, Indiana. She held the post for the remainder of the war. She was well liked by military men, who referred to her as "the Little Major."

After the war, Buckel returned to the practice of medicine and worked for a short time in Evansville, Indiana. She then moved to Boston, where she practiced at New England Hospital for Women and Children, founded by Marie Zakrzewska in 1862. Buckel was appointed resident physician there in 1868, specializing in respiratory ailments. In 1872, she took a two-year leave of absence from the hospital due to ill health. During that time, she traveled to Europe, observing surgery in clinics in Vienna and Paris. She returned to Boston in 1875 and was appointed attending surgeon. She resigned two years later, however, due to continuing health problems.

Buckel then moved to Oakland, California, where she opened a medical practice. In California, she also served as consulting physician at San Francisco's Pacific Dispensary for Women and Children, founded by Dr. Charlotte Brown in 1875.

Buckel took an active interest in the social and public health problems of her day. As early as 1871 she asked in an annual report for New England Hospital for Women and Children, "Can we not find some means to secure to infants a mother's care and love . . . by furnishing these mothers with some honest means of support . . . saving both mothers and children?" (quoted in Zakrzewska, p. 491). In Oakland, she was instrumental in getting home economics introduced to the schools, and she created and was president (1904–1909) of a pure milk commission. As president of the commission, she worked toward preventing milk from cows infected with tuberculosis from entering the milk supply. Buckel took a special interest in the welfare of orphaned children, and in 1901, she became a trustee and chairman at an Oakland home for orphaned and delinquent girls.

In 1906, Buckel moved to Piedmont, California, with longtime friend Charlotte Playter. She died there of arteriosclerosis on August 17, 1912. In 1914, a grant from her estate established a Buckel Foundation research fellowship at Stanford University for the study of child psychology.

See also Blackwell, Elizabeth; Blackwell, Emily; Brown, Charlotte Amanda Blake; Zakrzewska, Marie Elizabeth

Selected Additional Achievements

First woman admitted to the Alameda County Medical Association, 1878; founded local Agassiz Society to encourage children to study nature; founded a Chautauqua circle (an educational society); headed the biology section of the Oakland Ebell Society (a women's cultural and study club).

References

Brown, Adelaide. 1926. "The History of the Development of Women in Medicine in California." *Medical Woman's Journal* 33 (1):17–20. Reprinted from *California and Western Medicine* (May 1925).

Jensen, Joan M. 1971. "Buckel, Cloe Annette." In *Notable American Women, 1607–1950: A Biographical Dictionary*, edited by E.T. James, J.W. James, and P.S. Boyer. Cambridge: Belknap Press of Harvard University Press.

Martin, Margaret Elizabeth. 1940. "Dr. C. Annette Buckel, the 'Little Major.' " *California Historical Society Quarterly* (March):74–76.

Zakrzewska, Marie E. 1972. *A Woman's Quest: The Life of Marie E. Zakrzewska, M.D.* Edited by A. C. Vietor. New York: Arno Press.

LS

Burton, Pearlie (1904–1993)
Midwife

The career of midwife Pearlie Burton is representative of the work of many African Americans who practiced midwifery in the South between the world wars. She was born on April 21, 1904, in Hart County, Georgia, one of 15 children of Simon and Ollie (Stowers) Hunt. At the age of 18, she married Lafayette Burton. She wanted to be a nurse but could not afford the training. Instead, Burton apprenticed with her husband's mother, who was a midwife. The first baby that she delivered on her own was her brother's. After that success, she was called on, day and night, to deliver babies. She refused to be rushed when an overly anxious father-to-be came knocking at her door, particularly when she knew it was a woman's first child.

Burton delivered thousands of babies from the 1920s through the 1940s. She and other midwives met twice a month to discuss midwifery and health-related topics. She attended births in the homes of the mothers, in barns, and even in fields. When she arrived at an expectant mother's bedside, she would speak to her, perhaps tell her a joke to relax her, and would then don a white apron and rubber gloves in preparation for the birth. She might give the woman cane syrup and a glass of hot water to speed delivery but refused to use alcohol to dull the pain. She charged $5 and then $10 for a delivery but was often paid in goods or not at all.

In addition to midwifery, Burton and her husband farmed, raising such crops as cotton, sweet potatoes, and corn. Although the couple desperately wanted children, they were unable to have any of their own. Instead, they adopted many of the unwanted babies whom Burton delivered. In the 1940s they were the first African Americans to become foster parents for Hart County. In her later years, Burton taught Sunday school and volunteered at a local hospital. In 1991, she was recognized by the community as the Hart County Mother of the Year.

Burton died on March 12, 1993, in Royston, Georgia.

References

Dates of birth and death verified through *Social Security Death Index.* Online. http://www.ancestry.com/search/rectype/vital/ssdi/main.htm. 28 June 2000.

Greene, Melissa. 1987. "All the Hours of the Night: The Recollections of a Country Midwife." *Country Journal* 14 (November):59–63.

"Mrs. Pearlie Burton Is the '91 Hart Mother-of-Year." 1991. *Hartwell Sun* (May 8):1.

"Pearlie Burton." 1993. *Hartwell Sun* (March 17):5B.

LS

Butler, Ida de Fatio (1868–1949)
Nurse

Ida Butler was a prominent nursing and health care administrator who devoted much of her career to the American Red Cross. She was born in Watertown, New York, on March 18, 1868, the daughter of Major John Hartwell and Ida de M. Fatio Butler, a U.S. Civil War nurse. After the death of her mother, her grandfather, psychiatrist John S. Butler, raised her. John Butler instilled in Ida and her cousin, pioneering nurse Annie W. Goodrich, a desire to end human suffering. Butler received her early education in private schools in Connecticut.

In 1901, Butler earned a diploma from Hartford Hospital School of Nursing and then spent a short time as head nurse in a gynecological ward at the University of Pennsylvania Hospital in Philadelphia. In 1902, she began a long career at Hartford Hospital. Until 1918, she served the hospital in many capacities, most notably as the supervisor of the obstetric department. Concurrently, she taught classes in hygiene and care of the sick in Manchester, Connecticut.

Butler was a member of the American Red Cross Nursing Service since 1916. Two years later, after the outbreak of World War I, the Red Cross sent her to Lyons, France, where she directed nursing services at two children's hospitals, first at Hospital Violet and then at Hospital Holtzman. For her achievements, the French government awarded her the French Reconnaissance Medal. She was satisfied to learn 20 years later that the city of Lyons had established permanent child welfare programs based on the work that she had performed there.

Butler returned to the United States in 1919 and continued to work for the Red Cross as organizer and director of a home for convalescent victims of the influenza epidemic. The same year, she began a 15-week lecture tour for the Red Cross. Butler visited nearly 100 towns, supporting the employ-

ment of community and public health nurses and encouraging young women to enter nurse training schools.

In 1919, Butler began her work as an administrator for the American Red Cross. She was director of the nursing service of the organization's Foreign and Insular Division until 1920. That year she was appointed assistant director of the Red Cross, a position that she held until 1936. In this position, she maintained nurses' enrollment records with such meticulous detail that it was possible to assemble nurses quickly and efficiently for assistance during a disaster. Her enrollment records also facilitated the readiness of reserve nurses for the United States Army and Navy Nurse Corps.

Butler had decided to retire in 1936; however, the death that year of Red Cross director Clara Noyes postponed her plans. She served as director of the Red Cross for the next two years, during which time she assisted in the consolidation of several nursing functions of the Red Cross. Mary Beard was appointed director of this newly created unified nursing service in 1938.

Butler retired from the Red Cross in 1939. During her later years, she served as temporary secretary of the Nursing Council on National Defense (1940–1944). She was also chair of the Connecticut State Defense Council (1940) and the Connecticut State Nurses Council on National Defense during World War II. Additionally, she served as chair of the Red Cross Nursing Committee of Greater Hartford. Her work in that state earned her the Connecticut Distinguished Service Medal. Between 1940 and 1942 she was in charge of arrangements for the biennial nursing conventions held jointly by the American Nurses Association, the National League of Nursing Education, and the National Organization for Public Health Nursing.

In 1937, Butler received the Florence Nightingale Medal from the International Red Cross Committee of Geneva. She died in Hartford on March 11, 1949.

See also Beard, Mary; Goodrich, Annie Warburton; Noyes, Clara Dutton

References

"News about Nursing." 1938. *American Journal of Nursing* 38 (11):1278–1279.

"Obituary." 1949. *American Journal of Nursing* 49 (5):34, 36.

Pennock, Meta Rutter, ed. 1940. *Makers of Nursing History; Portraits and Pen Sketches of One Hundred and Nine Prominent Women.* New York: Lakeside.

Tao, Dorothy. 1988. "Ida de Fatio Butler." In *American Nursing: A Biographical Dictionary*, edited by V.L. Bullough, O.M. Church, and A.P. Stein. New York: Garland.

JSB

C

Calderone, Mary Steichen (1904–1998)
Physician

Mary Steichen Calderone, a sex education pioneer, made great inroads in the fields of birth control and human sexuality. She was born in New York City on July 1, 1904, the first of two daughters of painter and photographer Edward Steichen and Clara (Smith) Steichen. Calderone spent the first 10 years of her life in France, but when World War I broke out in 1914, her family returned to the United States. Shortly thereafter, her parents divorced, and Calderone was sent to live with a series of relatives and friends. Her early education was in schools in Connecticut and New York City.

Calderone entered the premedical curriculum at Vassar College in 1921, but she found the classes dull and achieved only mediocre grades. Consequently, in her senior year, she dropped out of the science program to concentrate on acting, music, and English. She graduated from Vassar in 1925 and studied acting at the American Laboratory Theater for three years before realizing that it was not her forte. In 1926, she married an actor, Lon Martin, with whom she had two daughters, the elder of whom died of pneumonia at the age of eight. The marriage ended in 1933, and Calderone, finding herself adrift, underwent psychoanalysis and a series of tests that indicated that she had a strong aptitude for science.

After briefly considering a doctoral program in nutrition, Calderone enrolled in medical school at the University of Rochester in New York. She graduated in 1939 and took a pediatric internship with Children's Medical Service at Bellevue Hospital in New York City. At this point, realizing that she did not want to spend many more years in hospital residencies that would further separate her from her growing daughter, she began a master of public health degree at Columbia University's School of Public Health. While at Columbia, she met her second husband, Dr. Frank Calderone, a district health officer. They married in 1941, and Calderone received her master's degree in 1942. She then had two more children and served part-time as a physician in the local public schools of Great Neck, New York.

The year that her husband retired (1953) Calderone reentered public life as medical director of the Planned Parenthood Federation of America. After some time, Calderone realized that the position had been offered to her because "most male physicians look[ed] upon it as a blind alley and professional suicide" (Calderone, p. 50). Under her direction, Planned Parenthood served as the testing ground for new methods of birth control.

In 1960 Calderone realized that she wanted to concentrate on the relationships that necessitate contraception and began to change the focus of her career away from family planning to sex education. During the next three years, she informally met with colleagues to study and discuss the current body of sex education and human sexuality research. The outcome was Calderone's proposal for the establishment of a voluntary, nonprofit educational health organization with the aim of establishing human sexuality as a part of a person's total health. Thus, in 1964, with financial support from Calderone's husband, the Sex and Information Education Council of the United States (SIECUS) was born, and Calderone resigned from Planned Parenthood.

Calderone served as executive director (1964–1975) and president (1975–1982) of SIECUS. SIECUS educates professionals and the public through publications, conferences, and consulting services on topics relating to human sexuality such as birth control, homosexuality, and masturbation. While at SIECUS, Calderone traveled extensively, giving lectures in person and on radio and television to students, parents, educators, and physicians. She believed that the best sex educators were parents, and her advice was to give children the simple facts of reproduction and masturbation in kindergarten and continue throughout elementary school. Her books about sex education, *The Family Book about Sexuality* (1981, with Eric W. Johnson) and *Talking with Your Children about Sex* (1984), are addressed to parents. In 1982, she left SIECUS to become an adjunct professor in the Program for Human Sexuality at New York University.

In the late 1980s, Calderone, a Quaker since her early 50s, retired to a Quaker community in Pennsylvania. She died October 24, 1998, in a nursing home in Kennett Square, Pennsylvania, after suffering from Alzheimer's disease for a decade.

Selected Additional Achievements

Calderone's many honors include the Annual Award for Distinguished Services to Humanity, Albert Einstein Medical Center (1966); Woman of Conscience Award, National Council of Women (1968); Humanist of the Year, American Humanist Association (1974); Elizabeth Blackwell Award for Distinguished Service to Humanity, Hobart and William Smith Colleges (1977); Margaret Sanger Award, Planned Parenthood Federation of America (1980); Edward Browning Award for Prevention of Disease, American Public Health Association (1980); Lifetime Achievement Award, Schlesinger Library, Radcliffe College (1983); and Living Legacy Award, Women's International Center, San Diego (1988). Calderone also received 12 honorary doctorates from prestigious schools, including Adelphi, Brandeis, Harvard, Hofstra, and the Woman's Medical College of Pennsylvania. Calderone's publications include *The First Picture Book: Everyday Things for Babies* (1930, as Mary Steichen Martin, with Edward Steichen), *The Second Picture Book* (1958, as Mary Steichen Martin, with Edward Steichen), *Abortion in the United States* (1958, editor), *Release from Sexual Tensions* (1960), and *Manual of Family Planning and Contraceptive Practice* (1964, rev. ed., 1970, editor).

References

Calderone, Mary S. 1973. "Physician and Public Health Educator." *Annals of the New York Academy of Sciences* 208:47–51.

Fox, Marisa. 1987. "A Candid Conversation with Dr. Mary Calderone." *Health* (May):75–78.

Moore, Gaylen, and Lynn Gilbert, eds. 1981. *Particular Passions: Talks with Women Who Have Shaped Our Times.* New York: Clarkson N. Potter.

"Obituary." 1998. *New York Times* (October 25): 52.

Reynolds, Moira Davison. 1994. *Women Advocates of Reproductive Rights: Eleven Who Led the Struggle in the United States and Great Britain.* Jefferson, N.C.: McFarland.

CMB

Callen, Maude Evelyn (1899–1990)
Nurse-midwife

Maude Callen was an African American nurse, midwife, and teacher who became famous for her work among the poor in rural South Carolina. Sources conflict as to her date of birth, but Social Security records indicate that she was born on May 8, 1899. She was orphaned when she was seven years old and raised by an uncle in Quincy, Florida.

Callen graduated from Florida A&M College and finished her nurse training at the Georgia Infirmary in Savannah, Georgia, around 1920. She continued her education with nurse-midwife training at the Tuskegee Institute in Alabama and with a course in the care of tuberculosis patients at the Homer G. Phillips Hospital in St. Louis, Missouri. She received special training in the care of premature infants from the South Carolina Division of Maternal and Child Health in the late 1930s.

In 1923, Callen moved to Pineville, South Carolina, as a missionary nurse for the Episcopal Church. Pineville had no paved roads, no telephones, no electricity, and no hospitals. Nutritional deficiencies, malaria, tuberculosis, and venereal diseases were rampant. Callen held classes in a one-room mission schoolhouse, where she taught women how to provide sound nutrition to their families on limited budgets. Eventually, she drove 36,000 miles each year to provide primary care for residents throughout the county. Callen made home visits and held clinics in schools and in churches to vaccinate children against smallpox, diphtheria, and typhoid, to check teeth and eyesight, and to educate residents about nutrition and health care. She worked to keep communicable diseases, such as tuberculosis, isolated by tracking down those who might have been exposed and arranging for the seriously ill to go to the state hospital.

At that time in the American South, midwives provided essentially the only pre- and postnatal care available to many African American mothers. Maternal and infant mortality rates in Berkeley County were among the highest in the nation because of the midwives' lack of formal training, poverty, and isolation, which limited access to physicians. Through a program cosponsored by the Episcopal Church and the state, in 1926 Callen began training midwives in an attempt to end old and ineffective traditions and to instill sanitary and scientific methods. She introduced the practices of registration, licensing, and wearing uniforms. She also accompanied the midwives on deliveries and delivered more than 1,000 babies herself. She used whatever supplies were available, including newspapers as a delivery pad, a fruit crate as a crib, and bottles of warm water around the sides of a box as an incubator.

In 1936, Callen became a public health nurse for the Berkeley County Health Department. With the help of a private physician, she then began the county's first prenatal and venereal disease clinics. During the 1940s, Callen was a principal in the Midwife Training Institutes organized by Dr. Hilla Sheriff, director of the state Division of Maternal and Child Health. Black lay midwives attended these two-week programs to receive medical training and to meet licensing requirements. Many of the midwives were illiterate, so Callen persuaded officials to send a teacher to the institutes to teach them how to fill out birth certificates and thereby eliminate one of the barriers to state licensing. The courses were popular and served to raise both the status of midwives and the standard of care that they offered.

Maude Callen retired in 1971. In September 1980, she volunteered to manage the Senior Citizens Nutrition Site, which was opened in her clinic. For the last decade of her life she served meals there to the 50 or so in attendance each day and then delivered more food to homebound residents in the community.

Callen was married and had one adopted son, Sinclair Richard Callen. She died January 22, 1990, and later that year was inducted into the South Carolina Hall of Fame.

Selected Additional Achievements

Pictorial essay in *Life* magazine (1951) prompted readers to donate $27,000, which was used to build the Maude E. Callen Clinic. Filmed for *On the Road with Charles Kuralt* (1980). Alexis de Tocqueville Society Award, United Way of America (1984); honorary degrees, Clemson University (1983), and the Medical University of South Carolina (1989).

References

Dates of birth and death verified through *Social Security Death Index*. Online. http://www.ancestry.com/search/rectype/vital/ssdi/main.htm. 29 June 2000.

Brown, J.M. 1999. "Maude Evelyn Callen, RN (1898–1990)." *Journal of the South Carolina Medical Association* 95 (3):120–121.

Hill, Patricia Evridge. 1997. "Maude E. Callen." In *Doctors, Nurses, and Medical Practitioners: A Bio-Bibliographical Sourcebook*, edited by L. Magner. Westport, Conn.: Greenwood Press.

Smith, W. Eugene. 1951. "Nurse Midwife Maude Callen Eases Pain of Birth, Life and Death." *Life* (December 3):134–145.

DTW

Chinn, May Edward (1896–1980)
Physician

May Chinn was one of the first African American women to practice medicine in New York City. She was born on April 15, 1896, in Great Barrington, Massachusetts, the only child of William Lafayette Chinn, son of a slave and a white plantation owner, and Lula Ann Chinn, daughter of a Chickahominy Indian mother and a slave father.

At age five, Chinn began her education at Bordentown Manual Training and Industrial School, a New Jersey boarding school for African American children. An infection of the jawbone forced her to leave during the first year. She then lived on jewelry tycoon Charles Tiffany's estate, where her mother was a maid. After one year, Chinn returned to New York to attend public school. She attended Morris High School but dropped out in the 11th grade for a factory job.

In 1917 Chinn entered Columbia University's Teachers College with plans to become a music teacher. However, she experienced discrimination against her race and sex by a professor in the music department. Disillusioned, Chinn took a course in hygiene in the meantime. She excelled in the class and chose medicine as her future career. She graduated in 1921 and enrolled in New York's Bellevue

Medical College (now New York University Medical College) the following year. Four years later, Chinn became the first African American woman to earn a medical degree from Bellevue. She received further education in the 1930s at New York Post-Graduate Hospital Medical School and earned a master of public health degree from Columbia University (1933).

Following her graduation from Bellevue, Chinn had been considered for a research fellowship by the Rockefeller Institute, until the institute learned that she was African American. Instead, she took a position as the first black female intern at Harlem Hospital and also became the first female member of the hospital's ambulance crew. She completed her internship in 1928 and the same year opened a private practice on the ground floor of a Harlem brownstone. The third floor served as an operating room for the adjoining Edgecombe Sanitorium, owned by seven male African American doctors. She worked at the sanitorium as the night-duty physician in return for living and office quarters.

Chinn's medical practice served the people of Harlem, who suffered from diseases caused by overcrowding, inadequate plumb-

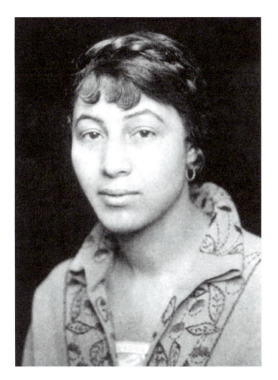

May Edward Chinn. Photograph courtesy of Ehrman Medical Library, New York University School of Medicine Archives.

ing, poor refrigeration, lack of prenatal care, and drug abuse. Since racism prevented her from having admitting privileges to local hospitals, she occasionally resorted to performing surgery in patients' homes. Not until 1940 did she earn the distinction of becoming the first African American woman granted admitting privileges to Harlem Hospital.

Over the course of her career, Chinn became especially interested in cancer. Denied research work in hospitals because of her race, she worked unofficially with resident physicians at Memorial Hospital who taught her to perform biopsies. Between 1928 and 1933, she assisted Dr. George Papanicolaou with the invention of his Pap smear (a method of detecting early signs of cervical cancer). As her reputation as a cancer researcher grew, other African American phy-

sicians began sending her biopsy samples for her to examine. In 1944, she took a position at the Strang cancer clinics, founded by Dr. Elise L'Esperance. Chinn worked at the Strang clinics until the age of 79, studying methods for determining cancer in asymptomatic patients. During this time, she was also on the staff of New York Infirmary for Women and Children (1945–1956).

In 1975, Chinn honored her predecessors by serving as a founder of the Susan Smith McKinney Steward Medical Society, named for New York's first African American woman physician. She retired from medical practice in 1977. She died on December 1, 1980.

See also L'Esperance, Elise Depew Strang; McKinney Steward, Susan Maria Smith

Selected Additional Achievements

Member, New York Academy of Sciences (elected 1954); citation, New York City Cancer Committee, American Cancer Society (1957); Society of Surgical Oncology (elected 1958); fellow, American Geriatrics Society (1959); medical membership, American Society of Cytology (1972); life member, American Academy of Family Physicians (1977); honorary doctor of science degree, Columbia University and New York University (1980); Distinguished Alumnus Award, Columbia University's Teachers College (1980).

References

Hayden, Robert C. 1999. "Chinn, May Edward." In *American National Biography*, edited by J.A. Garraty and M.C. Carnes. New York: Oxford University Press.

Maisel, Merry, and Laura Smart. *Women in Science: A Selection of 16 Significant Contributors.* 1997. San Diego: San Diego Supercomputer Center.

Newman, Laura. 1995. "May Edward Chinn." In *Notable Twentieth Century Scientists*, edited by E.J. McMurray. Detroit: Gale Research.

Shifrin, Susan. 1993. "Chinn, May Edward." In *Black Women in America: An Historical Encyclopedia*, edited by D.C. Hine, E. Barkley, and R. Terborg-Penn. Brooklyn, N.Y.: Carlson.

JSB

Clark, Nancy Talbot (1825–1901)
Physician

Nancy Talbot Clark was the second woman in the United States to graduate from a conventional male medical college, after Elizabeth Blackwell, and the first to seek membership in a state medical society. Clark was born on May 22, 1825, in Sharon, Massachusetts, the seventh of 10 children of Josiah and Mary (Richards) Talbot. Her early education was at the Sharon Academy, after which she taught in the Norwood, Massachusetts, schools. In 1845, she married Champion W. Clark, a dentist, and the couple moved to Baltimore. Within three years, Clark's infant daughter and her husband died. At the suggestion of an elderly female friend, she turned to the study of medicine.

In November 1850, Clark entered the medical program at Western Reserve University in Cleveland, Ohio. She was the first woman admitted to the school, which would later graduate noted physicians Emily Blackwell, Cordelia Greene, and Marie Zakrzewska. She graduated on March 3, 1852, moved to Boston, and established a successful medical practice. Within 10 months, she sought membership in the prestigious Massachusetts Medical Society because she wanted to "be publicly lifted from the rank of mere pretender" (quoted in Walsh, p. 151). The medical society rejected her application, and it would be nearly 30 years before a woman physician was admitted.

Undaunted, Clark sought additional medical training in Europe. She and her physician brother sailed to Europe in August 1854 for a year's study at La Maternité in Paris. She then returned to Boston and practiced for a year before marrying Amos Binney (July 1856), whom she had met on her way to Paris. After her marriage, she stopped practicing medicine. The couple had six children, two of whom died in childhood. During the Civil War, Amos Binney was commissioned in the paymaster's department, and the family moved to Baltimore. They also lived in Norfolk, Virginia, and New York City before returning to Boston. In 1874, Clark established a free dispensary for women and children, which she kept open for more than a year. At some point, the family moved to Newport, Rhode Island, where Amos Binney died in 1880. After her husband's death, Clark lived in several cities on the East Coast, as well as in Europe, before she died on July 28, 1901, in Haverford, Pennsylvania.

See also Blackwell, Elizabeth; Blackwell, Emily; Greene, Cordelia Agnes; Zakrzewska, Marie Elizabeth

References

Waite, Frederick C. 1931. "Dr. Nancy E. (Talbot) Clark: The Second Woman Graduate in Medicine to Practice in Boston." *New England Journal of Medicine* 205 (25):1195–1198.

Walsh, Mary Roth. 1977. *"Doctors Wanted: No Women Need Apply": Sexual Barriers in the Medical Profession, 1835–1975.* New Haven, Conn.: Yale University Press.

LS

Clayton, S. Lillian (1876–1930)
Nurse

Lillian Clayton was director of Philadelphia General Hospital School of Nursing for 15 years and a leader in professional nursing societies. She was born in 1876 in Kent County, Maryland. From an early age, she wanted to be a nurse and a missionary and began working at Children's Hospital in Philadelphia, when she was only 16.

In 1894, Clayton enrolled at Philadelphia General Hospital School of Nursing. The strict discipline there led her to leave the school, but an older sister convinced her to go back by telling her that she was being self-ish. She returned and graduated in 1896. While still in training, she had been appointed night supervisor at the hospital and kept the job until 1899. She then worked as a private-duty nurse and, to prepare for a missionary career, attended the Baptist Institute for Christian Workers. The Boxer Rebellion in China thwarted her plans for missionary work, however.

Instead, Clayton moved to Dayton, Ohio, where she worked with nurse Ella Crandall to modernize Miami Valley Hospital. Clayton's primary duty was directing the nursing school, and she spent much of her free time preparing for lectures and dissecting specimens. She was there until 1910, when she took courses at Columbia University's Teachers College in New York. From 1911 to 1914 she was a nursing teacher and administrator at Minneapolis City Hospital in Minnesota and was then the educational director of the Illinois Training School for Nurses in Chicago.

In 1915, Clayton became director of the Philadelphia General Hospital School of Nursing, a job that she considered her life's work. When she arrived, the hospital had several thousand patients yet employed almost no paid help. Male alcoholic patients were used to staff the hospital. Clayton did away with patient help, increased the number of graduate nurses working at the hospital from 20 to 156, and increased their salaries. She also brought in dieticians and developed physio- and occupational therapy and social service departments. When she arrived, the school had no full-time instructor, so she hired an educational director and eight full-time assistants. She also established a library of 1,000 volumes, organized a prenursing course and a student government association, and began offering postgraduate courses. With the help of the Rockefeller Foundation, the school became a center where many foreign students studied and observed. In 1920, Clayton's authority was expanded when she was made nursing director of all the hospitals under the Philadelphia Department of Health.

Although Clayton was not interested in professional nursing organizations at the beginning of her career, she later changed her mind and became involved in many activities. During the critical years of World War I, she was president of the National League of Nursing Education (1917–1919) and was on the Committee on Nursing of the General Medical Board of the Council of National Defense. She was a member of the Committee for the Study of Nursing Education, which produced the Winslow-Goldmark report (published as *Nursing and Nursing Education in the United States*) in 1923. The report led to the establishment of an experimental university school of nursing at Yale University. She was also chair of the American Nurses Association (ANA) Committee on Ethical Standards, which formulated a tentative Code of Ethics. She resigned that position to become president of the ANA in 1926, a position that she held until her untimely death.

On May 2, 1930, Clayton died from meningitis, after being ill for only 48 hours.

See also Crandall, Ella Phillips

Selected Additional Achievements

Pennsylvania State Board of Nurse Examiners; board president, *American Journal of Nursing*; National Organization for Public Health Nursing; National Committee on Red Cross Nursing Service; honorary master of nursing degree, Temple University. Bronze tablet presented to the city of Philadelphia in her honor (1928); Walter Burns Saunders Medal (1930); scholarship established in her honor, Philadelphia General Hospital School of Nursing (1947).

References

Bullough, Vern L. 1988. "S. Lillian Clayton." In *American Nursing: A Biographical Dictionary*, edited by V.L. Bullough, O.M. Church, and A.P. Stein. New York: Garland.

Goodrich, Annie W. 1930. "S. Lillian Clayton." *American Journal of Nursing* 30 (7):871–875.

"In Memoriam S. Lillian Clayton, 1874–1930." 1930. *American Journal of Nursing* 30 (6): 679–688.

Roberts, Mary M. 1954. "S. Lillian Clayton, 1876–1930." *American Journal of Nursing* 54 (11):1360–1363.

LS

Cleaves, Margaret Abigail (1848–1917)
Physician

Margaret Cleaves was an early American physician most noted for her work caring for mentally ill women. She was born in Columbus City, Iowa, on November 25, 1848, the third of seven children of John T. Cleaves, a physician and politician, and Elizabeth Stronach. She received her early education at home and in local schools. She later attended classes at the University of Iowa, but temporary financial constraints kept her from earning her baccalaureate degree. In 1870, she entered the University of Iowa's school of medicine, despite her family's objection to women physicians. She graduated at the head of her class on March 5, 1873.

In 1873, Cleaves became assistant physician at Iowa State Hospital (for the insane). In 1876, she established a private practice in Davenport, while continuing to serve as trustee for the State Hospital. The hospital appointed her as delegate to the National Conference of Charities and Corrections, where she presented a paper, "The Medical and Moral Care of Female Patients in Hospitals for the Insane" (Chicago, 1879). The following year, she became the first woman appointed by the governor of Iowa as state delegate to the National Conference of Charities and Corrections and the National Association for Protection of the Insane and the Prevention of Insanity (Cleveland, Ohio, 1880).

In 1880, Cleaves accepted a position as physician in charge of the Female Department of Harrisburg State Lunatic Hospital in Pennsylvania. Ill health forced her to resign this position in 1883. For the following two years, she traveled to several European countries, visiting insane asylums and attending lectures and clinics in general hospitals. She returned to Des Moines, Iowa, where for five years she operated a retreat for women suffering from mental and nervous afflictions. In 1889, she became the first woman to serve as chairman of obstetrics and gynecology at that year's Iowa State Medical Association annual meeting. In 1890, she moved to New York City to establish the New York Electro-Therapeutic Clinic Laboratory and Dispensary. She also taught electrotherapeutics at New York Post-Graduate Medical School and was professor of light energy at New York School of Physical Therapeutics.

Cleaves died in Mobile, Alabama, on November 13, 1917.

Selected Additional Achievements

Second woman member and secretary, Scott County Medical Society; second woman member, Iowa State Medical Society; first woman member, Iowa and Illinois Central District Medical Association. Member, Davenport Academy of Sciences, Missouri Valley Medical Association, Polk County Medical Society, Medical Society of the County of New York, and New York Electrical Society. Fellow, New York Academy of Medicine, American Electro-Therapeutic Association, Société Française d'Electrothérapie, and American Electro-Chemical Society. Contributor, *Journal of Nervous and Mental Disease* (1890's); editor, *Woman's Medical Journal* (1909); American editor of the English *Journal of Physiological Therapeutics*. Her most important medical work is *Light Energy: Its Physics, Physiological Action, and Therapeutic Applications* (1904, New York: Rebman).

References

Cleaves, Margaret. 1882. "Dr. Cleaves on the Treatment of Insanity by Women (transcript of speech given by Dr. Cleaves for the Conference of Charities, Boston, Mass., July 25, 1881)." *Journal of Social Science, Containing the Transactions of the American Association* (February): 101–103.

Cleaves, Margaret A. 1910. *The Autobiography of a Neurasthene as Told by One of Them.* Boston: Gorham Press.

Kelly, Howard A., and Walter L. Burrage, eds. 1928. *Dictionary of American Medical Biography: Lives of Eminent Physicians of the United States and Canada, from the Earliest Times.* New York: D. Appleton.

McGovern, Constance M. 1999. "Cleaves, Margaret Abigail." In *American National Biography*, edited by J.A. Garraty and M.C. Carnes. New York: Oxford University Press.

JSB

Cleveland, Emeline Horton (1829–1878)
Physician

Emeline Cleveland was a successful early woman physician who spent the majority of her medical career at Female (later, Woman's) Medical College of Pennsylvania in Philadelphia. She was born on September 22, 1829, in Ashford, Connecticut, the third of nine children of Chauncey and Amanda (Chaffee) Horton. In 1831, the family moved to a farm in Madison County, New York, and Cleveland's early education was at local schools and with private tutors.

Cleveland enrolled at Oberlin College in Ohio in the fall of 1850 and graduated three years later. Hoping to be a medical missionary, Cleveland registered at Female Medical College in October 1853. On March 8, 1854, she married the Reverend Giles Butler Cleveland, a lifelong friend. The couple planned a missionary career, but Giles Cleveland's poor health thwarted those plans. Upon Cleveland's graduation in March 1855, the pair settled in the Oneida valley of New York, where she established a private practice.

In the fall of 1856, Cleveland returned to Female Medical College as demonstrator of anatomy. Soon, she became professor of anatomy and histology, a position that she held until 1861. She also operated a private practice out of her home. In August 1860, Dr. Ann Preston of Female Medical College sent Cleveland to the School of Obstetrics at the Maternité of Paris to prepare for work at a new Woman's Hospital to be associated with Female Medical College. She earned a diploma in 1861 and briefly toured hospitals and lecture halls in London and Paris before returning to Philadelphia.

Upon her return in 1862, Cleveland became the chief resident at Woman's Hospital of Philadelphia. In this post, which she held until 1869, she initiated nurse training courses. She was also professor of obstetrics and diseases of women and children at Female Medical College (1862–1878), and she continued her private practice. Her surgical skills were superior. She was the first woman

to perform an ovariotomy in Philadelphia and one of the first female ovariotomists in the United States.

From 1872 to 1874, Cleveland was dean of Woman's Medical College (the name having been changed in 1867). Her tenure as dean was short due to her frail health, but even in the year of her death, 1878, Cleveland was active with the college and with her hospital duties. That year, she was also appointed gynecologist of the Department for the Insane at Pennsylvania Hospital, making her one of the first women to be on staff at a public institution. Cleveland died of tuberculosis on December 8, 1878. She had a son, Arthur, in February 1865, who also became a physician.

See also Preston, Ann

Selected Additional Achievements

Despite her successes, Cleveland was not permitted entrance into the prestigious medical soci-

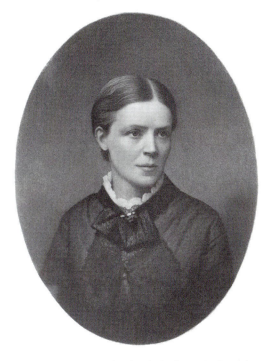

Emeline Horton Cleveland. Archives & Special Collections on Women in Medicine, MCP Hahnemann University.

eties of her day. One of her papers, "A Complicated Case of Vesico-Vaginal Fistula," was read before the Philadelphia Obstetrical Society by a male colleague and later published in the society's *Transactions* (1877).

References

Alsop, Gulielma Fell. 1950. *History of the Woman's Medical College, Philadelphia, Pennsylvania, 1850–1950.* Philadelphia: Lippincott.

Morantz, Regina Markell. 1984. "Cleveland, Emeline (Horton)." In *Dictionary of American Medical Biography,* edited by M. Kaufman, S.

Galishoff, and T.L. Savitt. Westport, Conn.: Greenwood Press.

Papers Read at the Memorial Hour: Commemorative of the Late Prof. Emeline H. Cleveland, M.D. 1879. Philadelphia: Woman's Medical College of Pennsylvania.

Ward, Patricia Spain. 1971. "Cleveland, Emeline Horton." In *Notable American Women, 1607–1950: A Biographical Dictionary,* edited by E.T. James, J.W. James, and P.S. Boyer. Cambridge: Belknap Press of Harvard University Press.

LS

Cole, Rebecca J. (1846–1922)
Physician

Rebecca Cole, the first African American woman to graduate from Woman's Medical College of Pennsylvania in Philadelphia and the second African American woman in the United States to receive a medical degree, after Rebecca Crumpler, was a pioneer in the field of medical social services. She was born on March 16, 1846, in Philadelphia. She graduated from Philadelphia's Institute for Colored Youth (now Cheyney University) in 1863 and the following year entered Woman's Medical College of Pennsylvania (now MCP Hahnemann University). She earned her M.D. in 1867, becoming the first African American woman to graduate from the college. Her graduation thesis was titled, "The Eye and Its Appendages" (1867).

After graduation Cole accepted a position as resident physician at New York Infirmary for Women and Children. The infirmary, established by Dr. Elizabeth Blackwell, was the first hospital in the United States to be entirely owned and operated by women physicians. In her autobiography, *Pioneer Work in Opening the Medical Profession to Women* (1895), Blackwell describes Cole's promotion from resident physician to sanitary visitor: "In addition to the usual departments of hospital and dispensary practice . . . we established a sanitary visitor. This post was filled by [Cole], whose special duty it was to give simple, practical instruction to poor mothers

on the management of infants and the preservation of the health of their families" (p. 183).

Cole eventually settled in Philadelphia to establish a private practice. She continued to support public health education as a means of improving living conditions in poor communities. To combat diseases caused by overcrowding, she advocated cubic space air laws, which would legislate the number of tenants whom landlords could allow in one dwelling. She was well aware that her work in poor communities was important to eliminate the belief that the African American neighborhood was by definition unhealthy and crime-ridden. In an article that she wrote for *The Woman's Era* (1896), she described her work in these neighborhoods as an effort "to attack vice, disease and crime . . . for they have no complexion" (p. 5).

Cole died in Philadelphia on August 14, 1922.

See also Blackwell, Elizabeth; Crumpler, Rebecca Davis Lee

Selected Additional Achievements

Private practice in Columbia, South Carolina; superintendent, Government House for Children and Old Women, Washington, D.C. Established a Woman's Directory Center to give medical and legal aid to women (1873) and cofounded the National Association of Colored Women (1896).

References

Black Women Physicians Collection, Special Collections on Women in Medicine, Archives and Special Collections, MCP Hahnemann University, Philadelphia.

Blackwell, Elizabeth. 1895. *Pioneer Work in Opening the Medical Profession to Women*. London: Longmans, Green.

Cole, Rebecca. 1896. "First Meeting of the Woman's Missionary Society of Philadelphia." *The Woman's Era* (October/November): 4–5.

Galloway-Wright, Brenda. 1993. "Cole, Rebecca J." In *Black Women in America: An Historical Encyclopedia*, edited by D.C. Hine, E. Barkley, and R. Terborg-Penn. Brooklyn, N.Y.: Carlson.

JSB

Comfort, Anna Amelia Manning (1845–1931)
Physician

Anna Manning Comfort is credited with being the first female physician to practice in Connecticut. She was later a successful gynecologist in Syracuse, New York. She was born in Trenton, New Jersey, on January 19, 1845, one of at least two daughters of Elizabeth (Price) Manning and Alfred G. Manning, founder and first president of Brown University.

After receiving her academic education in Boston, Comfort matriculated with the first class of the New York Medical College and Hospital for Women (Homeopathic) in 1863, founded by her aunt, Dr. Clemence Lozier. In addition to her regular studies, Comfort was able to obtain gynecological training at Bellevue Hospital, in spite of riotous protests by male medical students and professors against women who studied at Bellevue. She graduated in 1865.

The following year Comfort established a medical practice in Norwich, Connecticut, and is thought to be the first female physician in that state. Her sister, Emily Manning Smith, took over the Connecticut practice when Comfort returned to New York City (1870) to assume a practice left by the death of her cousin, Charlotte Lozier. Comfort also lectured at her alma mater and was elected chair of the science committee of the woman's club Sorosis.

On January 19, 1871, she married George Fisk Comfort, a founder of the New York Metropolitan Museum of Art. The following year, the couple moved to Syracuse, where George founded and was dean of the Syracuse University College of Fine Arts. After setting aside her medical career to care for the couple's young children, Comfort established a successful practice specializing in gynecology. During her career, she traveled twice (1887 and 1891) to Europe to study in hospitals and other medical institutions.

Like many of the early female physicians, Comfort supported women's right to higher education. In 1874, she and her husband published *Woman's Education and Woman's Health Chiefly in Reply to Dr. Edward Clarke's "Sex in Education."* The Comforts attacked Clarke's theory that higher education was detrimental to women's health and instead concluded: "As far as the general subject of the higher education of women is concerned, there is no question but that its tendency is to promote the physical health of her sex" (p. 155).

Comfort retired from her Syracuse practice in 1901. She died on January 11, 1931.

See also Lozier, Clemence Sophia Harned

References

Comfort Family Papers, Syracuse University Archives and Records Management, Syracuse, N.Y.

Comfort, George F., and Anna Manning Comfort. 1874. *Woman's Education and Woman's Health Chiefly in Reply to Dr. Edward Clarke's "Sex in Education."* Syracuse, N.Y.: Thos. W. Durston.

The National Cyclopaedia of American Biography. 1891. Vol. 3. New York: James T. White.

Willard, Frances E., and Mary A. Livermore. 1967. *A Woman of the Century: Fourteen Hundred-*

Seventy Biographical Sketches Accompanied by Portraits of Leading American Women in All Walks of Life. Reprint ed., Detroit: Gale Research. Original ed., Buffalo, N.Y.: Charles Wells Moulton, 1893.

JSB

Corbin, Hazel (1894–1988)
Nurse

As a longtime director of New York City's Maternity Center Association, Hazel Corbin had a major impact on programs devoted to improving prenatal and maternity care in the United States. She was born on August 31, 1894, in Nova Scotia, Canada, the daughter of John Winton and Susan (Mason) Corbin. When World War I broke out, Corbin decided to become a nurse and studied at Brooklyn Hospital in New York, graduating in 1917.

From 1918 to 1922 Corbin was a staff nurse at the Maternity Center Association (MCA), which was founded in 1918 to combat high maternal and infant death rates. She became assistant director of the MCA in 1922 and general director the next year, a position that she held until her retirement in 1965. She helped to establish the Lobenstine Midwifery Clinic and School in 1931, the first American school of nurse-midwifery. In 1934, the school became part of the MCA. Corbin was also instrumental in developing nurse-midwife certification programs at the State University of New York Downstate Medical Center, as well as at Columbia, Yale, and Johns Hopkins Universities.

During Corbin's tenure as director, the MCA disseminated a great deal of information to nurses, nurse-midwives, and prospective parents on maternal and child health. In addition to books and pamphlets, the MCA created the first major exhibit on childbearing for the 1939–1940 World's Fair, the first nationwide television series on childbearing (1954), and the first film on family life and sex education, *From Generation to Generation* (1959).

Corbin died on May 18, 1988, in New Smyrna Beach, Florida.

Selected Additional Achievements

The MCA established the Hazel Corbin Fund for the study of nurse-midwifery upon Corbin's retirement. *Getting Ready to Be a Father* (1945). Martha May Eliot Award, American Public Health Association (1966); Medal for Distinguished Service, MCA (1968).

References

Fowler, Glenn. 1988. "Hazel Corbin, Health Expert, Is Dead at 93." *New York Times* (May 20):B6.

Maternity Center Association. *Yesterday and Today*. Online. http://www.maternity.org/yesterday.html. 3 November 2000.

Stein, Alice P. 1992. "Hazel Corbin." In *American Nursing: A Biographical Dictionary*, edited by V.L. Bullough, L. Sentz, and A.P. Stein. New York: Garland.

Who's Who of American Women: A Biographical Dictionary of Notable Living American Women. 1961. 2nd ed. Chicago: Marquis-Who's Who.

LS

Craighill, Margaret (1898–1977)
Physician

In 1943, Margaret Craighill became the first woman doctor to be commissioned as an officer in the Medical Corps of United States Army. She was born on October 16, 1898, in Southport, North Carolina, the daughter of Colonel W. E. Craighill. She began her education in private schools in Alabama and West Virginia and graduated from Portland

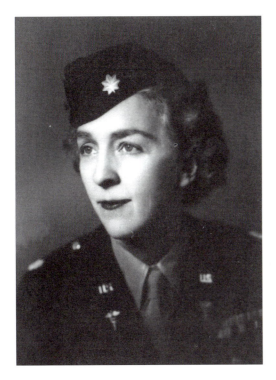

Margaret Craighill. National Library of Medicine.

High School in Maine. She earned two degrees in general science from the University of Wisconsin, a B.A. in 1920 and an M.S. in 1921. She spent the next year at the Chemical Warfare Service in Maryland studying the effect of war gases on animals. In 1924, she earned an M.D. from Johns Hopkins Medical School in Baltimore.

From 1924 to 1925, Craighill interned in gynecology and surgery at Johns Hopkins Hospital. The following year, she was assistant in pathology at Yale Medical School. She returned to Johns Hopkins in 1926 as assistant resident in gynecology until 1928. For six months that year she was a radiologist at Howard A. Kelly Hospital in Baltimore. She then moved to Greenwich, Connecticut, to serve as assistant in general surgery at Bellevue Hospital (1928–1937). She also maintained a practice in obstetrics and gynecology and worked as assistant surgeon and attending gynecologist at Greenwich Hospital (1928–1941). Between 1940 and 1942, she was assistant gynecologist at Philadelphia

General Hospital. In 1940, Craighill was appointed dean of Woman's Medical College of Pennsylvania in Philadelphia.

Craighill became active in war issues during the early years of World War II. She was a strong supporter of the Sparkman-Johnson Bill (H.R. 1857), which proposed granting women physicians the right to serve in the Medical Corps of the United States Army and Navy. Additionally, she was chairman of the Committee on Medical Schools for the Philadelphia Council of Defense and chairman of the Advisory Council for the Bryn Mawr College School of Nursing. These two committees were responsible for developing a program of medical preparedness for the military. From 1941 to 1944, Craighill was vice chairman, Committee on Women Physicians, Procurement and Assignment Service, War Manpower Commission.

In 1943, after the passage of the Sparkman-Johnson Bill, Craighill became the first woman physician to officially join the military. Commissioned as a major in the Army Medical Corps, she took a temporary leave (1943–1946) from Woman's Medical College to begin her duties in Washington, D.C. On May 10, 1943, she was sworn in the army as liaison officer for the Women's Army Corps, Office of the Surgeon General of the Army. She worked in the Department of Preventive Medicine as an adviser regarding the medical issues of 90,000 women army personnel.

In January 1944, Craighill was appointed as the first consultant to the Women's Health and Welfare Unit in the Office of the Surgeon General. The unit was responsible for setting medical standards for enlistment, providing medical care after enlistment, and recommending preventive health care measures. Until she took over these duties, this task was handled on a part-time basis by a medical corps officer whose policy was to give women the same physical examinations as men. Thus, Craighill's first directive was to initiate a program of standardized gynecological exams for women and for monthly examinations thereafter. She also initiated mental health screening for women, which, up to that time, was severely inefficient due to a lack of standardized testing procedures and insufficient training of examiners.

In fulfillment of her duties, Craighill traveled 56,000 miles to army installations around the world, recommending improvements for women's working and living conditions. Craighill's work shattered the belief that American women were unfit for work in the harsh conditions overseas. In November 1945, she was awarded the Legion of Merit for initiating notable improvements in the health of members of the Women's Army Corps and was promoted to lieutenant colonel. In 1946 she was released from active duty, but she continued to serve as consultant to the Veterans Administration regarding the medical care of women veterans.

Craighill returned to Woman's Medical College in 1946 but resigned later the same year. From 1946 to 1948, she was resident in psychiatry at Winter Veterans Administration Hospital in Topeka, Kansas, as a Menninger School of Psychiatry fellow. In 1949, she was appointed chief of service of the Menninger Psychiatric Clinic, in charge of the medical care of women veterans at the hospital. Afterward, she returned to private practice in Greenwich and New Haven, Connecticut, and was chief psychiatrist at the Connecticut College for Women in New London.

Craighill died at her home in Southbury, Connecticut, in July 1977.

Selected Additional Achievements

Member, Fairfield County and Connecticut State Medical Societies; fellow, New York Academy of Medicine, American Medical Association, and American College of Surgeons; diplomate, American Board of Gynecology and Obstetrics; member, American Medical Women's Association, and Obstetrical Society of Philadelphia. She was awarded the Elizabeth Blackwell Citation in 1949.

References

Date of birth and degree information provided by the Alumni Records Office of the University of Wisconsin System Office in Madison. August 18, 1998.

"Colonel Margaret D. Craighill." 1946. *Medical Woman's Journal* 53 (5):33–34.

"First Woman Commissioned Officer in the Medical Corps, U.S. Army." 1943. *Medical Woman's Journal* 50 (6):140–141.

Henderson-Smathers, Irma. 1951. "Medical Women of North Carolina." *Medical Woman's Journal* 58 (2):33–34.

"Obituary." 1977. *New York Times* (July 26):32.

Poulos, Paula Nassen, ed. 1996. *A Woman's War Too: U.S. Women in the Military in World War II.* Washington, D.C.: National Archives and Records Administration.

Treadwell, Mattie E. 1954. *The Women's Army Corps, the United States Army in World War II: Special Studies.* Washington, D.C.: Office of the Chief of Military History, Department of the Army.

JSB

Crandall, Ella Phillips (1871–1938)
Nurse

Ella Crandall was instrumental in the development of the field of public health nursing. She was born on September 16, 1871, in Wellsville, New York, one of two daughters of Herbert A. and Alice (Phillips) Crandall. In 1872 the family moved to Dayton, Ohio, where Crandall graduated from high school (1890). Several years later, she became interested in nursing and completed a two-year course at Philadelphia General Hospital School of Nursing, graduating in 1897.

Crandall then returned to Dayton and worked at local hospitals before beginning work with nurse Lillian Clayton at Dayton's Miami Valley Hospital (1899). The two women transformed the hospital, which had been staffed in the old style by German Protestant deaconesses, into a modern institution and founded a nursing school there. From 1908 to 1909, Crandall was also on the executive council of the American Society of Superintendents of Training Schools for

Nurses. In 1909, she left Ohio and took a supervisory position at Lillian Wald's famed Henry Street Visiting Nurse Service in New York City. At the same time, she took courses at the New York School of Philanthropy (later, the New York School of Social Work). She left Henry Street in 1910 to become a faculty member at Teachers College, Columbia University. There she helped advance public health nursing by developing courses in district nursing and health protection.

Crandall was a member of the joint American Nurses Association and American Society of Superintendents of Training Schools for Nurses commission that studied the need for a specialty organization for public health nurses. Based on the commission's recommendations, the National Organization for Public Health Nursing (NOPHN) was founded in 1912, with Crandall as executive secretary. She set high standards for membership in the NOPHN by requiring that members be graduates of a two-year hospital nursing school with at least 50 beds. She established the NOPHN headquarters in New York City and quickly expanded the association's staff from 1 to 20. She also traveled around the country to establish contact with nurses in the field and helped to make the Cleveland Visiting Nurse Association magazine into the NOPHN's professional journal, *Public Health Nurse* (later, *Public Health Nursing*). In 1917, Crandall was instrumental in winning a $30,000 grant for the NOPHN from the Rockefeller Foundation.

During World War I, Crandall moved to Washington, D.C., to be executive secretary of three national committees for the Council of National Defense and to serve on the Nursing Committee of the American Red Cross; through these organizations she helped coordinate the nation's nursing efforts. In 1920, she resigned her position as executive secretary of the NOPHN and turned her attention to programs for poor women and children. She was executive secretary of the Committee to Study Community Organization for Self Support for Health Work for Women and Young Children and director of the nursing service of New York's Association for Improving the Condition of the Poor, as well as associate director of the American Child Health Association. In 1927 she was named executive secretary of the Payne Fund, established by future congresswoman Frances Payne Bolton to promote the education of youth for peace.

Crandall died 10 years later from pneumonia on October 24, 1938, in New York City.

See also Clayton, S. Lillian; Wald, Lillian D.

Selected Additional Achievements

Articles in the professional nursing literature; *Organization and Administration of Public Health Nursing* (1914). Board of Directors, American Nurses Association (1913–1916, 1918–1920).

References

"Ella Phillips Crandall." 1938. *American Journal of Nursing* 38 (12):1406–1408.
Gault, Alma E. 1971. "Crandall, Ella Phillips." In *Notable American Women, 1607–1950: A Biographical Dictionary*, edited by E.T. James, J.W. James, and P.S. Boyer. Cambridge: Belknap Press of Harvard University Press.
Mernitz, Kenneth S. 1988. "Ella Phillips Crandall." In *American Nursing: A Biographical Dictionary*, edited by V.L. Bullough, O.M. Church, and A.P. Stein. New York: Garland.

LS

Crumpler, Rebecca Davis Lee (1831–1895)
Physician

Rebecca Crumpler was the first African American woman to earn a medical degree in the United States. In spite of this achievement, very little is known about her life and career. She was born to Absolum Davis and Matilda Webber on February 8, 1831, in

Delaware. She was raised in Pennsylvania, however, by an aunt who was known for her nursing abilities.

By 1852, Crumpler was living in Charlestown, Massachusetts, where she worked as a nurse for local doctors. She apparently learned the art of healing from her aunt, as formal training did not exist for nurses at that time. In 1860, with recommendations from the physicians who employed her, she applied and was admitted to New England Female Medical College in Boston. She graduated in 1864. She practiced medicine in Boston for a time, specializing in the treatment of women and children. She then "travelled to the British Dominion" for more medical training (Crumpler, p. 2).

Sometime after the Civil War, Crumpler moved to Richmond, Virginia, where she treated black patients through an agreement with the Freedmen's Bureau. She also married Arthur Crumpler around this time. By 1869, she was back in Boston practicing medicine. In 1883, she compiled her journal entries into *A Book of Medical Discourses*, with the hope that the "book shall be as a primary reader in the hands of every woman" (pp. 3–4). The work contained practical advice on the medical care of women and children.

Crumpler died on March 9, 1895, in Hyde Park, Massachusetts.

References

"Ahead of Her Time: Doctress Rebecca Lee Crumpler." 1995. *Bostonia* (Summer):60.

Black Women Physicians Collection, Special Collections on Women in Medicine, Archives and Special Collections, MCP Hahnemann University, Philadelphia.

Crumpler, Rebecca. 1883. *A Book of Medical Discourses*. Boston: Cashman, Keating.

Pfatteicher, Sarah K.A. 1999. "Crumpler, Rebecca Davis Lee." In *American National Biography*, edited by J.A. Garraty and M.C. Carnes. New York: Oxford University Press.

LS

Cushier, Elizabeth (1837–1932)
Physician

Elizabeth Cushier was a leading woman surgeon in America at the end of the nineteenth century. She was born in 1837, one of seven surviving children, and received her early education in both private and public schools. At age 16, she moved with her family from New York to Little Falls, New Jersey. Her mother died in 1869, and Cushier assumed responsibility for the household duties until her father remarried a year later.

Cushier decided to study medicine in 1868 after reading a medical article on the influence of the ganglionic system in producing sleep. She wrote in her short autobiography: "I knew nothing of the Ganglionic System . . . but the article looked most interesting, if one could only understand it! This meant, I knew, a knowledge of physiology, and physiology suggested medicine and its study. I knew that there were a few women physicians but I had never met one, and the thought of taking up the study of medicine seemed chimerical; however, it became a fixed idea" (quoted in Thelberg, p. 86).

At the encouragement of friends, she entered a women's homeopathic college in New York City. She received practical instruction in anatomy and physiology but was disappointed with the school's academic standards. Cushier left the homeopathic college after one year to enter Woman's Medical College of the New York Infirmary for Women and Children. The college and infirmary were established by physicians Elizabeth and Emily Blackwell to provide superior medical education to women physicians and to offer women medical treatment by highly trained physicians of the same sex. After her graduation in 1872, Cushier spent one year at the infirmary as intern and extern and a second year as resident physician. After an 18-month trip to Zurich to study histology, she returned to the infirmary as resident physician and professor of obstetrics.

Cushier also maintained a private practice, specializing in gynecological surgery. Her most rewarding case was one in which a woman, diagnosed by other physicians as a cancer victim, came to her for treatment. Cushier examined the patient and discovered a pessary embedded in the vaginal wall. She was able to remove the pessary, but it had buried itself in such a way as to require complicated surgery to repair the area. Cushier wrote that it was "the most difficult piece of work I had ever done . . . [and with] much anxiety I awaited the result, which proved successful" (quoted in Thelberg, p. 91).

A large part of Cushier's importance to women in medicine was her work as one of the early administrators of New York Infirmary. In an 1881 trustee's report, she noted that the "increase in the number of [women] who have received assistance and relief in the Infirmary, proved convincingly the necessity for the existence of our institution" (quoted in Daniel, p. 171). Regarding the educational benefits for women physicians, she reported that "the school has kept pace with the most advanced medical schools of the country, among which the Harvard Medical School and others have adopted a course somewhat similar" (quoted in Daniel, p. 168).

In 1899, Woman's Medical College of the New York Infirmary closed its doors when Cornell University Medical School began accepting women. The infirmary building was used to expand Woman's Hospital, where Cushier continued her work in gynecology and surgery. A year after the closing of the college, she and Emily Blackwell gave up their practices to travel to Europe. They returned the next year and settled in Montclair, New Jersey, and had a summer home in York Cliffs, Maine. Failing eyesight kept Cushier out of active medical practice in her later years; however, she was able to "rejoice in the progress of women in Medicine, and in the growth and usefulness of the New York Infirmary for Women and Children" (quoted in Thelberg, p. 94). Cushier died in 1932.

See also Blackwell, Elizabeth; Blackwell, Emily

References

Brody, Irwin A. 1955. "The Decision to Study Medicine." *New England Journal of Medicine* 252 (4):130–134.

Daniel, Annie Sturges. 1941. " 'A Cautious Experiment': The History of the New York Infirmary for Women and Children and the Woman's Medical College of the New York Infirmary; Also Its Pioneer Founders, 1853–1899." *Medical Woman's Journal* 48 (6):167–173.

L'Esperance, Elise S. 1949. "Influence of the New York Infirmary on Women in Medicine." *Journal of the American Medical Women's Association* 4 (6):255–261.

Thelberg, Elizabeth B., ed. 1933. "Autobiography of Elizabeth Cushier." In *Medical Women of America: A Short History of the Pioneer Medical Women of America and of a Few of Their Colleagues in England* by Kate Campbell Hurd-Mead. New York: Froben Press.

JSB

D

Daniel, Annie Sturges (1858–1944)
Physician

As director of the Out-Practice department of New York Infirmary for nearly 60 years, Annie Daniel helped to significantly improve the health, living, and working conditions of New York's poor. Daniel was born in Buffalo, New York, on September 21, 1858, the daughter of John M. and Miranda (Sturges) Daniel. Both parents died while Daniel was young, and she was raised by relatives in Monticello, New York.

Daniel matriculated at the Woman's Medical College of the New York Infirmary for Women and Children, founded by Dr. Elizabeth Blackwell in 1868. Following her graduation in 1879, she spent one year as pharmacist at the infirmary and a second year as intern. In 1881, Blackwell appointed Daniel as physician in charge of the infirmary's newly founded Out-Practice department and dispensary. In this position, Daniel provided medical services to the poor, mostly immigrant tenement population on New York's East Side for approximately 60 years.

Specializing in women and children's health, Daniel visited thousands of East Side families and quickly became convinced of the relationship between preventable illness and low wages. She responded by teaching wives and mothers the basics of nutrition and hygiene. She was especially concerned with home manufacturing, a practice that created a sweatshop environment in the home. She blamed home manufacturing for creating unsanitary, overcrowded conditions and supported legislation for its prohibition. She became a beloved member of the tenement community and her patients dubbed her the Angel of the Lower East Side.

By 1889, course work in the Out-Practice department was a requirement at Woman's Medical College. As teacher of student physicians and nurses, Daniel had an impact on the future of preventive medicine. She taught a course on the "normal child" as the basis for understanding abnormal children. This course would later inspire her student, S. Josephine Baker, to lead the establishment of the Bureau of Child Hygiene at the New York Department of Health. Daniel's reputation as an authority on tenement life and preventive medicine grew beyond that of the college. She was appointed as investigator for the New York State Tenement House Commission (1884), studied home sweatshop conditions for a congressional committee (1892), and testified before another New

York tenement commission on the ill effects of home manufacturing (1894). Her report for the Women's Prison Association of New York was instrumental in legislation requiring sex-segregated prison facilities and to the appointment of female matrons to supervise the women prisoners (1888).

Daniel continued her work with the Out-Practice department into her 80s. The services provided by the department were even more critical during the depression, when the number of home visits doubled, and the number of patients at the department's infirmary increased by 50 percent. By the time of her retirement in the 1940s, Daniel had seen the successful passage of legislation for improved housing conditions and for the prohibition of home manufacturing. She was also an active suffragist and a member of the Working Women's Society. She died of arteriosclerosis in New York City on August 10, 1944.

See also Baker, S. [Sara] Josephine; Blackwell, Elizabeth

Selected Additional Achievements

Daniel published the "Report of Out-Practice of the N.Y. Infirmary for Women and Children" (1891) and a history of New York Infirmary, "A Cautious Experiment," serialized in the *Medical Woman's Journal* (May 1939 to December 1942). Other publications include "The Wreck of the Home: How Wearing Apparel Is Fashioned in the Tenements" (*Charities* [April 1, 1905]) and "The City's Health-Living Conditions" (*Municipal Affairs* [June 1898]).

References

"Doctoring the Poor for 35 Years." 1914. *New York Times* (March 15):Section 6.

Lubove, Roy. 1999. "Daniel, Annie Sturges." In *American National Biography*, edited by J.A. Garraty and M.C. Carnes. New York: Oxford University Press.

Perry, Marilyn Elizabeth. 1971. "Daniel, Annie Sturges." In *Notable American Women, 1607–1950: A Biographical Dictionary*, edited by E.T. James, J.W. James, and P. S. Boyer. Cambridge: Belknap Press of Harvard University Press.

JSB

Darrow, Anna Albertina Lindstedt (1876–1959)
Physician

Anna Darrow was one of the first women physicians to successfully practice in Florida. She was born in Jasper County, Indiana, on September 16, 1876, to Per Jon and Emma (Lundin) Lindstedt. She received her early education in Chicago schools. In 1896, she married Charles Ray Darrow, and the couple eventually had two children, Richard Gordon and Dorothy Anna. In 1905, she and her husband earned doctor of osteopathy degrees from Kirksville College of Osteopathy in Missouri. Darrow also studied at Jenner Medical College and earned an M.D. with honors from Chicago College of Medicine and Surgery in 1909.

Darrow practiced medicine in Chicago until 1912, when she and her family moved to rural Okeechobee, Florida. Her husband was surgeon for the Florida East Coast Railway,

while Darrow earned the distinction of being the first woman physician in the area. At least one of the local male doctors was unimpressed with her achievement. Discontented with "having 'Dr. Anner' quoted to him as an authority on how to treat sick folks," he threatened to "run the 'petticoat doctor' out of town" ("Darrow," p. 753). A licensed pharmacist, Darrow and her husband also operated a drugstore in Okeechobee (1912–1922). She served as sanitary inspector for the community and provided medical care to the Seminole Indians in the surrounding Everglades.

The Darrows left Okeechobee in 1922. They lived in Stuart, Florida, until Charles Darrow died in 1926. Darrow then moved to Ft. Lauderdale, where she founded and was on the medical staff (1927–1949) of

Broward General Hospital. She was also active in the Broward County Medical Association and was a charter member of the South Florida Branch of the American Medical Women's Association. In 1949, she retired to her daughter's home in Coral Gables, Florida. Darrow died on July 22, 1959.

Selected Additional Achievements

Member, General Foundation of Women's Clubs, Women's Club of Okeechobee, American Medical Association, American Medical Women's Association, Southern Medical Association, Florida State Medical Association, and Business and Professional Women's Club of Ft. Lauderdale. In 1947, she won second prize from the American Medical Art Exhibition for her 1920 painting depicting a close call with a rattlesnake on her way to deliver twins in the Florida Everglades.

References

"Darrow, Old Doc Anna: As Told by Dr. Anna." 1968. *Journal of the Florida Medical Association* 55 (8):749–756.

Hendricks, Anne M. 1960. "Memorial to Anna R. Darrow, M.D." *Journal of the American Medical Women's Association* 15 (1):75–76.

The National Cyclopaedia of American Biography. 1965. Vol. 48. New York: James T. White.

JSB

Davis, Frances Elliott (1882–1965)
Nurse

Frances Elliott Davis was the first African American nurse officially enrolled in the American Red Cross. She was born on April 28, 1882, near Shelby, North Carolina, to Emma Elliott, a white heiress, and Darryl Elliott, a part black and part Cherokee Indian sharecropper. Due to racism and prejudice against interracial couples in the South, her father fled for his life soon after Davis' birth. Her mother died when she was five, and Davis spent the next several years being passed from one foster family to another before ending up in Pittsburgh with a family that treated her as a maid.

When she was a teenager, Davis sought work outside her foster home and began working for the Joseph Reed family. The family paid for her secondary and normal school education at Knoxville College in Tennessee. She graduated in 1907 with a teaching degree, even though she wanted to be a nurse. She took a job as a practical nurse at the college's School Hospital before illness forced her to accept a job at the Henderson Normal Institute in North Carolina. She saved enough money to attend nursing school and entered Freedmen's Hospital Training School for Nurses in Washington, D.C., in the spring of 1910, graduating three years later.

Davis then worked as a private-duty nurse in Washington, D.C., for three years. Next, she applied to the American Red Cross (ARC) and was the first African American nurse selected to take the ARC Town and Country Nursing Service course at Teachers College, Columbia University in New York. She completed the course and did fieldwork at the Henry Street Visiting Nurse Service in New York City. In July 1917, she was sent by the ARC Town and Country Nursing Service to Jackson, Tennessee, where she provided nursing and midwifery service and taught hygiene and prenatal care.

When the United States became involved in World War I, Town and Country nurses were automatically enrolled as ARC nurses and made eligible for service with the Army Nurse Corps (ANC). Because of her race, Davis was initially excluded from the ARC program. In July 1918, she became the first black nurse to be enrolled with the ARC and was given badge number 1-A, with the letter A identifying her as African American. The ANC continued to refuse black nurses until after the armistice, however. Davis worked with recovering soldiers for the ARC Public Health Service (formerly the Town and Country Service) in Tennessee in 1918. That year, she also became a victim of the influenza epidemic, and the illness permanently damaged her heart.

In 1919, Davis moved to Tuskegee, Alabama, to become director of nurses' training at John A. Andrew Memorial Hospital. Not long afterward, she was asked to organize the first training school for African American nurses at Dunbar Hospital in Detroit. She saw the first class graduate and pass state board exams, and then she began working for the Detroit Visiting Nurses' Association. On December 24, 1921, she married William A. Davis, a musician; the next year the couple's only child was stillborn. In 1923, Davis returned to her job at Dunbar Hospital and obtained funding from a philanthropist to upgrade the nursing program there. When the medical staff tried to take charge of the funds, she resigned in 1927. In 1929, she was awarded a Rosenwald Fellowship to work on her bachelor's degree at Teachers College, but poor health prevented her from completing it. Davis then moved to Inkster, Michigan, near Detroit, where she helped

distribute food at the Ford Motor Plant, worked with the health department and the Visiting Nurse Association, served on the school board, and developed a day nursery. From 1945 to 1951, she was on staff at the Eloise Hospital in Wayne County in Inkster.

Davis died from a heart attack on May 2, 1965, in Mount Clemens, Michigan, a few days before she was to be honored at an American Red Cross national convention.

References

DelBene, Susan B., and Vern L. Bullough. 1988. "Frances Elliot [*sic*] Davis." In *American Nursing: A Biographical Dictionary*, edited by V.L. Bullough, O.M. Church, and A.P. Stein. New York: Garland.

Elmore, Joyce Ann. 1980. "Davis, Frances Elliott." In *Notable American Women: The Modern Period: A Biographical Dictionary*, edited by B. Sicherman and C.H. Green. Cambridge: Belknap Press of Harvard University Press.

Pitrone, Jean Maddern. 1969. *Trailblazer: Negro Nurse in the American Red Cross*. New York: Harcourt, Brace, and World.

LS

Davis, Mary E.P. (ca. 1840–1924)
Nurse

Mary Davis had a great influence upon nursing education and upon the professionalization of nursing. She was born around 1840 in New Brunswick, Canada, to John Davis, an officer in the British army, and Charlotte (McFarland) Davis. Little is known of her family situation or early education.

Davis graduated from Boston Training School for Nurses at Massachusetts General Hospital in 1878, where she remained as a graduate nurse until the next year. Afterward, she worked as a private-duty nurse and was a public health nurse in and around Boston. She then became superintendent of the University of Pennsylvania Hospital and Training School for Nurses (1889–1899), where she reorganized and expanded the school and established a three-year nursing course.

In 1893, Davis attended the nursing congress of the World's Fair in Chicago, where she met with several nursing leaders. This group eventually formed the American Society of Superintendents of Training Schools for Nurses of the United States and Canada (now the National League for Nursing). Davis served as vice president (1894–1895) and president (1896). In her presidential address of the society's third annual convention in Philadelphia, she proposed a universal standard of training for nurses and outlined the necessary qualifications of a supervisor. Throughout her career, she was an outspoken advocate of improved nursing education.

In 1897, the society formed a second national nursing organization named the Nurses' Associated Alumnae of the United

States and Canada (from 1911, the American Nurses Association). Davis' major contribution to the future of the Associated Alumnae was as chair of its committee on periodicals (1899–1902). In January 1900, she and a committee of prominent nursing leaders began the work of establishing a journal published by nurses for nurses. Determined to ensure the journal's complete financial, and therefore editorial, independence, she created a joint-stock company. She also collected the first subscriptions and contracted a publisher and printer. In October 1900, the first issue of the *American Journal of Nursing* was published. That year, Davis became first president of the *Journal*'s Board of Directors, while Sophia Palmer was first editor in chief. Until 1909, Davis worked as the *Journal*'s business manager, steering the publication through its early tough financial times.

In 1895, Davis helped form her alma mater's Alumnae Association, which became one of the first associations to join the national Associated Alumnae. She also contributed to the establishment (1903) of the Massachusetts Nurses Association. She declined the opportunity to be the association's first president, choosing instead to chair the legislative committee, which, for the next seven years, lobbied for the enactment of nurse registration laws. She then served as president from 1911 to 1913.

At various times during her career, Davis was superintendent of Boston State Hospital in Dorchester, Massachusetts, where she established a nurse training school, and was superintendent of the Washington [D.C.] Training School for Nurses. She also established central directories of nurses in Washington, D.C. (1909), Boston (1912), and Philadelphia. During World War I, she was an examiner for American Red Cross classes.

Davis died in Norwood, Massachusetts, on June 9, 1924. In 1940, the library at Massachusetts General Hospital was renamed the Palmer-Davis Library, in honor of both Davis and Sophia Palmer. She was inducted into the American Nurses Association Hall of Fame in 1982.

See also Palmer, Sophia French

References

American Journal of Nursing Company. 1975. *The American Journal of Nursing and Its Company: A Chronicle, 1900–1975.* New York: American Journal of Nursing Company.

Birnbach, Nettie. 1992. "Mary E.P. Davis." In *American Nursing: A Biographical Dictionary*, edited by V.L. Bullough, L. Sentz, and A.P. Stein. New York: Garland.

Hawkins, Joellen Watson. 1988. "Davis, Mary E.P." In *Dictionary of American Nursing Biography*, edited by M. Kaufman. New York: Greenwood Press.

Riddle, Mary M. 1920. "Twenty Years of the Journal." *American Journal of Nursing* 21 (1): 6–12.

JSB

Delano, Jane Arminda (1858/62–1919)
Nurse

Jane Delano is most noted for her work with the American Red Cross during World War I. Delano was born on March 12, 1858 (some sources say 1862) in Townsend, New York, the younger of two daughters of George and Mary Ann (Wright) Delano. Her early education was at local schools and the Cook Academy in Montour Falls, New York. She taught school for two years but was inspired to become a nurse when a friend went to India as a missionary nurse.

Delano entered Bellevue Hospital Training School for Nurses in New York City in 1884 and was made a head nurse at the hospital upon graduation two years later. In 1888 and 1889 she was superintendent at two hospitals, first in Jacksonville, Florida, during a yellow fever epidemic and then in Bisbee, Ar-

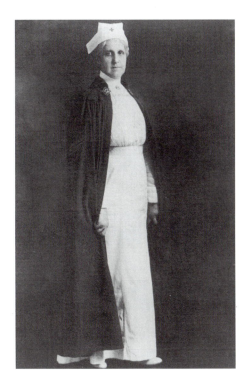

Jane Arminda Delano. National Library of Medicine.

izona, during an outbreak of typhoid. She became instructor and assistant superintendent of nurses at the University of Pennsylvania Hospital nursing school in Philadelphia in 1890, where she helped to expand the curriculum and to improve the nurses' living conditions. She also founded the school's alumnae association. After resigning in 1896, she took classes at the University of Buffalo Medical School for a short time and was one of the first students at the New York School of Civics and Philanthropy.

For two years (1900–1902) Delano worked with delinquent girls at the House of Refuge on Randall's Island in New York. A trustee of the institution was so impressed by her selflessness that he provided for her in his will, which eventually allowed her to work without pay. From 1902 to around 1907, Delano was superintendent of training schools at Bellevue and Allied Hospitals in New York. There she insisted that the nurses be referred to as nurses rather than "girls," required students to witness an autopsy as part of their training, im-

proved their diets, and initiated social and cultural activities for them.

In 1909, Delano took on three jobs that put her at the center of American nursing activity. She became president of the Nurses' Associated Alumnae (renamed the American Nurses Association in 1911), an office that she held until 1912, was made chair of the National Committee on Red Cross Nursing Service, and was appointed superintendent of nurses for the Army Nurse Corps (ANC). Delano accepted the ANC superintendency to promote the corps' relationship with the American Red Cross. As superintendent, she surveyed hospitals in Hawaii, the Philippines, China, and Japan, and to attract more nurses to the corps, she secured increased pay and other benefits for ANC nurses. Under her leadership, American Red Cross nurses were designated the reserve nurses for the army. Wanting to devote her time to the Red Cross and having received her inheritance, she resigned from the ANC in 1912.

Delano joined the Red Cross (New York state branch) in 1899, during the Spanish-American War, and became interested in enrolling nurses for service with the organization at that time. After a 1905 restructuring of the Red Cross, its leaders sought a closer relationship with the nation's nurses to ensure the availability of trained nurses in times of disaster or war. One result was the establishment of the National Committee on Red Cross Nursing Service, with Delano as chair. Her primary task was to develop and implement a plan to enroll qualified nurses in the American Red Cross Nursing Service.

Through Delano's efforts, the Red Cross was able to send nurses overseas when war broke out in Europe in 1914. Commenting on the success of these nurses, Delano stated in the 1915 annual report of the Red Cross, "*We* have learned that women can be mobilized without confusion; that their chances of illness when carefully selected seem to be no greater than men's; that they face danger with equanimity" (quoted in Dock, p. 227). When the United States entered World War I in April 1917, the Red Cross was able to supply 8,000 nurses for service.

American entrance into the war made the need for nurses acute. Although Delano had worked diligently to ensure qualified nurses for the American Red Cross Nursing Service, she believed that the war created an emergency that necessitated the use of trained aides. Her plan was opposed by Annie Goodrich and others in the nursing profession who proposed an Army School of Nursing to meet the need. Although the War Department sided with Goodrich, Delano continued her nurse recruitment efforts and by the end of the war had mobilized 20,000 nurses. In the spring of 1918 the Red Cross created a Department of Nursing, and Delano was named director.

In January 1919, Delano sailed to France to inspect postwar conditions there. She soon fell ill and died in Savenay on April 15 of mastoiditis. Delano was eventually buried in Arlington National Cemetery. A sculpture stands outside the Washington, D.C., headquarters of the Red Cross in tribute to Delano and the other 296 Red Cross nurses who died during World War I.

See also Goodrich, Annie Warburton

Selected Additional Achievements

Numerous articles in nursing journals and a monthly column on Red Cross nursing in the *American Journal of Nursing* (1911–1919); *American Red Cross Textbook on Elementary Hygiene and Home Care of the Sick* (with Isabel McIsaac, 1913). Distinguished Service Medal, United States; Distinguished Service Medal, American Red Cross; American Red Cross Medal of Merit; American Nurses Association Hall of Fame (1982).

References

Clarke, Mary A. 1934. *Memories of Jane A. Delano*. New York: Lakeside.

Dock, Lavinia L., Sarah Elizabeth Pickett, Clara D. Noyes, Fannie F. Clement, Elizabeth G. Fox, and Ann R. Van Meter. 1922. *History of American Red Cross Nursing*. New York: Macmillan.

Gladwin, Mary E. 1931. *The Red Cross and Jane Arminda Delano*. Philadelphia: W.B. Saunders.

Nichols, Jeannette P. 1971. "Delano, Jane Arminda." In *Notable American Women, 1607–1950: A Biographical Dictionary*, edited by E.T. James, J.W. James, and P.S. Boyer. Cambridge: Belknap Press of Harvard University Press.

Reeves, Connie L. 1999. "Delano, Jane Arminda." In *American National Biography*, edited by J.A. Garraty and M.C. Carnes. New York: Oxford University Press.

Sabin, Linda E. 1988. "Jane Arminda Delano." In *American Nursing: A Biographical Dictionary*, edited by V.L. Bullough, O.M. Church, and A.P. Stein. New York: Garland.

LS

Deming, Dorothy (1893–1972)
Nurse

Dorothy Deming was a nurse and a leader in national public health organizations. She was born on June 8, 1893, in New Haven, Connecticut, the youngest of three children of Clarence and Mary Bryan (Whiting) Deming. Her early education was in private schools, and she later earned a bachelor's degree from Vassar (1914).

After her mother's death in 1914, Deming began volunteer work at the New Haven Visiting Nurse Association. Her experiences there, combined with the outbreak of World War I, inspired her to study nursing at New York City's Presbyterian Hospital School of Nursing in preparation for service overseas. By the time she graduated in 1920, the war had ended, and she went on to study at the Henry Street Visiting Nurse Association. After a short time as a private-duty nurse, she was on staff at the New Haven Visiting Nurse Association (1922–1923). Afterward, she returned to Henry Street as supervisor of the association's Harlem Center and as field director of its Manhattan Branch. Around 1924, she became director of the Holyoke Visiting Nurse Association.

In 1927, Deming became assistant to the director of the National Organization for

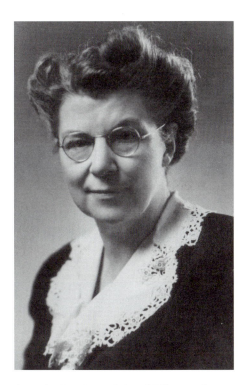

Dorothy Deming. National Library of Medicine.

Public Health Nursing (NOPHN), while concurrently serving as assistant to the editor of *Public Health Nursing*, the organization's journal. From 1935 to 1942, she was director general and journal editor. Under her leadership, the NOPHN became a clearinghouse for information on public health. The organization also provided professional consulting services to public health agencies; these services were especially valuable during the critical years of the Great Depression and World War II.

Deming left the NOPHN to join the American Public Health Association (1942–1952) to assist in the development of civil service merit examinations. During this time, she was also a consultant for the National Health Council's study of voluntary health agencies. Her work with these national organizations allowed her to study public health on a national level. She put her knowledge to paper and published several books, as well as articles in the *American Journal of Nursing*. In her publications, she analyzed the important health issues of her day, such as the effect of World War II on public health and the use of practical nurses.

Deming published several fictional nursing novels to encourage young women to take up the "challenge of effective instruction of the public in ways to keep well and prevent illness" (quoted in Block and Rothe, p. 168). Her first novel, *Penny Marsh: Public Health Nurse* (1938), was so popular that many high schools started Penny Marsh Clubs for future nurses. Deming's professional peers praised the books for accurately portraying the education, skills, and duties required of a nurse. By 1962, Deming had published at least 20 novels about nursing.

Deming died in Winter Park, Florida, in January 1972.

Selected Additional Achievements

Home Nursing (1942); *The Practical Nurse* (1947); and *Careers for Nurses* (1947).

References

Biographical Sketches from the National League of Nursing Education. 1940. New York: National League of Nursing Education.

Block, Maxine, and Anna Rothe, eds. 1944. *Current Biography 1943: Who's News and Why*. New York: H.W. Wilson.

Friedman, Alice Howell. 1988. "Deming, Dorothy." In *Dictionary of American Nursing Biography*, edited by M. Kaufman. New York: Greenwood Press.

Thom, Leslie. 1988. "Dorothy Deming." In *American Nursing: A Biographical Dictionary*, edited by V.L. Bullough, O.M. Church, and A.P. Stein. New York: Garland.

JSB

Dickey, Nancy Wilson (1950–   )
Physician

Nancy Dickey, a Texas physician, became the first female president of the American Medical Association in June 1998. She was born in Clark, South Dakota, on September 10, 1950, one of four daughters of Ed Wilson. When Dickey was nine, the family moved to Sacramento, California. Five years later, they settled in Katy, Texas, a small town outside Houston.

Dickey made the decision to become a doctor early in life. However, her high school counselor told her that it was impossible to be both a doctor and a wife and mother. Dissuaded, Dickey majored in psychology, rather than premedicine, at Stephen F. Austin State University in Houston. There she met her husband, Franklin Dickey, who encouraged her to pursue her medical education. After graduating in 1972, she enrolled at the University of Texas Medical School in Houston, where she was only one of seven women in a class of 50. Although she did not believe that being in a minority was a disadvantage, there was an occasion when she and the other women walked out of a dermatology presentation when the professor included slides from men's magazine centerfolds.

Dickey earned her medical degree in 1976 and then rose through the ranks at the Medical School's Memorial Hospital System Department of Family Practice. She completed postgraduate work (1976–1979) and was then appointed to a family practice residency as director of patient education (1979–1982). She served as clinical associate professor (1987–1991) and associate professor (1991–1995).

Dickey, who was the founding program director of the Family Practice Residency of the Brazos Valley, has been active in the American Medical Association (AMA) since 1977. She was first elected to its Board of Trustees in 1989. She also served as secretary-treasurer (1993–1994); vice-chair of the board (1994–1995); and chair of the board (1995–1997). In June 1998, she assumed her yearlong role as the first woman president of the AMA. Of this accomplishment, she said, "It's kind of nice to be celebrated as the first, but what I really want to do is make sure we've opened the right doors and left them open for other women to follow. If there isn't a continued rise in the number of women physician voices in organized medicine, then we will not have accomplished very much" (quoted in Mitka, p. 19).

Dickey's other goals as the AMA president included increasing patient advocacy, establishing insurance for all Americans, and improving the health care delivery system. Dickey currently lives in College Station, Texas, where she is president of the Texas A&M University System Health Science Center. She and her husband have three children, Danielle, Wilson, and Elizabeth.

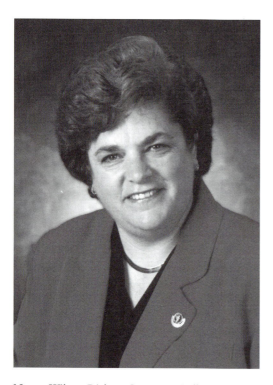

Nancy Wilson Dickey. Courtesy, College of Medicine, Texas A&M University, College Station, Texas.

Selected Additional Achievements

Member, American Academy of Family Physicians (1977–), Texas Academy of Family Physicians (1977–); vice president, Texas Medical Association (1986–1987); Distinguished Alumnus, University of Texas Medical School at Houston (1987); Outstanding Alumnus, Stephen F. Austin State University (1989). Dickey has served as a reviewer for the *Journal of the American Medical Association* and on the editorial advisory boards of *Patient Care*, *Medical World News*, *Medical Ethics Advisor*, and *Archives of Family Medicine*.

References

Dickey, Nancy W. N.d. Curriculum Vitae.
Dickey, Nancy W. 1998. "Packing My Bag for the Road Ahead." *Journal of the American Medical Association* 280 (12):1045.
Mitka, Mike. 1998. "Standing up for Docs." *American Medical News* 41 (21):19.

JSB

Dimock, Susan (1847–1875)
Physician

Susan Dimock was among the best educated and most skilled of the early American women surgeons; her great promise remained tragically unfulfilled because of her early death, but her achievements helped to make a place for women in the medical profession. She was born on April 24, 1847, in Washington, North Carolina, to Henry and Mary Malvina (Owens) Dimock. She received her early education at her mother's school and later at Washington Academy. In her Latin courses, Dimock studied a Latin pharmacopoeia that sparked an interest in medicine. The family doctor, Dr. Solomon Satchwell, nurtured this interest by lending Dimock medical texts and by allowing her to accompany him on calls.

Dimock's studies were interrupted when Union soldiers occupied her hometown during the Civil War. When her father died in 1864 during the occupation, she and her mother moved to Massachusetts. There, Dimock taught school, yet still desired to study medicine. She obtained a reading list of medical works from Dr. Marie Zakrzewska, founder of the New England Hospital for Women and Children. In 1866, Dimock began clinical training at New England Hospital under Zakrzewska and Dr. Lucy Sewall. The following year, Dimock and pioneering English female physician Sophia Jex-Blake were rejected by Harvard Medical School, which had not yet accepted any women. In the meantime, Dimock attended clinics at Massachusetts General Hospital and at the Eye and Ear Infirmary.

In 1868, on the suggestion of Zakrzewska, Dimock applied to the University of Zurich medical school, which had just begun admitting women. She was accepted and graduated with honors from the five-year course in just three years. Her thesis, "Ueber die verschiedenen Formen des Puerperalfiebers" ("The Different Forms of Puerperal Fever") (1871), was considered an intelligent discussion of puerperal fever and received praise from her professors. After graduation, she undertook another year of clinical study in Vienna and Paris and returned to Boston with an excellent medical education. In 1872, she began a three-year appointment at New England Hospital for Women and Children. As attending physician, Dimock performed most of the surgeries and was soon considered a most capable surgeon. She also administered the hospital's nurse training program, one of the first nurse training schools to be organized in the United States.

After her term as attending physician was completed, Dimock accepted a renewal on the condition that she be allowed a five-month leave for further training in Europe. In April 1875, Dimock set sail on the steamship *Schiller*. On May 7 the ship wrecked on the Scilly Islands off the coast of England, killing almost everyone on board, including Dimock. Her remains were recovered from the wreck and returned to Boston for burial, at which eight distinguished male Boston physicians were pallbearers. In her memory, the Susan Dimock Free Bed was established at New England Hospital. She was also made an honorary member of the North Carolina Medical Society. In a memorial tribute, Dr. Mary Putnam Jacobi wrote that Dimock's deserved reputation as a surgeon was of "great value . . . in the difficult enterprise of hewing out for woman an equal place in the medical profession" (Dimock, p. 154).

See also Jacobi, Mary Corinna Putnam; Sewall, Lucy Ellen; Zakrzewska, Marie Elizabeth

References

Bonner, Thomas Neville. 1999. "Dimock, Susan." In *American National Biography*, edited by J. A. Garraty and M. C. Carnes. New York: Oxford University Press.

[Cheney, Ednah Dow]. 1875. *Memoir of Susan Dimock: Resident Physician of the New England Hospital for Women and Children*. Boston: [J. Wilson Press].

Dimock, Susan. 1875. "A Case of Congenital Anal Occlusion of an Unusual Kind, with an Obituary of the Author by Mary Putnam Jacobi, M.D." *Medical Record* (May 22):153–155.

Ingebritsen, Shirley Phillips. 1971. "Dimock, Susan." In *Notable American Women, 1607–1950: A Biographical Dictionary*, edited by E.T. James, J.W. James, and P.S. Boyer. Cambridge: Belknap Press of Harvard University Press.

The National Cyclopaedia of American Biography. 1926. Vol. 19. New York: James T. White.

JSB

Dix, Dorothea Lynde (1802–1887)
Nurse

Dorothea Dix is best known for her efforts to reform treatment of the mentally ill, but she was also the superintendent of Union army nurses during the American Civil War. She was born on April 4, 1802, in Hampden, Maine, the first of three children of Joseph and Mary (Biglow) Dix. At the age of 14, she moved to Worcester, Massachusetts, to live with relatives and opened the first of several schools there. When her father died in 1821, she assumed responsibility for one of her brothers and moved to Boston, where she opened another school and later began teaching at the city's Female Monitorial School. In addition to teaching, she earned a living by writing works such as her elementary science textbook, *Conversations on Common Things* (1824). Bouts of ill health interrupted her teaching career, forcing her to take extended breaks, but she continued to publish.

On March 28, 1841, Dix taught a Sunday school class at the Middlesex County House of Correction in East Cambridge, Massachusetts. She also toured the facilities, noting that about 12 mentally ill inmates at the jail had no fire for heat. The visit sparked her interest in the treatment of the mentally ill, who were frequently restrained and isolated from the public in jails and almshouses. In June 1842, she began a tour of such institutions throughout Massachusetts and gathered information that culminated in her *Memorial to the Legislature of Massachusetts* (January 1843). The 30-page document described the need for a hospital for the mentally ill and the horrific way they were kept "in *cages, closets, cellars, stalls, pens! Chained, naked, beaten with rods*, and *lashed* into obedience!" (quoted in Brown, p. 89). The *Memorial* resulted in the Massachusetts legislature providing funds for the mentally ill at Worcester State Hospital. Following this success, Dix moved on to other states, and by August 1845, she had traveled 10,000 miles and visited 500 almshouses, 300 county jails, 18 state penitentiaries, and numerous hospitals.

Dix's efforts resulted in most states' taking some action to reform treatment of the men-

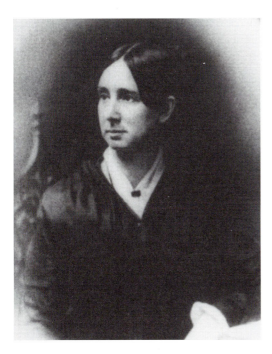

Dorothea Lynde Dix. National Library of Medicine.

tally ill. Among her major successes was the New Jersey legislature's approving a proposal to establish a new hospital at Trenton. Over the next few years, she continued touring state facilities and working for reform. As she traveled alone throughout the country, her crusade made her a nationally known and respected figure. In 1848, she moved to Washington, D.C., where she lobbied Congress to fund mental hospitals from the sale of public lands. Federal support proved elusive, however, and Dix spent six difficult years in Washington before Congress passed her measure. When President Franklin Pierce vetoed the bill, a disappointed Dix left the United States to recuperate in Europe.

Dix was influential in reform campaigns for the mentally ill in Scotland and on the continent and returned to the United States in the fall of 1856 to continue her reform efforts. When the Civil War broke out, she volunteered her services to the Union army and on June 10, 1861, was appointed superinten-

dent of women nurses. As superintendent, she was the first woman to hold a position of federal executive authority. Her mission was to appoint and supervise nurses, and she eventually trained about 180 women for medical duty. She also stockpiled supplies and issued instructions to volunteer sewing societies. She set strict guidelines as to who could be a nurse; she refused Catholic nuns and applicants younger than 30 and declared that nurses should be unattractive. Her methods and austere manner quickly made her unpopular with women who wished to serve, other humanitarian organizations vying for power, and army doctors. As a result, in October 1863 the secretary of war took away her authority to appoint nurses. She refused to resign, however, and served until the war's end. At that point, she resumed her travels across the country and her crusade for the mentally ill.

In October 1881, Dix retired to the Trenton, New Jersey, hospital that she had helped establish. She died there on July 18, 1887.

Selected Additional Achievements

Hymns for Children (1825); *Meditations for Private Hours* (1828); *A Garland of Flora* (1829); *American Moral Tales for Young Persons* (1832); *Remarks on Prisons and Prison Discipline* (1845). Awarded two national flags for her work during the Civil War (1866); honorary doctoral degree, Wells College, Aurora, New York (1870); American Nurses Association Hall of Fame (1976).

References

Brown, Thomas J. 1998. *Dorothea Dix: New England Reformer*. Cambridge: Harvard University Press.
Marshall, Helen E. 1971. "Dix, Dorothea Lynde." In *Notable American Women, 1607–1950: A Biographical Dictionary*, edited by E.T. James, J.W. James, and P.S. Boyer. Cambridge: Belknap Press of Harvard University Press.
Wood, Andrew G. 1999. "Dix, Dorothea Lynde." In *American National Biography*, edited by J.A. Garraty and M. C. Carnes. New York: Oxford University Press.

LS

Dixon Jones, Mary Amanda (1828–1908)
Physician

Mary Dixon Jones was one of the first American women physicians to establish herself as a successful gynecological surgeon. She was born on February 17, 1828, in Dorchester County, Maryland, to Noah and Sarah (Turner) Dixon. In 1845, she graduated from Wesleyan Female College in Wilmington, Delaware, with the first honors given from that institution. The following year, she was appointed chair of belles lettres and physiology at Wesleyan. In 1850, she went on to a similar position at Baltimore Female College and two years later accepted the principalship of a ladies' seminary in Maryland. In 1854, she married John Q.A. Jones, a lawyer. The couple had three children, Henry, Charles, and Mary. Charles would also become a physician and his mother's lifelong colleague.

During her teaching career, Dixon Jones studied medicine under Henry F. Askew in Wilmington, Delaware, and Thomas E. Bond Jr., a prominent Baltimore physician and surgeon. Eventually, Dixon Jones entered the sectarian Hygeio-Therapeutic College in New York, graduating in 1862 with the highest honors of her class. Following graduation, Dixon Jones set up a successful private practice in Brooklyn, New York. Ten years into her practice, she decided to pursue a mainstream medical education. This decision was probably inspired by her inability to treat female patients with serious gynecological disorders. At the age of 44, she entered Woman's Medical College of Pennsylvania in Philadelphia and attended surgical clinics at Blockley Hospital. At Woman's Medical, she heard lectures by Emeline Cleveland, professor of obstetrics and diseases of women and the first woman to perform an ovariotomy in Philadelphia. Dixon Jones received her second medical degree in 1873, graduating with the highest scores in the history of the school. Subsequently, she passed a three-month preceptorship under Dr. Mary Putnam Jacobi,

perhaps the most highly regarded woman physician at that time.

In 1876, Dixon Jones returned to Brooklyn to reestablish her practice. She also studied with microscopist and surgeon Charles Heitzman. With his assistance, she identified two diseases, endothelioma, cancer of the uterine lining; and gyroma, cancerous tumor of the ovary. In 1882, she became chief medical officer at the Women's Dispensary and Hospital in Brooklyn and took courses in surgery at the New York Postgraduate Medical School under Benjamin Franklin Dawson, with whose assistance she performed her first laparotomy. During the following decade, she developed her surgical skills and published several articles describing her successful treatment of difficult gynecological cases.

In 1886, Dixon Jones went to Europe with her son Charles to visit the major hospitals and witness operations performed by prominent physicians. The year after her return from Europe, she successfully performed a new and innovative surgery to remove a cancerous uterus. The same year, she became the first American physician to perform a successful hysterectomy for fibroid tumors. She also made important discoveries on the nature of cancerous diseases (see her article "Carcinoma on the Floor of the Pelvis," *Medical Record* [March 11, 1893]) and new observations regarding the anatomy of fallopian tubes and diseases of the ova.

Dixon Jones' spectacular career ended just as dramatically. She asked the *Brooklyn Eagle* to feature her hospital in its paper; the *Eagle* instead produced a series of 24 lurid articles alleging financial and medical malpractice by Dixon Jones. The scandal culminated in 1890 with the sensational case of the *People v. Mary A. Dixon Jones and Charles Dixon Jones, Physicians*. Dixon Jones was cleared of any legal charges, but her attempt to regain her reputation in an even more spectacular libel suit was unsuccessful. Historian of medicine Regina Morantz-Sanchez claims that as a result of the trial, Dixon Jones' "surgical career was cut short, and her promise as a voice in shaping the direction of . . . gynecology [was] abruptly terminated before it could be fulfilled" (p. 189).

Dixon Jones retreated to New York City, where she became editor of the *Woman's Medical Journal*. She spent the rest of her career writing articles on pathology, using specimens collected over her years as a surgeon. She died in New York in 1908.

See also Cleveland, Emeline Horton; Jacobi, Mary Corinna Putnam

Selected Additional Achievements

Dixon Jones published over 50 medical articles and many letters to the editor of medical journals.

She was associate editor of the *Philadelphia Times and Register* and the *American Journal of Surgery and Gynecology.*

References

Kelly, Howard A., and Walter L. Burrage, eds. 1928. *Dictionary of American Medical Biography: Lives of Eminent Physicians of the United States and Canada, from the Earliest Times.* New York: D. Appleton.

Morantz-Sanchez, Regina. 1999. *Conduct Unbecoming a Woman: Medicine on Trial in Turn-of-the-Century Brooklyn.* New York: Oxford University Press.

Watson, Irving A. 1896. "Jones, Mary Amanda Dixon." In *Physicians and Surgeons of America: A Collection of Biographical Sketches of the Regular Medical Profession.* Concord, N.H.: Republican Press Association.

JSB

Dock, Lavinia Lloyd (1858–1956)
Nurse

Lavinia Dock was a leader in American nursing as well as an advocate for women's rights. She helped to professionalize nursing through her involvement in the formation of three nursing organizations and her contributions to the nursing literature. She was born on February 26, 1858, in Harrisburg, Pennsylvania, the second of six children of Gilliard and Lavinia Lloyd Bombaugh Dock. Her parents had inherited property, which allowed the Docks and their children to live a comfortable lifestyle. Her early education was at a girls' school in Harrisburg.

Dock had not considered nursing until reading an 1882 article in *Century Magazine* that described it as a new profession for women. Two years later, she entered Bellevue Hospital Training School for Nurses in New York City and graduated in 1886. After graduation, she worked as a visiting nurse for the Grace Church of New York City and for the United Workers social organization in Norwich, Connecticut. She then went to assist nursing leader Jane Delano at a yellow fever epidemic in Jacksonville, Florida, in 1888. The next year, Dock helped during the

Johnstown, Pennsylvania, flood and met Clara Barton, founder of the American Red Cross. For a short time in 1889 she was night supervisor at Bellevue Hospital in New York. During that period, she wrote *Text-book of Materia Medica for Nurses* (1890), the first manual on pharmacology for nurses. A popular aspect of the work was the recipes Dock included to help make medicines more palatable, and more than 100,000 copies of the book sold.

In November 1890 Dock became assistant superintendent of nurses at the new Johns Hopkins Training School for Nurses in Baltimore. There she worked under nursing leader Isabel Hampton Robb. Dock taught first-year classes and did much of the ward instruction. In 1893, Dock and Robb attended the Conference of Charities, Correction, and Philanthropy associated with the Chicago World's Fair, and Dock spoke of the need to separate medical and nursing lines of authority. From this meeting, the American Society of Superintendents of Training Schools for Nurses of the United States and Canada was born; Dock served as secretary of the organization from 1896 to 1903. The society was the first national nursing organization in the United States, and it continues today as the National League for Nursing.

After the conference, Dock remained in Chicago for two years, becoming superintendent of the Illinois Training School for Nurses. When her father died, she returned to her hometown to allow her sister to further her education. In 1896, Dock moved into New York City's Henry Street Settlement, founded by Lillian Wald to provide health care for the poor. At Henry Street, Dock met nurses who practiced with little interference from physicians and was exposed to the plight of the working class. In an autobiographical essay that remained unpublished until long after her death, Dock wrote, "I never began to *think* until I went to Henry Street" (1977, p. 24). While in New York, she was also a part-time instructor for the nursing program of Teachers College, Columbia University.

Dock's research into the structure of women's societies and of the American Medical Association provided a model for the Nurses' Associated Alumnae of the United States and Canada, founded in 1896. The Associated Alumnae, renamed the American Nurses Association in 1911, was the first general membership organization for nurses, and it continues to exist today. In 1899, Dock attended meetings of the International Council of Women and joined British nursing leader Ethel Gordon Fenwick in establishing the International Council of Nurses. Dock served as secretary of the organization for 22 years (1900–1922).

Dock was also a contributing editor to the *American Journal of Nursing*, the first nurse-owned and operated publication. In the inaugural issue of the journal (October 1900) Dock wrote an influential article, "What We May Expect from the Law" (pp. 8–12), in which she advocated legislation to control nursing practice. Dock's monthly "Foreign Department" columns brought the international world of nursing to the attention of

American nurses until her retirement from the journal in 1922.

Dock helped to preserve nursing history by writing the multivolume work *A History of Nursing*. She traveled to libraries in Europe to collect information on the history of her profession, and the first two volumes of the work were published in 1907, with two more in 1912. Although nursing leader Adelaide Nutting is listed as a coauthor, Dock actually wrote all but two chapters of the important work. She and Isabel Stewart later published an abridged version, *A Short History of Nursing*, that went into several editions (1st ed. 1920).

Dock was one of the early nurses to campaign against venereal disease and for birth control. In 1910, she wrote *Hygiene and Morality*, in which she condemned "the double standard [that] tacitly permits men to indulge freely and unchecked in sexual irregularity without consequent loss of social standing, but . . . dooms the women who are necessarily involved in these irregularities to social ostracism and even to complete degradation" (pp. 60–61).

Dock resigned from the Henry Street Settlement in 1916 to devote more time to furthering women's economic, social, and political freedom. She was a member of the New York Women's Trade Union League and appealed to her fellow nurses to feel a sisterhood with other working women. She was an ardent supporter of woman suffrage and was jailed several times for her suffragist activities. In 1922, she moved to Fayetteville, Pennsylvania, to live with her five sisters. In her later years, increasing deafness kept her at home. Dock broke her hip in a fall in 1956 and died that year on April 17 in Chambersburg, Pennsylvania.

See also Barton, Clarissa Harlowe [Clara]; Delano, Jane Arminda; Nutting, [Mary] Adelaide; Robb, Isabel Adams Hampton; Stewart, Isabel Maitland

Selected Additional Achievements

Numerous articles in American and British nursing publications; *Short Papers on Nursing Subjects*

(1900); *The History of American Red Cross Nursing* (with others, 1922). American Nurses Association Hall of Fame (1976). Recipient of the Lavinia Dock Fund, International Council of Nurses (Atlantic City, N.J., 1947).

References

Bradford-Burnam, Mary Ann. 1998. "Lavinia Lloyd Dock: An Activist in Nursing and Social Reform." Doctoral diss., Ohio State University.

Dock, Lavinia L. 1910. *Hygiene and Morality: A Manual for Nurses and Others, Giving an Outline of the Medical, Social, and Legal Aspects of Venereal Diseases.* New York: G. P. Putnam's Sons.

Dock, Lavinia L. 1977. "Lavinia L. Dock: Self-Portrait." *American Journal of Nursing* 25 (1): 22–26.

James, Janet Wilson. 1980. "Dock, Lavinia Lloyd." In *Notable American Women: The Modern Period: A Biographical Dictionary*, edited by B. Sicherman and C.H. Green. Cambridge: Belknap Press of Harvard University Press.

James, Janet Wilson, and Alice P. Stein. 1988. "Lavinia Lloyd Dock." In *American Nursing: A Biographical Dictionary*, edited by V.L. Bullough, O.M. Church, and A.P. Stein. New York: Garland.

Roberts, Mary M. 1956. "Lavinia Lloyd Dock— Nurse, Feminist, Internationalist." *American Journal of Nursing* 56 (2):176–179.

LS

Dodge, Eva Francette (1896–1990)
Physician

Eva Dodge, an obstetrician and gynecologist, is best known for her work in developing programs for maternal and child health care. She was born in New Hampton, New Hampshire, on July 24, 1896, the daughter of George Francis Dodge, a physician, and Winnie Josephine (Worthen) Dodge. She received her preliminary education at the New Hampton Literary Institute and then graduated from Ohio Wesleyan University in 1919.

In 1925, Dodge became the fifth woman to earn an M.D. from the Medical School of the University of Maryland. She then became the first woman to serve a rotating internship (1925–1926) and residency in obstetrics (1926–1927) at the University Hospital of her alma mater. In 1927, she moved to San Francisco, where she worked for private physicians and was resident in charge of the maternity clinic at Children's Hospital. She left California in 1928 to serve as acting professor of obstetrics at the Woman's Christian Medical School in Shanghai, China. She left China in 1929 and then toured European medical clinics and completed postgraduate study in Vienna, Austria, until 1931.

In 1932, Dodge established a private practice in obstetrics and gynecology in Winston-Salem, North Carolina, and thus became the first woman physician of that city. She also organized and directed (1933–1937) a maternity clinic at the City Memorial Hospital and was chief of the obstetrics staff (1934–1937). Since medical care was not readily available to county residents outside Winston-Salem, she led the organization of the County Maternity Clinic at Baptist Hospital and eventually helped establish three more similar clinics.

In 1937, Dodge became an obstetrics consultant to the Alabama Bureau of Maternal and Child Health. In this position she directed and organized maternity clinics in 57 counties for patients whose babies were delivered by midwives. Partly as a result of her work, the state's high maternal mortality rate decreased by half. She took a three-month leave (1940) to consult for the Maternal and Child Health Bureau of the Puerto Rico Health Department. The following year, she took a second leave as consultant to the Children's Bureau of the U.S. Department of Labor. After returning to Alabama, she was director (1942–1943) of the Consultants for Public Health Maternity Clinics training program. World War II interrupted the program, and Dodge began an assignment as associate medical director (1943–1945) of the Planned Parenthood Federation of America in New York. In this capacity, she instituted maternity care and birth control instruction for working women in the eastern United States. Concurrently, she integrated Planned Parenthood services for the Mississippi State Health Department.

In 1945, Dodge began her career with the department of obstetrics and gynecology at the university of Arkansas School of Medicine in Little Rock (now University of Arkansas for Medical Science). She stayed at the university until 1964, advancing from the rank of assistant professor to associate professor (1947) and full professor (1960). She was acting head of her department between 1948 and 1949. Outside of her teaching duties, Dodge coordinated with county maternity clinics and midwife programs to improve the quality and access to maternity care. She also maintained a private practice and taught nurses (1945–1947) at St. Vincent's Infirmary and at Baptist Hospital, both in Little Rock.

Dodge retired on June 30, 1964, and became the first female professor emerita at the University of Arkansas Medical School and only the second professor of the school to earn such recognition. After her retirement, she assisted the Texas Health Department's Maternal and Child Health Division in organizing a comprehensive maternity care clinic (1964–1965). She was director of the Health, Education and Welfare Department's Maternal and Infant Care Project #3 in Detroit (1964–1966) and of the East Arkansas Family Planning Project of the Arkansas State Health Department (1969–1972). She remained active internationally as representative (1956–1964) for the Pan American Medical Women's Alliance on the medical advisory board of Medico, an organization founded to supply medical personnel to underdeveloped countries. During the winter of 1962–1963, she visited Medico installations in the Middle and Far East. In 1969, she made a United Nations tour of four African countries, visiting family-planning projects, and took a similar tour of the South Pacific the following year.

Eva Dodge died in March 1990.

Selected Additional Achievements

Diplomate, National Board of Medical Examiners; fellow, American College of Surgeons, American College of Obstetrics and Gynecology, and American Medical Association; organizer, Arkansas Branch, American Medical Women's Association. Honorary member, Bolivian Obstetric and Gynecology Society; charter member, Alabama Obstetrical and Gynecological Society; president, Pan American Medical Women's Alliance (1962–1964); vice-president and secretary, American Medical Women's Association. Her publications include *Manual for Education for Responsible Parenthood* (with William Hollister, 1952) and several articles on obstetrics and gynecology. The University of Arkansas Junior Branch of the American Medical Women's Association was named in her honor (1958). Her many awards include an honorary L.H.D. from Ohio Wesleyan University (1969).

References

Death date provided by the Alumni Department, College of Medicine, University of Arkansas for Medical Sciences, Little Rock.

"Eva F. Dodge, M.D." 1964. *Journal of the American Medical Women's Association* 19 (10): 870–872.

Kittredge, Elizabeth. 1960. "Eva F. Dodge, M.D." *Journal of the American Medical Women's Association* 15 (11): 1096.

The National Cyclopaedia of American Biography. 1972. Vol. 50. Clifton, N.J. James T. White.

JSB

Dolley, Sarah Read Adamson (1829–1909)
Physician

Sarah Adamson Dolley was the third woman in the United States to earn a medical degree, after Elizabeth Blackwell and Lydia Folger Fowler, and the first to serve as an intern at an American hospital. Dolley was born on March 11, 1829, in Chester County, Pennsylvania, the third of five children of Charles and Mary (Corson) Adamson. Many members of her mother's family were physicians, including her uncle, Dr. Hiram Corson. Dolley's early education was at a Friends' school in Philadelphia. At age 18, she discovered a copy of an anatomy text in her uncle's office and was captivated by the study of medicine. At first, Corson discouraged her medical study, but eventually he accepted her as an apprentice in his office.

Dolley applied to several medical schools in Philadelphia, but none would accept her. At the time, there were virtually no medical schools accepting women, and the women's medical schools had not yet opened. Finally, a new sectarian school, Central Medical College in Syracuse, New York, advertised that it would accept women when it opened in November 1849. The college was the first medical school in the United States to adopt a policy of coeducation, and Dolley was one of a handful of women in its first class. Central Medical soon moved to Rochester, New York, and Dolley graduated there on February 20, 1851. After finishing her degree, her uncle and another physician helped her secure an unpaid internship at Blockley Hospital in Philadelphia, making Dolley the first woman intern in an American hospital.

After completing her internship, she married Dr. Lester Clinton Dolley, a professor of anatomy and surgery from Central Medical College, on June 9, 1852. The couple returned to Rochester and practiced medicine together for the next 20 years. Dolley devoted her part of the practice to the care of women and children. The Dolleys had two children, one of whom died in infancy. Their surviving child, Charles Sumner Dolley,

would also become a physician. Sarah Dolley was instrumental in getting women physicians appointed to the staffs of local hospitals in the Rochester area and in getting a New York state law passed that required women's institutions to have a female physician on staff.

During the winter of 1869–1870, Dolley traveled to Paris for postgraduate training. In 1872, Lester Dolley died, and soon after, Sarah left Rochester to teach at the Woman's Medical College of Pennsylvania in Philadelphia. She was professor of obstetrics there during the winter of 1873–1874. In 1875, she again traveled to Europe and studied at the Hôpital des Enfants Malades in Paris, as well as in clinics in Prague and Vienna. In 1886, she was elected the first president of the Provident Dispensary Association in Rochester. The association had been formed by women physicians to provide care for indigent women and children.

In 1887, Dolley helped to organize and found the Practitioner's Society (renamed the Blackwell Medical Society in 1906), the first incorporated scientific society of women physicians. At a 1907 banquet in honor of Dolley's 78th birthday, the Blackwell Medical Society joined with four other medical associations to form the Women's Medical Society of New York State. The society was organized to "encourage greater activity in organized work and to cultivate social relations and mutual helpfulness among women physicians" (Dolley, p. 62). Dolley died not long afterward, on December 27, 1909, in Rochester. Her death was attributed to old age.

See also Blackwell, Elizabeth; Fowler, Lydia Folger

Selected Additional Achievements

Member, Monroe County (New York) Medical Society; organized and headed the Rochester Society of Natural Sciences (1879); helped organize the Rochester Woman's Educational and Industrial Union (1893); president of the Ignorance Club, a Rochester business and professional women's society named in mockery of a similar male club.

References

Dolley, Sarah R. A. 1908. "Address." *Woman's Medical Journal* 18 (April):62–65.
Miller, Genevieve. 1971. "Dolley, Sarah Read Adamson." In *Notable American Women, 1607–1950: A Biographical Dictionary*, edited by E.T. James, J.W. James, and P.S. Boyer. Cambridge: Belknap Press of Harvard University Press.
Waite, Frederick C. 1932. "Dr. Lydia Folger Fowler: The Second Woman to Receive the Degree of Doctor of Medicine in the United States." *Annals of Medical History* 4 (new series) (3):290–297.
"Women's Medical Society of New York State; Doctor Sarah Adamson Dolley." 1908. *Woman's Medical Journal* 18 (April):86–87.

LS

Duckering, Florence West (1869–1951)
Physician

Florence West Duckering was a Boston physician and one of the first women to be admitted to the American College of Surgeons. She was born in Sussex, England, on August 22, 1869, the daughter of Thomas, a farmer, and Eliza (West) Duckering. She received her early education at a private school and later completed a course in nursing at a London hospital. She left England in 1895 for Boston, and in 1897 she entered Tufts College Medical School.

Duckering earned her medical degree cum laude in 1901. She spent the following two years at Massachusetts Women's Hospital as extern and later as resident surgeon and superintendent. In 1903, she established a medical practice, which she maintained until her retirement. The same year, she became assistant surgeon at New England Hospital for Women and Children, founded by Dr. Marie Zakrzewska in 1862. There, she advanced to senior surgeon by the end of her first year. She also worked with the Fayette Street Dispensary, an affiliate of New England Hospital.

In 1913, Duckering became one of the first woman fellows of the American College of Surgeons, founded the same year by a group of American and Canadian surgeons. During the two world wars, she volunteered with the American Red Cross and for the American Women's Hospitals, a medical relief organization directed by Dr. Esther Lovejoy. She was also a volunteer for the Medical Service Corps and was a member of the Council of National Defense. Her career was an inspiration to her niece, Florence A. Duckering, who would also graduate with an M.D. from Tufts (1937) and practice medicine in Boston.

Duckering retired in 1946, spending her later years in St. Petersburg, Florida, and New Hampshire. She died in Peterborough, New Hampshire, on October 25, 1951.

See also Lovejoy, Esther Pohl; Zakrzewska, Marie Elizabeth

References

Bernard, Marcelle. 1952. "Women Fellows of the American College of Surgeons." *Journal of the American Medical Women's Association* 7 (9): 342.
The National Cyclopaedia of American Biography. 1955. Vol. 40. New York: James T. White.

JSB

Dyke, Eunice Henrietta (1883–1969)
Nurse

Eunice Dyke was the first director of public health nursing at the Toronto Department of Public Health. In this role, she built a public health department that soon became a model for other departments in Canada and beyond. She was born on February 8, 1883, the fifth of six children of Samuel Allerthorn, a pastor, and Jennie (Ryrie) Dyke. She grew up in Toronto, where she graduated from Parkdale Collegiate. She went on to normal school and afterward taught kindergarten in a private school.

In 1905, Dyke entered the Johns Hopkins Training School for Nurses in Baltimore and worked as a district nurse. Her studies were interrupted for one year while she recuperated from tuberculosis at the Muskoka Sanatorium in Ontario. After her recovery, she graduated from Johns Hopkins (1909) and began her career as a private-duty nurse, first in Baltimore and then in Canada. In May 1911, Toronto's medical officer of health, Dr. Charles Hastings, appointed her as a tuberculosis nurse at the city's Department of Health.

The department's nurses worked in specialized divisions that often resulted in a duplication of efforts, with more than one nurse visiting the same family to address different health problems. This changed in 1914, when Dyke became head of the department's Division of Public Health Nurses (later, the Division of Public Health Nursing). She reorganized the division into eight health districts in which the nurses "specialized in homes rather than diseases" (quoted in Royce, p. 49). The nurses worked out of district offices that allowed them to become knowledgeable of health concerns in their areas. This system put an end to multiple visits to one family by more than one nurse and dramatically reduced the time that nurses spent traveling to patients' homes. To avoid further overlap of efforts, Dyke also coordinated with other municipal departments and outside social service organizations, such as the Victorian Order of Nurses. Such efficiency allowed her to address each new public health concern as it arose.

Dyke earned acclaim in Canada and abroad for her ability to reorganize or expand the division as needed. In 1917, she and Dr. Hastings went to New York to study public health nursing but were told that they did not need training since other cities were building public health programs based on Toronto's model. Dyke's renown had reached an international level by 1924, when she spent four months in Paris as a consultant in public health nursing for the League of Red Cross Societies.

Another hallmark of Dyke's career was her dedication to the education of nurses. When she became director, there were no formal training programs for public health nurses. As early as 1913, she introduced a probationary period as well as a series of in-service educational programs. In 1915, Dyke herself took a course in public health nursing at Boston's Simmons College. By 1921, she required that new nurses have a certificate of completion from a one-year course in public health at the University of Toronto. In 1926, the course was expanded to four years.

In November 1932, after 21 years at her post, Dyke was fired. Her dismissal centered around the death of an infant caused by the alleged neglect of one of the department's nurses. Dyke retained public support during the scandal and in 1933 was honored at a public reception. Later that year, she began a short fellowship at the International Health Division of the Rockefeller Foundation in New York City. She then went to Ottawa, where she accepted a six-month appointment as secretary of the Division on Maternity and Child Hygiene of the Canadian Council on Child and Family Welfare. At the close of her appointment, she returned to Toronto, where she formed and directed the Second Mile Club (1937), Canada's first senior citizens' organization. Dyke, who suffered from cancer, spent the last years of her life in a

Toronto nursing home. She died there on September 1, 1969.

References

Emory, Florence H.M. 1945. *Public Health Nursing in Canada: Principles and Practice.* Toronto: Macmillan.

MacDougall, Heather. 1990. *Activists and Advocates: Toronto's Health Department, 1883–1983.* Toronto: Dundurn Press.

Royce, Marion V. 1983. *Eunice Dyke, Health Care Pioneer: From Pioneer Public Health Nurse to Advocate for the Aged.* Toronto: Dundurn Press.

JSB

E

Eliot, Martha May (1891–1978)
Physician

Martha May Eliot, the first woman president of the American Public Health Association (1947), was also on the faculty of the Yale University Medical School and a leader in worldwide public health affairs. She was born in Dorchester, Massachusetts, on April 7, 1891, the daughter of Christopher Rhodes and Mary Jackson (May) Eliot and cousin to poet T.S. Eliot. She received her early education at local public and private schools and graduated from Radcliffe College in 1913. Although her parents hoped that their daughter would choose a teaching career, she decided to pursue medicine. She applied to Harvard Medical School but was unsuccessful, as the school had not yet begun accepting women. Instead, Eliot entered Johns Hopkins University Medical School in Baltimore, where she earned her medical degree with honors in 1918.

After completing an internship at Peter Bent Brigham Hospital in Boston, Eliot served as resident at St. Louis Children's Hospital (1919–1920). She hoped to stay another year at St. Louis but left as a result of opposition by the male staff to a female senior resident. She returned to Boston, where she was assistant in the Children's Clinic of Massachusetts General Hospital

(1920–1921) and also established a private practice in pediatrics. In 1921, Edward A. Park, who was then developing a pediatric department at Yale University Medical School, asked Eliot to serve as the department's chief resident. She accepted and continued there as instructor (1923–1927), assistant clinical professor (1927–1932), associate clinical professor (1932–1935), professor (1935–1949), and thereafter as lecturer. She assisted Park in two studies on the treatment of the childhood disease rickets, first at Yale and then for the U.S. Public Health Service in Puerto Rico. With Park, Eliot co-authored an article on rickets published in the medical text *Practice of Pediatrics* (1938).

Concurrent with her work at Yale, Eliot served as director of the Division of Child and Maternal Health of the U.S. Children's Bureau (1924–1934). In 1934 she was appointed assistant chief of the bureau. In this capacity, she wrote the children's section of the Social Security Act and afterward administered the Social Security programs that applied to child and maternal health and welfare. After the United States entered World War II, she took a leading role in the enactment of the Emergency Maternity and

Infant Care (EMIC) program. This federal program distributed free health care to about 1.5 million wives and children of military men serving abroad. The EMIC program led to similar permanent legislation providing medical care for needy pregnant women and their children.

Eliot's public health work was not limited to U.S. borders. In 1935, she was the U.S. representative for the League of Nations Advisory Commission for the Protection and Welfare of Children and Young People in Geneva, Switzerland. The following year the league's Health Organization appointed her to an international committee to study child health and nutrition programs in Europe. After her promotion to associate chief of the Children's Bureau in 1941, the U.S. War Department and the Advisory Committee of National Defense to England appointed her as the only woman of a five-member commission to observe methods of evacuating children in areas at risk for bombing. Her work resulted in a bureau report, *Civil Defense Measures for the Protection of Children* (1942).

In 1946, Eliot was vice chairman of the U.S. delegation to the first World Health Conference in New York City. The delegation drafted the constitution establishing the World Health Organization (WHO), and Eliot has the distinction of being the only woman signer of that document. In addition to her duties at the bureau, she served as chief medical consultant (1947–1949) to the United Nations International Children's Emergency Fund (UNICEF). In this role, she visited 13 European countries to survey the living conditions of children. The trip resulted in child health and food supply programs for children in many war-torn European countries.

Eliot left the Children's Bureau in 1949 to serve as assistant director of WHO but was called back by presidential appointment as

the bureau's chief. She did, however, continue her work with UNICEF as the U.S. representative to the executive board (1952–1957). Upon her retirement from the bureau in 1956, Eliot accepted a professorship and position as department head at the Harvard School of Public Health. She left Harvard in 1960 to travel to Asia and Africa on behalf of WHO and UNICEF to study and teach maternal and child health education.

Eliot spent her later years as head of the Massachusetts Committee for Children and Youth (1959–1971). She died in Cambridge, Massachusetts, on February 14, 1978.

Selected Additional Achievements

President, National Conference on Social Welfare (1949); first woman elected president (1947) and first woman to receive the Sedgwick Memorial Medal, American Public Health Association (1958); first woman admitted to the American Pediatric Society, later earning its highest prize, the Howland Medal. She was awarded the Lasker Award (1948), and the American Public Health Association established an annual award in her name (1964). Fellow, American Medical Association, American Academy of Pediatrics, and American Institute of Nutrition. Member, National Organization for Public Health Nursing, Society for Research in Child Development, the National Committee for Mental Hygiene, and the Connecticut and Massachusetts medical societies. Eliot received eight honorary degrees and published many articles in professional journals for the Children's Bureau.

References

The National Cyclopaedia of American Biography. 1981. Vol. 60. Clifton, N.J.: James T. White.
Rothe, Anna, and Constance Ellis, eds. 1949. *Current Biography: Who's News and Why, 1948.* New York: H.W. Wilson.
Wolfe, Richard J. 1999. "Eliot, Martha May." In *American National Biography*, edited by J. A. Garraty and M. C. Carnes. New York: Oxford University Press.

JSB

Erickson, Hilda Anderson (1859–1968)
Midwife

Hilda Erickson, a midwife, is considered the last of Utah's immigrant pioneers. She was born on November 11, 1859, in Ledsjo, Sweden, one of five children of Pehr and Maria Kathrina (Larsson) Andersson. The family was Lutheran, the national religion of Sweden, but converted to the Church of Jesus Christ of Latter-Day Saints when Erickson was a child. In 1866, the family emigrated to Utah to join the Latter-Day Saints, settling in Grantsville, Utah, where Erickson attended school and took in sewing and tailoring work.

On February 23, 1882, she married John A. Erickson, also a Swedish immigrant, in Salt Lake City. The couple had two children, Amy (1884) and Perry (1890). In 1883, the couple joined a mission on the Goshute Indian Reservation in Ibapah (then called Deep Creek Valley), Utah. At the mission, Erickson served as nurse and midwife to expectant mothers and was secretary of the mission Sunday school. In 1885, she went to Salt Lake City to study obstetrics at Deseret Hospital. The following year, she received a license and certificate in obstetrics and returned to Ibapah, where she helped both Native American and white women deliver their babies. To reach her patients, she traveled sidesaddle on her horse, sometimes up to 25 miles, across the sparsely settled mission. During this time, she also served as physician for minor medical problems and became known for her ability to pull a bad tooth.

Around 1898, the Ericksons left the mission to purchase a 320-acre cattle ranch, called the "Last Chance Ranch." In 1925, Erickson established a general store in Grantsville, which she managed for over 21 years. She renewed her midwifery certification every year until at least the age of 90. She died in Salt Lake City on January 1, 1968. Today, a bronze monument showing Erickson riding sidesaddle stands in front of the Grantsville City Hall.

References

Carter, Kate. 1952. *Treasures of Pioneer History, Vol. I-VI.* Salt Lake City: Daughters of Utah Pioneers.

"Hilda Anderson Erickson—Pioneer." 1963. In *Our Pioneer Heritage*, edited by K.B. Carter. Vol. 6. Salt Lake City: Daughters of Utah Pioneers.

Tanaka, Julynn Ann. 1997. *Hilda A. Erickson: Last Surviving Utah Pioneer.* Tooele: Settlement Canyon Chapter of the Sons of Utah Pioneers.

JSB

Ernst, Eunice Katherine MacDonald [Kitty] (1926–)
Nurse-midwife

Kitty Ernst has worked for the foremost nurse-midwifery programs in the United States and has helped to develop continuing education and support organizations for nurse-midwives. She was born in Weston, Massachusetts, on July 21, 1926. When she was in the first grade, she became ill and was cared for by a public health nurse. From that time, Ernst knew that she wanted to be a nurse. In 1947, she received a diploma from the Waltham Hospital School of Nursing in Waltham, Massachusetts, and was then on staff at the hospital.

In 1949 and 1950, Ernst was a nurse for the University of Chicago Clinics. She moved to rural Leslie County, Kentucky, in 1951 and became the night nurse for medicine, surgery, and pediatrics at the Frontier Nursing Service (FNS) hospital. The FNS was founded by pioneering nurse-midwife Mary

Breckinridge in 1925. Ernst's previous experience in hospital obstetrics wards led her to believe that she never wanted to be involved in obstetrical nursing. After being present at a home birth with the FNS midwives, however, Ernst changed her mind. She says that witnessing the home birth helped her understand "the difference between giving birth, . . . and being delivered, which is what [she] had been exposed to as a student nurse" (National Association of Childbearing Centers, *Generations Library*). She received a certificate in nurse-midwifery in 1951 and then began working as a nurse-midwife and public health nurse for the FNS.

From 1954 to 1958, Ernst was a nurse-midwife for the Maternity Center Association (MCA) in New York City. During this time, she also earned a bachelor's degree in education from Hunter College (1957). In 1959, she earned a master's degree in public health from Columbia University and was then made assistant professor at the university's nursing school (1959–1961). In the 1960s, she focused her energies on her family and was self-employed as an educator, lecturer, and consultant on nurse-midwifery. In 1971, she took a refresher course in nurse-midwifery at King's County Hospital in Brooklyn, New York. Around this time, she developed a family-centered maternity program for the Salvation Army Booth Maternity Center in Philadelphia. She also developed continuing education courses for nurse-midwives, consulted with agencies and universities interested in nurse-midwifery programs, and, with nurse-midwife Ruth Lubic, developed the MCA Childbearing Center as an alternative to home birth.

In 1979 Ernst conducted an on-site survey of 14 freestanding birth centers around the country, which convinced her of the need for a support and networking system for the centers. Continuing that work, she became director of the Cooperative Birth Center Network (CBCN), an MCA program designed to assess the needs of freestanding birth centers (1981–1983). While working on this project, Ernst was in a serious car ac-

cident that prevented her from commuting to the MCA in New York. Thus, the CBCN was relocated to Ernst's hometown of Perkiomenville, Pennsylvania. In 1983 the CBCN was renamed the National Association of Childbearing Centers (NACC), with Ernst serving as director until 1993. The NACC collects and disseminates information for nurse-midwives and childbearing families and sets national standards for birth centers. Ernst was also director of the Community-Based Nurse-Midwifery Education Pilot Program, a distance learning program designed to prepare nurse-midwives for work in birth centers (1988–1991).

Since 1989, Ernst has been a faculty member of Case Western Reserve University's Frances Payne Bolton School of Nursing. She is also the Mary Breckinridge Chair of Midwifery at the Frontier School of Midwifery and Family Nursing (1991–   ) and is director of the NACC Consulting Group (1993–   ).

She is married to Albert T. Ernst and has three children.

See also Breckinridge, Mary; Lubic, Ruth Watson

Selected Additional Achievements

Numerous articles in the nursing and nurse-midwifery literature. President (1961–1963), vice president (1981–1983), American College of Nurse-Midwives (ACNM). Martha May Elliot Award for Exceptional Health Service to Mothers and Children, American Public Health Association (1981); Hattie Hemschemeyer Award, ACNM (1988); Recognition of Outstanding Service, NACC (1992); MCA Medal for Distinguished Service (1993); lifetime fellow, ACNM (1994); Professional Achievement Award, NACC (1996).

References

Biographical Directory of the American Public Health Association, 1979. 1979. New York: R.R. Bowker.
Ernst, Eunice Katherine MacDonald. 2000. Curriculum Vitae.
Frontier School of Midwifery and Family Nursing. *Academic Faculty.* Online. http://www.midwives.org/fac-direct-acad.htm. 10 November 2000.
National Association of Childbearing Centers.

FAQ's on Birth Centers. Online. http://www.birthcenters.org/faqbirthcenters/. 10 November 2000.

National Association of Childbearing Centers.

Generations Library. Online. http://www.birthcenters.org/generationslibrary/. 10 November 2000.

LS

F

Fagin, Claire Mintzer (1926–   )
Nurse

Claire Fagin is a leader in American nursing whose early research helped to reform pediatric psychiatric nursing practice. She was born on November 25, 1926, in New York City, the younger of two daughters of Harry and Mae (Slatin) Mintzer. The family lived in four of New York's five boroughs before she was five years old and then settled in the Bronx, where her father was a grocer. She attended Hunter College in New York City for a year, before transferring to the nursing program at Wagner College on Staten Island during World War II. She decided to study nursing after noticing advertisements for the U.S. Cadet Nurse Corps, believing that it would allow her to take an active part in the war effort.

While in school, Fagin became interested in psychiatric nursing. Working at a tuberculosis hospital and seeing the great psychological needs of children with the disease deepened her interest in the field. She earned her bachelor's degree in 1948 and went to work at Bellevue Hospital's adolescent psychiatric ward. After two years, she took a leave of absence from Bellevue to earn a master's degree. She was awarded a National Institute of Mental Health Fellowship to study at Teachers College, Columbia University,

under Hildegard Peplau, a pioneer in the theory and practice of psychiatric nursing.

After finishing her master's degree in 1951, Fagin intended to return to Bellevue but found that she would be a supervisor, which at the time, "was a very traditional role . . . unconnected with patient care" (Fagin, 1988, p. 100). Instead, she took a yearlong position as a psychiatric nurse consultant to the National League of Nursing Education. Next, she was assistant chief of the psychiatric nursing service at the Clinical Center, National Institutes of Health, where she was responsible for the children's unit and in-service education. From 1956 to 1958, she was the research project coordinator of the Children's Hospital Department of Psychiatry in Washington, D.C., as well as an instructor in psychiatric mental health nursing at New York University (NYU).

In 1952, she married Samuel Fagin. When the couple adopted a baby boy in 1958, she chose to be a stay-at-home mother. By 1960, Fagin decided to earn her doctorate and was accepted at NYU. She graduated in 1964, and her dissertation, "The Effects of Maternal Attendance during Hospitalization on the Behavior of Young Children" (published in 1966), was partially inspired by her son's hospitalizations and her earlier experience working with children with tuberculosis. The work received national attention and helped to change hospital visiting policies for young children. The Fagins adopted a second boy in 1963, and the next year Fagin returned to NYU as an associate professor, where she directed a child psychiatric nursing program.

In 1969, Fagin accepted an offer to become chair and professor of the new nursing department at Herbert H. Lehman College in New York City. At Lehman, she developed an innovative undergraduate program to prepare nurses to be primary care practitioners and worked to recruit and retain minority students. She left Lehman in 1977 to become professor and Margaret Bond Simon Dean of the University of Pennsylvania School of Nursing, a position that she would hold until 1992. Under her leadership, the school prospered and became one of the highest rated nursing programs in the United States. She was also interim president of the University of Pennsylvania for one year (1993–1994), the first woman to hold the office in the university's history.

Fagin has published numerous books and articles in the nursing literature on topics such as nursing leadership and policy, nursing education, the cost-effectiveness of nursing, and health care reform. She has also promoted nursing in the national media and the popular press and believes that "the health of our health care system depends on nurses" (Fagin, 1999, p. 7). She currently lives in New York and is professor and dean emerita at the University of Pennsylvania, a consultant in academic and health care leadership, and program director of the John A. Hartford Foundation's "Building Academic Geriatric Capacity."

See also Peplau, Hildegard E.

Selected Additional Achievements

Fellow, American Academy of Nursing; member, Institute of Medicine, National Academy of Science. President, American Orthopsychiatric Association (1985–1986), National League for Nursing (1991–1993). Numerous awards, including 10 honorary doctorates; Honorary Recognition Award, American Nurses Association (1988); Hildegard E. Peplau Award, American Nurses Association (1994); Lillian D. Wald Spirit of Nursing Award, Visiting Nurse Service of New York (1994); Living Legend, American Academy of Nursing (1998).

References

Fagin, Claire. 1988. "Claire Fagin." In *Making Choices, Taking Chances: Nurse Leaders Tell Their Stories*, edited by T.M. Schorr and A. Zimmerman. St. Louis: C.V. Mosby.

Fagin, Claire M. 1999. "Nurses, Patients and Managed Care." *New York Times* (March 16):F7.

Fagin, Claire M. June 28, 2000. Interview with author via e-mail.

Fagin, Claire M. June 2000. Curriculum Vitae and Brief Biography.

Who's Who of American Women 1999–2000. 1998. 21st ed. New Providence, N.J.: Marquis Who's Who.

LS

Foley, Edna Lois (1878–1943)
Nurse

Edna Foley was a leading public health nurse, and served as director of the Chicago Visiting Nurses Association for 25 years. She was born in Hartford, Connecticut, to William R. and Matilda (Baker) Foley on December 17, 1878. She received her early education in local schools and earned a B.A. from Smith College in Northampton, Massachusetts, in 1901.

After graduating from the nursing program at the Hartford Hospital Training School for Nurses in 1904, Foley held several nursing positions. She was head nurse at Hartford Hospital (1904–1905), chief nurse of Children's Hospital in Albany, New York (1905–1906), night supervisor of Children's Hospital in Boston, (1906–1907), and a Boston municipal tuberculosis visiting nurse

(1907–1909). She also completed postgraduate work at the Boston School of Social Work (1908). She relocated to Chicago to work for the Chicago Tuberculosis Institute (1909–1911) and was then superintendent of the city's Municipal Tuberculosis Nurses.

In 1912 Foley began her most notable work as superintendent of the Chicago Visiting Nurses Association (VNA). During her tenure with the VNA, she studied visiting nurses associations around the country and the world and integrated the best practices of each into the Chicago institution. Her work earned both her and the Chicago VNA a place of importance in the nursing world. Nurses from all over the country applied for positions at the VNA or sought her expertise. Many nurses who worked under her went on to establish new VNAs or improve existing organizations. Her book *Visiting Nurse Manual* (1914) was in such demand by nurses and other workers in the social services that it went into two more editions (1915, 1919).

In June 1919 Foley took leave from the VNA to succeed Mary Gardner as chief nurse of the American Red Cross Tuberculosis Commission for Italy. During her tenure overseas, Foley oversaw the training of visiting nurses to care for tuberculosis patients and the establishment of tuberculosis clinics. When the American Red Cross completed its nursing activities for Italy in December 1919, she returned to the VNA, where she remained for the next 17 years.

Throughout her career, Foley championed the advancement of public health nursing. In 1912, she chaired the meeting that led to the formation of the National Organization for Public Health Nursing. She became the organization's first vice president and was president from 1920 to 1921. She became director of the National Society for the Study and Prevention of Tuberculosis (1916) and of the Chicago Tuberculosis Institute (1931). She actively supported the importance of VNAs, the continuing education of nurses, and the improvement of nursing worldwide. She also advocated increased educational and professional opportunities for African American nurses.

Foley retired to New York City in 1937. She died of a stroke on August 4, 1943.

See also Gardner, Mary Sewall

Selected Additional Achievements

Author of many articles in professional journals; editor, department of public health, *American Journal of Nursing*; member, Red Cross, Chicago Board of Charities (1911), the National Committee on Red Cross Nursing Service, executive committee, National Tuberculosis Association (1920); honorary doctor of science degree, Smith College (1928); first Citizen Fellowship award, Chicago Institute of Medicine (1934); Florence Nightingale Medal (1937). The 47th street annex of the VNA was named the Edna L. Foley Substation.

References

Davis, Audrey. 1988. "Edna Lois Foley." In *American Nursing: A Biographical Dictionary*, edited by V.L. Bullough, O.M. Church, and A.P. Stein. New York: Garland.

Dock, Lavinia L., Sarah Elizabeth Pickett, Clara D. Noyes, Fannie F. Clement, Elizabeth G. Fox, and Ann R. Van Meter. 1922. *History of American Red Cross Nursing*. New York: Macmillan.

"Foley, Edna L." 1943. *American Journal of Nursing* 43 (9):876.

Hawkins, Joellen Watson. 1988. "Foley, Edna Lois." In *Dictionary of American Nursing Biography*, edited by M. Kaufman. New York: Greenwood Press.

JSB

Follansbee, Elizabeth A. (1839–1917)
Physician

Elizabeth Follansbee is credited with being the first woman to practice medicine in southern California. She was born in Pillston, Maine, on December 9, 1839, the granddaughter of Roger Sherman, a signer of the Declaration of Independence. She received her early education at schools in Brooklyn, New York, Boston, and France. Afterward, she taught at the Green Mountain Institute and at the Hillsdale Seminary in Montclair, New Jersey.

In 1875, Follansbee became one of the first two women admitted to the Medical Department of the University of California. After one year, she continued her studies at the University of Michigan and at the Woman's Medical College of Pennsylvania in Philadelphia. She graduated from Woman's Medical in 1877 and then completed an internship at New England Hospital in Boston.

Follansbee began her medical career in San Francisco, where she established a private practice. She also helped Dr. Charlotte Brown reorganize the Pacific Dispensary for Women and Children into Women's and Children's Hospital, the only female-founded hospital on the West Coast at that time. In 1883, she relocated to Los Angeles and resumed her practice. Two years later, she became the first female faculty member at a California medical school when she was appointed as professor of pediatrics at the University of Southern California. In addition, she taught at the Los Angeles County Hospital, where she also served as pediatrician. During her tenure, Follansbee was instrumental in obtaining internships for her students at Women's and Children's Hospital.

Follansbee was member of the Los Angeles County Medical Association, the Southern California Medical Society, the Medical Society of California, and the American Medical Association. In 1908, she became professor emerita at the University of Southern California. She died on August 22, 1917, in Los Angeles County Hospital.

See also Brown, Charlotte Amanda Blake

References

Kress, George H. 1910. *A History of the Medical Profession of Southern California with a Historical Sketch.* 2nd ed. Los Angeles: Press of the Times-Mirror Print.

Mall, Janice. 1985. "Becoming a Doctor in the 19th Century." *Los Angeles Times* (July 21):6.

Martin, Helen Eastman. 1979. *The History of the Los Angeles County Hospital, 1878–1968, and the Los Angeles County-University of Southern California Medical Center, 1969–1978.* Los Angeles: University of Southern California Press.

Mason-Hohl, Elizabeth. 1943. "Early California and Its Medical Women." *Medical Woman's Journal* 50 (4):89–91.

"Obituary." 1917. *Journal of the American Medical Association* 69 (11):929.

JSB

Fowler, Lydia Folger (1822–1879)
Physician

In June 1850, Lydia Folger Fowler became the second woman in the United States to earn a medical degree, after Elizabeth Blackwell. She was born on May 5, 1822, in Nantucket, Massachusetts, the sixth of seven children born to Gideon and Eunice (Macy) Folger. Fowler was educated at local schools and spent a year (1838–1839) at Wheaton Seminary in Norton, Massachusetts, where she later taught (1842–1844). A distant relative, the father of the woman astronomer Maria Mitchell, also taught Fowler and encouraged her early interest in science. She was an eager student and received more comprehensive training than most young women of her day.

On September 19, 1844, she married Lorenzo Niles Fowler, a phrenologist from New York City. Lorenzo, his brother, sister, and her husband were major proponents of phrenology, a pseudoscience that relied on the shape of a person's skull to judge his or her character and mental ability. Through public lectures and their publishing house, Fowler and Wells, Lorenzo and family touted their beliefs in phrenology. Lydia Fowler joined her husband on lecture tours soon after their marriage. By 1847, she was giving her own lectures to women on phrenology, anatomy, physiology, and hygiene. Also that year, Fowler and Wells published two of her books: *Familiar Lessons on Physiology* and *Fa-*

miliar Lessons on Phrenology. Both books gave frank and simple explanations of human physiology and hygiene; they were very popular and were reprinted many times. In 1848, Fowler and Wells published Lydia's third volume in the series, *Familiar Lessons in Astronomy.*

In order to further her knowledge of health and physiology, in November 1849 Fowler enrolled at Central Medical College in Syracuse, New York, leaving her young daughter, born in 1846, at home in the care of a housekeeper. Central Medical College was a new sectarian medical school and the first in the United States to adopt a policy of coeducation. The school would also graduate Sarah Adamson Dolley and Rachel Brooks Gleason, the third and fourth women in the United States to earn medical degrees. Central Medical soon moved to Rochester, New York, and Fowler graduated there in June 1850. She gave birth to a second daughter two months later. After graduation, she became principal of the Female Department and demonstrator of anatomy to the female students at Central Medical College.

In 1851, Fowler was appointed professor of midwifery and diseases of women and children at the college, making her one of the first woman professors in an American medical college. Also in 1851, she presented an address on obstetrics to the New York State Eclectic Medical Society; it was the first address given by a woman to an organized group of medical men in the United States. Fowler's professorial appointment was short-lived as Central Medical College was dissolved in 1852. Undaunted, she established a private medical practice in New York City, which lasted until 1863. She practiced from morning to midafternoon in her own office and in the late afternoon at her husband's phrenological office.

In addition to practicing medicine, Fowler continued lecturing to women on health topics. Biographer Madeleine Stern described Fowler's medical philosophy as being founded on temperance, hydropathy, and the "complete, unrestrained development of the whole woman" (1977, p. 1138). In 1854, Fowler taught an eight-week course at Met-

ropolitan Medical College, and by 1860 she and her husband had logged over 30,000 miles lecturing across North America.

In 1860, the couple traveled to England. While abroad, Fowler cared for her daughters (a third had been born in 1856), lectured, and studied medicine in London and Paris. A letter written to the editors of the *Water-Cure Journal* reveals some of the difficulty that a woman in medicine faced during her time. In the letter, Fowler wrote that a French physician had admitted to her that French medical schools were free and open for study, "but not for woman." To this she replied, "This old ditty I have heard all my life. . . . There is no sex in science, and God, who made the brain, and gave an intellectual lobe to woman, has never declared that woman should bury her talents in a napkin" (p. 62). Eventually, the doctor relented and allowed her to study with his class.

In 1862 the Fowlers returned home, and Lydia Fowler resumed her medical practice. She also taught midwifery that year at the New York Hygeio-Therapeutic College, a school that pioneering women physicians Mary Dixon Jones and Mary Walker would attend. By 1863, however, the Fowlers returned to England, and Lydia Fowler continued her lectures. She also lectured throughout Europe and in Turkey, Egypt, and Palestine. Throughout the 1870s, her career flourished, but her life was cut short when she contracted pneumonia in the course of her work among London's poor. She died of the disease on January 26, 1879.

See also Blackwell, Elizabeth; Dixon Jones, Mary Amanda; Dolley, Sarah Read Adamson; Gleason, Rachel Brooks; Walker, Mary Edwards

Selected Additional Achievements

Secretary, two national women's rights conventions (1852, 1853); delegate, New York Daughters of Temperance (January 1852); president, women's temperance mass meeting in New York City (1853); honorary secretary, British Women's Temperance Association. In addition to her books, Fowler also published at least three journal articles: "Medical Progression," *Syracuse Medical & Surgical Journal* 6 (1854):200–202; "Female Medical Education," *Journal of Medical Reform*

1 (1854):43–45; and "Suggestions to Female Medical Students," *Journal of Medical Reform* 1 (1854):127–130; as well as a temperance novel, *Nora, the Lost and Redeemed* (1863); a compilation of her lectures on child care, *The Pet of the Household and How to Save It* (1865); and a book of poems, *Heart-Melodies* (1870).

References

Blake, John B. 1971. "Fowler, Lydia Folger." In *Notable American Women, 1607–1950: A Biographical Dictionary*, edited by E.T. James, J.W. James, and P.S. Boyer. Cambridge: Belknap Press of Harvard University Press.

Fowler, Lydia Folger. 1861. "Letter from Mrs. Dr. Fowler." *Water-Cure Journal* 32 (September):62–63.

Stern, Madeleine B. 1971. *Heads and Headlines: The Phrenological Fowlers.* Norman: University of Oklahoma Press.

Stern, Madeleine B. 1977. "Lydia Folger Fowler, M.D.: First American Woman Professor of Medicine." *New York State Journal of Medicine* 77 (June):1137–1140.

Waite, Frederick C. 1932. "Dr. Lydia Folger Fowler: The Second Woman to Receive the Degree of Doctor of Medicine in the United States." *Annals of Medical History* 4 (new series) (3):290–297.

LS

Franklin, Martha Minerva (1870–1968)
Nurse

Martha Franklin was an African American nurse whose efforts to promote racial equality in nursing resulted in the founding of the National Association of Colored Graduated Nurses. She was born on October 29, 1870, in New Milford, Connecticut, one of three children of Henry J. and Mary E. (Gauson) Franklin. She was raised in Meriden, Connecticut, and graduated from the city's high school in 1890.

In 1895, Franklin entered the Woman's Hospital Training School for Nurses in Philadelphia and graduated in December 1897, the only black woman in the class. She then returned to Meriden and worked as a private-duty nurse for several years before moving to New Haven, Connecticut, where she continued her private-duty work. On June 17, 1908, she became one of the first nurses to pass the Connecticut state registration exam. During this time, segregation and discrimination were a constant reality for black nurses. In most states, African Americans could not be members of state nursing associations and were thus prevented from being members of the national nursing organization, the American Nurses Association. Blacks were also excluded from admission to many nursing schools, forcing the establishment of separate schools.

Concerned with the situation, Franklin sent 500 letters to black nurses around the country in the fall of 1906, inquiring about their experiences. Although the response rate was slow, she persisted with her study and recognized that many black nurses were as concerned as she was about their status. She believed that with collective action the nurses could combat racial discrimination and bias and thus mailed 1,500 letters suggesting that black nurses gather for a meeting. Nurse Adah Thoms, who was serving as president of the Lincoln Hospital School of Nursing Alumnae Association, was among those who responded favorably to Franklin's call to action. Thoms invited Franklin and other interested nurses to New York City, and in August 1908, more than 50 African American nurses came together to discuss their situation. Franklin proposed the formation of an organization for black graduate registered nurses in order to combat discrimination in the profession, to promote leadership and networking among black nurses, and to promote standards in administration and education.

After three days of discussion, the women established the National Association of Colored Graduate Nurses (NACGN), with 26 charter members, and elected Franklin president of the association. She was reelected to the presidency in 1909 and was asked to serve a third term but refused. Instead, she was designated the honorary president for life and was named the NACGN'S permanent historian. By 1940 membership in the NACGN had grown to 12,000, and a national registry was established for black nurses. The American Nurses Association began admitting black women in 1948, and the NACGN officially disbanded three years later.

In the 1920s Franklin moved to New York City and enrolled in a postgraduate program at Lincoln Hospital. She became a registered nurse in New York and worked as a school nurse in the New York City public schools. From 1928 to 1930, she took additional courses in nursing education at Teachers College, Columbia University.

Franklin died in New Haven, Connecticut, on September 26, 1968. She was one of the first nurses elected to the American Nurses Association Hall of Fame in 1976.

See also Thoms, Adah Belle Samuels

References

Davis, Althea T. 1988. "Martha Minerva Franklin." In *American Nursing: A Biographical Dictionary*, edited by V.L. Bullough, O.M. Church, and A.P. Stein. New York: Garland.

Davis, Althea T. 1999. *Early Black American Leaders in Nursing: Architects for Integration and Equality*. Sudbury, Mass.: Jones and Bartlett.

Friedman, Alice Howell. 1988. "Franklin, Martha Minerva." In *Dictionary of American Nursing Biography*, edited by M. Kaufman. New York: Greenwood Press.

LS

Freeman, Ruth Benson (1906–1982)
Nurse

Ruth Freeman was a prominent educator, speaker, and author in the field of public health nursing. She was born on December 6, 1906, in Methuen, Massachusetts, the oldest of three children of Wilbur Milton and Elsie (Lawson) Freeman. In 1924, Freeman entered Mt. Sinai Hospital School of Nursing in New York. She married Anselm Fisher in 1927, shortly after her graduation from nursing school. They had one daughter, Nancy Ruth.

Immediately following graduation, she accepted a position as staff nurse at Henry Street Visiting Nurse Service in New York City. There, she became committed to nursing through her contact with patients and their families and with prominent members of the nursing profession, such as Lillian Wald. While working at Henry Street, she attended Columbia University's program for nurses and earned a B.S. (1934) and a M.A. (1939). She earned a doctor of education degree from New York University in 1951.

Freeman left Henry Street in 1937 to become nursing instructor at New York University (NYU). She taught at NYU until 1941, when she became professor of public health nursing at the University of Minnesota School of Public Heath. In Minnesota, she learned the necessity of providing an education that went beyond theoretical nursing. For example, the program served many older students from rural areas of Manitoba, Canada. Freeman learned from the Manitoba deputy director of health and welfare that the nurses were returning from the program incapable of doing their jobs well. She went to Manitoba and discovered that the problem was that their education focused on nursing theory rather than experience. As a result, Minnesota changed its teaching methods, and Freeman began to form different ideas about nursing education.

Freeman left Minnesota in 1946 to serve as administrator of nursing services at the American Red Cross in Washington, D.C. During this time, she was also consultant to the National Security Resources Board, which was developing a nursing program in preparation for national emergencies.

In 1950, the Johns Hopkins School of Hygiene and Public Health invited Freeman to establish its nursing program. Rather than establishing a separate nursing department, students enrolled in existing health care courses, not specialized courses for nurses. Freeman considered the development of a multidiscipline, multidepartment nursing program at Johns Hopkins to be her main contribution to nursing. In addition to being program coordinator, she was professor of public health administration (1950–1962), professor of public health (1962–1971), and professor emerita (1971–1982).

As president of the National League for Nursing (1955–1959), Freeman encouraged ordinary citizens to participate in nursing issues since they would someday rely upon a nursing program for health care. The goal of citizen participation was to bring patient and nurse together in a "full and respected partnership [to] move toward the best possible health for the individual and for the community" (Freeman, 1959, p. 16).

Freeman died of Alzheimer's disease on December 2, 1982, in Cockeyesville, Maryland.

See also Wald, Lillian D.

Selected Additional Achievements

Techniques of Supervision in Public Health Nursing (1945), *Public Health Nursing Practice* (1950), *Administration in Public Health Services* (1960), and *Community Health Nursing Practice* (1970). President, Minnesota Nurses' Association (1944–1946); fellow and member of Executive Board, American Public Health Association (1950–1951); Pearl McIver Award for distinguished work in public health nursing (1958); president, National Health Council (1959–60); Bronfman Prize from American Public Health Association for excellence in public health (1972); honorary fellow, American Academy of Nursing (1981).

References

Evory, Ann, ed. 1979. *Contemporary Authors.* Vols. 41–44. Detroit: Gale Research.

Freeman, Ruth B. 1957. "Meeting Nursing Needs through Citizen Participation." *Nursing Outlook* 5 (1):43–44.

Freeman, Ruth B. 1959. "Nursing, Patients and Progress." *Nursing Outlook* 7 (1):16–18.

Lawrence, Joy T. 1988. "Ruth Benson Freeman (Fisher)." In *American Nursing: A Biographical Dictionary*, edited by V.L. Bullough, O.M. Church, and A.P. Stein. New York: Garland.

Safier, Gwendolyn. 1977. *Contemporary American Leaders in Nursing: An Oral History.* New York: McGraw-Hill.

JSB

Führer, Charlotte Heise (1834–1907)
Midwife

Charlotte Führer's life and career shed interesting light on the changing tale of midwifery in mid-Victorian Canada. She was born in Hanover, Germany, in 1834. Little is known about her life before May 1853, when she married Ferdinand Adolph Führer; the couple eventually had six children. Shortly after their marriage, the Führers immigrated to New York, where Ferdinand opened a German import business. The venture soon failed, and the Führers returned to Germany. To help support the family, Führer decided to become a midwife and then return to America. She believed that expectant American women would rather be attended by a female midwife than a male physician.

Although Führer claimed that she received a diploma from the University of Hamburg, there is evidence only that she studied under an obstetrician (1856–1859) at a maternity hospital in Hamburg. In the summer of 1859, the Führers again immigrated to North America, this time to Montreal. Upon arrival, Führer established a thriving midwifery practice in the city, which would last until shortly before her death. She attended women in their homes and established a maternity residence where women could give birth. She aided married and unmarried women from both the working and middle classes. When a child was born out-of-wedlock, she often handled the adoption of the baby or placed it in an orphanage.

Führer's position as midwife made her a confidante and confessor to women who found themselves pregnant out-of-wedlock. Although she aided these women, she held Victorian ideals of sexuality and in 1881 wrote *The Mysteries of Montreal: Being Recollections of a Female Physician*, "to warn others from taking that first false step which so often leads to future misery and bitter remorse" (Führer, p. 37). The book, which she claimed to be case histories, is a sensational account of women and men whose inability to control their sexual desires leads to their downfall.

Around the turn of the century, Führer and her husband retired to their daughter's home. She died of cancer on November 5, 1907, in Montreal.

References

Führer, Charlotte. 1984. *The Mysteries of Montreal: Memoirs of a Midwife*. Edited by W.P. Ward. Reprint and expanded ed. Vancouver: University of British Columbia Press. Original ed., *The Mysteries of Montreal: Being Recollections of a Female Physician*. Montreal: John Lovell and Son, 1881.

Kenneally, Rhona Richman. 1994. "Heise, Charlotte." In *Dictionary of Canadian Biography: Volume 13, 1901–1910*, edited by R. Cook. Toronto: University of Toronto Press.

LS

G

Gannt, Love Rosa Hirschmann (1875–1935)
Physician

Rosa Gannt was an American physician who practiced in South Carolina and North Carolina. She was born on December 29, 1875, in Camden, South Carolina, the third of six children of Solomon and Lena (Debhrina) Hirschmann. After completing her early education in Charleston public schools, she enrolled in the Medical College of the State of South Carolina in 1898. She graduated in 1901, one of the first two women to earn a degree from the Medical College. She completed postgraduate work at the Eye and Ear Clinic of New York University and at the New York Ophthalmalic and Aural Institute.

Gannt returned to South Carolina to become resident physician at Winthrop College in Rock Hill. She left this position in 1905 to marry Robert Joseph Gannt, a lawyer from Spartanburg, South Carolina. As Spartanburg's first female physician, she operated a private practice as an ear, eye, nose, and throat specialist. She was also director of Spartanburg Baby Hospital and held staff positions at Spartanburg General Hospital and at the Mary Blake Clinic.

Gannt's other medical activities reveal her concern for public health. She established and led the Spartanburg Health League and was active in the Spartanburg Anti-Tuberculosis Association and in the Public Health and Legislation Committees of the South Carolina Federation of Women's Clubs. In 1918, she established a state reform school for girls in Campobello, South Carolina, and was chair of that institution for 10 years. She also served for five years on the South Carolina Board of Public Welfare and ran a free clinic, paying a nurse with her own money. Gannt worked with the South Carolina Medical Association and the State's Federation of Women's Clubs to see the 1920 passage of legislation requiring physical examinations of school children. She also led campaigns to teach the public about the health dangers of houseflies, rats, and shared drinking cups.

The outbreak of World War I offered Gannt the opportunity to use her medical skills on a larger scale. She served as director of recreational activities for soldiers at Camp Wadsworth, served on the Spartanburg Selective Service Board, was acting surgeon for the U.S. Public Health Service, and was a medical examiner of pilots for the U.S. Department of Commerce. Additionally, she organized about 500 women to serve in medical and volunteer organizations on behalf of soldiers.

During the war, Gannt joined the Medical Women's Association (now the American Medical Women's Association). As president of the association (1931–1932), she persuaded the American Women's Hospitals (AWH) to expand its overseas public health efforts to include work in the United States. The AWH, an arm of the American Medical Women's Association (AMWA), was led by Dr. Esther Lovejoy and existed to provide medical relief in war-torn countries. The AWH began its stateside work in Spartanburg County and in nearby Polk County, North Carolina. This was the first public health service established in the southern Appalachians, then suffering from an outbreak of pellagra, a disease caused by malnutrition. Under Gannt's direction, the AWH provided information on immunization, nutrition, and prenatal care and established obstetrical and hospital facilities. Gannt relocated to Polk County in 1927, where she continued to direct public health operations and served on the staff of St. Luke's Hospital in Tryon, North Carolina. She also continued to maintain her Spartanburg practice.

In 1935, Gannt underwent an operation for cancer at the Woman's Medical College Hospital in Philadelphia. She died of an embolism on November 16 of the same year.

See also Lovejoy, Esther Pohl

Selected Additional Achievements

Secretary, Spartanburg Medical Society (1909–1918); twice read papers before the Southern Medical Association; board-certified, American Board of Ophthalmology; member, North and South Carolina Medical Societies; legislative chairman, South Carolina Equal Suffrage League (1914–1915). Her publications on the physical examination of schoolchildren appeared in the *Journal of the South Carolina Medical Association* (September 1911), in *Pediatrics* (June 1911), and in *Southern Medical Journal* (April 1913).

References

Biographical Sketch. Vertical file. Special Collections on Women in Medicine, Archives and Special Collections, MCP Hahnemann University, Philadelphia.

"Dr. Rosa L. Gannt." 1951. *Medical Woman's Journal* 58 (2):34–35.

Leland, Thomas M. 1987. "L. Rosa Gannt, M.D." *Journal of the South Carolina Medical Association* 83 (11):620.

Lemmon, Sarah McCulloh. 1971. "Gannt, Love Rosa Hirschmann." In *Notable American Women, 1607–1950: A Biographical Dictionary*, edited by E.T. James, J.W. James, and P.S. Boyer. Cambridge: Belknap Press of Harvard University Press.

Newsom, Elizabeth Young. 1999. "Gannt, Love Rosa Hirschmann." In *American National Biography*, edited by J.A. Garraty and M.C. Carnes. New York: Oxford University Press.

JSB

Gardner, Mary Sewall (1871–1961)
Nurse

Mary Gardner was a leader in the field of public health nursing in the first half of the twentieth century. She was born in Newton, Massachusetts, on February 5, 1871, the only child of Mary (Thornton) and William Sewall Gardner. Her early education was with a French governess as well as at private schools. Her desire to be of service to the community led her to the field of nursing, and in 1901, she enrolled at the Newport (Rhode Island) Hospital Training School for Nurses, graduating in 1905.

Gardner then became director of nurses of the Providence (Rhode Island) District Nursing Association (PDNA). In order to improve the PDNA, she visited similar associations, including Lillian Wald's Henry Street Visiting Nurse Service in New York City. Among Gardner's innovations with the PDNA were the establishment of a record-keeping system, the institution of regular meetings, and the introduction of uniforms. She was also a firm believer in continuing education and offered the PDNA nurses in-

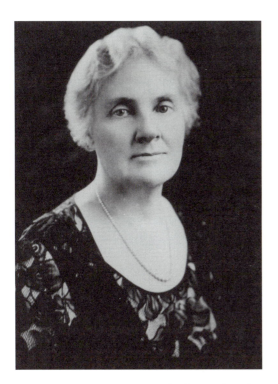

Mary Sewall Gardner. National Library of Medicine.

first textbook on the subject. The book was translated into several languages and was so popular that she issued new editions in 1924 and 1936.

During World War I, Gardner took a leave of absence from the PDNA to serve as director of the American Red Cross Town and Country Nursing Service (later, the Bureau of Public Health Nursing) but was soon sent to Italy to serve as director of the American Red Cross Tuberculosis Commission (1918–1919). In 1921, she traveled to Eastern Europe to study child welfare for the American Red Cross.

After retiring from the PDNA, Gardner wrote two fictional books on nursing, *So Build We* (1942) and *Katherine Kent* (1946). She died in Providence on February 20, 1961.

See also Wald, Lillian D.

Selected Additional Achievements

Honorary Master of Arts, Brown University (1918); Walter Burns Saunders Medal (1931); American Nurses Association Hall of Fame (1986).

References

Kantrov, Ilene, and Kate Wittenstein. 1980. "Gardner, Mary Sewall." In *Notable American Women: The Modern Period: A Biographical Dictionary*, edited by B. Sicherman and C.H. Green. Cambridge: Belknap Press of Harvard University Press.

Nelson, Sophie C. 1953, 1954. "Mary Sewall Gardner." *Nursing Outlook* 1, 2 (December, January):37–39, 668–670.

Reeves, Connie L. 1999. "Gardner, Mary Sewall." In *American National Biography*, edited by J.A. Garraty and M.C. Carnes. New York: Oxford University Press.

LS

service training programs. She remained with the PDNA until her retirement in 1931, when she was made honorary director.

In addition to her work in Rhode Island, Gardner served on the committee that created the National Organization of Public Health Nursing (NOPHN). She was named the first secretary of the NOPHN (1912–1913) and was then president of the organization (1913–1916). As president, she was instrumental in the growth of the NOPHN's journal, *Public Health Nurse* (later, *Public Health Nursing*). In 1916, she published a book, *Public Health Nursing*, which was the

Gaskin, Ina May (1940–   )
Midwife

Ina May Gaskin is often referred to as the mother of authentic midwifery. Her ideal of a woman-centered system of childbirth care is presented in her book *Spiritual Midwifery*,

now in its third edition. Born in Marshalltown, Iowa, on March 8, 1940, Gaskin began her journey into midwifery in 1970 while traveling across the United States on a lecture tour with her husband, Steven, a spiritual leader, and hundreds of his followers.

Their caravan of converted school buses had stopped in a parking lot at Northwestern University in Evanston, Illinois, and Steven was about to give a speech when one of the members went into labor. Because the cost of a hospital birth was beyond the caravan community's financial resources, Gaskin, with no midwifery training, volunteered to help with the birth. The ensuing labor lasted only three hours, and the outcome for both the infant and the mother was positive. The success of this event led the members of the caravan to turn to Gaskin for assistance with the several births that followed during their two-year cross-country campaign. Upon arrival at their final destination of Summertown in rural Tennessee, the caravan established an alternative community, the Farm, and Gaskin established the Farm Midwifery Center for the community's obstetrical needs.

Gaskin received an undergraduate education at the University of Iowa, where she graduated summa cum laude (1962). After an assignment as a secondary school English teacher in Kuala Trengganu, Malaysia (1963–1965), with the U.S. Peace Corps, she returned to the United States and obtained an M.A. in English from Northern Illinois University (1966). She then went on to become a teacher of English as a second language for the Office of Economic Opportunity in San Francisco.

After the birth of the first child on the caravan, Gaskin felt that she had "a definite calling to be a midwife," even though her formal education had not prepared her "for anything so real life as birth" (Gaskin, p. 22). She is a self-educated midwife and employs the principles that she learned from her husband: respecting life's force, truth, and holiness; managing spiritual energy; being compassionate; not being afraid; and helping people relax. She also draws upon her own five birth experiences, including the death of her prematurely born son. In addition, compassionate doctors have helped educate and train her. Dr. Louis La Pere visited the caravan when it passed through Rhode Island

and gave Gaskin and her assistants instruction on emergency childbirth. He also taught them sterile technique and gave them some necessary medications and Gaskin's first obstetrics textbook. Once settled in Tennessee, Gaskin found guidance from Dr. John O. William Jr., who attended the home births of the nearby Old Order Amish community. Williams so strongly believed in Gaskin's midwifery abilities that he entrusted her to provide the Amish with childbirth care in the late 1980s.

The validity of Gaskin's approach is documented in *The American Journal of Public Health* (Durand). A comparison of 1,707 births attended by Gaskin and her midwives on the Farm between 1971 and 1989 and the 1980 U.S. National Natality/National Fetal Mortality Survey reveals that Gaskin's midwifery techniques are not necessarily less safe than hospital, physician-assisted deliveries for relatively low-risk pregnancies. The study also shows that the percentage of assisted births (i.e., use of cesarean section, forceps, or vacuum extractor) on the Farm was 2.11 percent, while the national rate was 26.6 percent. Gaskin attributes this discrepancy to the compassionate prenatal and childbirth care provided to the mothers in her community.

Gaskin, the current president of Midwives' Alliance of North America, as well as the current editor of *The Birth Gazette*, continues to direct the Farm Midwifery Center. Gaskin is also involved in national health care reform with the goal of establishing the Farm Midwifery Center's woman-centered philosophy of childbirth care as the norm for national obstetrical care.

References

Chester, Penfield. 1997. *Sisters on a Journey: Portraits of American Midwives.* New Brunswick, N.J.: Rutgers University Press.

Durand, A.M. 1992. "The Safety of Home Birth: The Farm Study." *The American Journal of Public Health* 82:450–452.

Gaskin, Ina May. 1990. *Spiritual Midwifery.* 3rd ed. Summertown, Tenn.: Book Publishing.

Lorente, Carol Wiley. 1995. "Mother of Midwifery: Ina May Gaskin Hopes to Birth a Local Movement of Midwives." *Vegetarian Times* (July):194.

Trosky, Susan M., ed. 1990. *Contemporary Authors*. Vol. 129. Detroit: Gale Research.

CMB

Gault, Alma Elizabeth (1891–1981)
Nurse

Alma Gault was a nurse, educator, and administrator known primarily for her work at Meharry Medical College School of Nursing, a historically black institution in Nashville, Tennessee. She was born in Fernwood, Ohio, on September 28, 1891, to Davison Stewart and Nancy Emma (Stark) Gault. In 1910 she graduated from Wells High School in Steubenville, Ohio. She received a bachelor's degree in philosophy from the College of Wooster in Wooster, Ohio, in 1916.

Gault attended the Vassar Training Camp for Nurses in 1918 and continued her nursing education at Philadelphia General Hospital School of Nursing. After she graduated in 1920, she became a head nurse at Philadelphia General Hospital. She later held clinical nursing positions with the Ohio State Department of Health and Johns Hopkins Hospital in Baltimore. She held positions as a public health nursing educator at the Illinois Training School and at the Cook County School of Nursing in Chicago. She served as director of the Union Memorial Hospital School of Nursing in Baltimore and director of nursing service at Memorial Hospital in Springfield, Illinois.

From 1944 to 1953, Gault served as dean at Meharry. During her tenure there, she developed an accredited diploma school of nursing and a baccalaureate program. Meharry became the first historically black institution to hold membership in the American Association of Collegiate Schools of Nursing. Nationally, the school was rated in the top one-third of nursing schools. Gault was able to use her position as a white administrator of an African American school to become active in social causes, including desegregation, school lunch programs, and day-care centers.

In 1953, Gault accepted a position as an associate professor in the nursing school at Vanderbilt University in Nashville. She was also acting dean. Although she retired in 1959, she later served as dean of the school from 1965 to 1967. During this time, the first black nursing student enrolled at Vanderbilt. When she retired as dean in 1967, the mayor of Nashville proclaimed May 21 of that year as Alma Gault Day. The North Central Tennessee League for Nursing organized this honor. She continued public service after her retirement, working to establish a multiphasic screening program as a member of the Senior Citizens, Inc. of Nashville.

Gault died on July 12, 1981, in Columbus, Ohio.

Selected Additional Achievements

Several articles, primarily on nursing education. American Nurses Association Hall of Fame (1984). Member, American Nurses Association, National League for Nursing, Tennessee Board of Nursing, Tennessee Council on Aging, American Association of University Women.

References

American Nurses Association. *The Hall of Fame Inductees: Alma Elizabeth Gault*. Online. http://www.ana.org/hof/gaulae.htm. 30 June 2000.

Baldwin, Patricia E. 1988. "Alma Elizabeth Gault." In *American Nursing: A Biographical Dictionary*, edited by V.L. Bullough, O.M. Church, and A.P. Stein. New York: Garland.

Donaldson, Mary Louise. 1985. *A History of the Vanderbilt University School of Nursing 1909–1984*. Nashville, Tenn.: Vanderbilt University.

DTW

Geister, Janet Marie Louise Sophie (1885–1964)
Nurse

Janet Geister was a researcher and writer who held several key leadership positions in professional nursing organizations. She was one of the few nursing leaders to champion the cause of private-duty nurses, the most populous group of nurses until World War II. She was born on June 17, 1885, in Elgin, Illinois, the fifth child of Jacob Christian Henry and Sophie (Witte) Geister. As a child, Geister suffered from diphtheria and other illnesses that would trouble her throughout life. She graduated from high school in 1902 and was conflicted as to whether she wanted to be a physician, journalist, or nurse.

Geister pursued a writing career in Chicago for a short time but eventually entered Elgin's Sherman Hospital School of Nursing. After graduating in 1910, she worked as a private-duty nurse before entering the Chicago School of Civics and Philanthropy summer program in 1912. On the strength of her performance, she was conditionally accepted to the school's regular program and lived at Hull House, a settlement house in Chicago. She earned a certificate in social work from the program in June 1914.

Geister remained in Chicago and was a social service worker for Cook County Hospital and then an instructor of nurses, assistant to the superintendent, and emergency supervisor of the Chicago Visiting Nurses Association. In 1917, Julia Lathrop, chief of the federal Children's Bureau, hired her to investigate the high rate of infant mortality in northern Montana. In 1918, Geister began writing for public health journals on methods of supervision and education of public health nurses and worked on the "Save 100,000 Babies" campaign. The same year, she helped design a mobile health care unit to be used in rural areas, which was extremely popular and revealed the health needs of rural children.

In October 1919, Geister became field secretary for the National Organization for Public Health Nursing (NOPHN). She was also involved in the Winslow-Goldmark study of nursing education and a hospital survey in Cleveland, Ohio. In 1921, a diagnosis of uterine cancer and subsequent radium treatment interrupted her career. After recovering, Geister applied for the position of educational secretary of the NOPHN but was rejected because she lacked a college degree in nursing.

From 1923 to 1927, Geister was executive secretary of the Foundation Committee on Dispensary Development, a major study of New York City dispensaries. During this time, she also conducted an independent survey of 1,400 private-duty nurses in two districts of the New York State Nurses' Association. Private-duty nurses were independent practitioners and accounted for 70 percent of the American Nurses Association (ANA) membership in 1926. At the 1926 ANA convention, Geister presented a paper based on her research that helped nursing leaders and the public better understand the role of the private-duty nurse. Her research was published in the *American Journal of Nursing* and showed that the income of the private-duty nurse was "about even with that of charwomen, servants, and unskilled labor" (Geister, 1926, p. 519). As a result of her study, Geister became the champion of rank-and-file nurses, leading ANA president Lillian Clayton to offer her the position of director at ANA headquarters in August 1926.

Geister's goals as director were to bolster ANA public relations with the newly forming state associations and to deal with the private-duty nursing problem. She believed that the creation of a central registry and independent group practices to provide community nursing services, as well as ANA sponsorship of continuing education, would save private-duty nursing. Her beliefs conflicted with those of ANA leaders, however, who were more concerned with improving professional status by raising educational standards than dealing with existing nurses. On January 30, 1933, she was asked to resign and did so, effective March 31.

In June 1933, Geister became an associate

editor and, later, editor (1941) of *Trained Nurse and Hospital Review*, to which she contributed a column, "Plain Talk." She resigned in 1946 due to ill health but the next year began writing "Candid Comments" for the journal *RN*, which she continued until October 1956. Despite poor health Geister continued to write, make speeches, and participate in professional nursing organizations until her death on December 8, 1964, in Evanston, Illinois.

See also Clayton, S. Lillian

Selected Additional Achievements

More than 300 professional articles, including a 1948 article, "The Hospital and the Nurse," *Modern Hospital* 71 (August):59–61, which won her that publication's Gold Medal in 1949. Life membership, Illinois League of Nursing; honorary member, Student Nurse Association of Illinois; American Nurses Association Hall of Fame (1984).

References

Deforge, Virginia M. 1986. "Janet Marie Louise Sophie Geister, 1885–1964: Health Care Revolutionary." Doctoral diss., Boston University.

Geister, Janet M. 1926. "Hearsay and Facts in Private Duty." *American Journal of Nursing* 26 (July):515–528.

Geister, Janet M. 1964. "This I Believe about My Half-Century in Nursing." *Nursing Outlook* 12 (March):58–61.

LS

Gleason, Rachel Brooks (1820–1905)
Physician

Rachel Brooks Gleason was the fourth woman in the United States to earn a medical degree. She was born in Winhall, Vermont, on November 27, 1820, and was educated in local schools, including Townsend Academy. She was a teacher until 1844, when she married Silas O. Gleason, a graduate of Castleton Medical College; the couple had two children.

In 1847, the Gleasons briefly owned Greenwood Springs, a water cure facility in New York. Water cure practitioners believed that internal and external applications of water, along with fresh air, proper nutrition, and exercise, cured and prevented disease. Later that year, they established, in partnership with two others, the Glen Haven Water Cure near Scott, New York. Gleason was in charge of the female patients, work that inspired her to formally study medicine.

Gleason attended Central Medical College in Syracuse, New York, a sectarian medical school that was the first in the United States to adopt a policy of admitting women. She entered the college for its first session on November 5, 1849. Among her classmates were Lydia Folger Fowler and Sarah Adamson Dolley, the second and third American women to earn medical degrees, after Elizabeth Blackwell. In January 1850, the college moved to Rochester, New York. Gleason, who was also on the college's teaching staff, graduated on February 20, 1851.

Following her graduation, the Gleasons worked for a short time at the Forest City Water Cure near Ithaca, New York. In 1852, they established the Elmira Water Cure in Elmira, New York. An 1882 circular describes its services: "Hot and Cold water Baths, Electricity, Swedish Movements, the Health Lift and Light Gymnastics. . . . The Cure is furnished with Turkish and Russian Baths, which are used with great success in many cases. . . . Ladies are under the care of Dr. Rachel B. Gleason." From 1893 to 1903, the establishment was known as the Gleason Sanitarium and after 1904 as the Gleason Health Resort.

The popularity of Gleason's "parlor talks" to women on physiology and hygiene inspired her to write *Talks to My Patients, Hints on Getting Well and Keeping Well* (1870). The book was designed as a home medical reference "to guide in those matters of delicacy with which women's life is so replete" (p. vi). In most of her published work, she stressed that inactivity, improper nutrition, and the organ-compressing fashions of the day were the cause of "women's rapid physical deterioration" (1853, p. 7). In one of her many essays on the topic of dress reform, she wrote, "Every woman who has a waist to correspond with the fashion plates, usually has her interior organs in such a shocking and disgusting situation . . . [as to] . . . interrupt their healthful functions" (1856, pp. 3–4).

Gleason used her position as a successful and well-known female physician to help other women enter the profession. Her sister, Zippie Brooks Wales, an 1873 graduate of Woman's Medical College of Pennsylvania, and Frances Rutherford received clinical experience at the Water Cure. Gleason's daughter, Adele, earned a medical degree from the University of Michigan in 1875 and worked with her mother at the Elmira Water Cure. The value of this opportunity for clinical experience was especially important since very few hospitals and clinics would admit women for study. She also financed the medical education of several women students.

Gleason wrote many articles for the *Water-Cure Journal*, the *Herald of Health*, and the *Syracuse Medical and Surgical Journal*. She died in her daughter's home in Buffalo, New York, on March 17, 1905.

See also Blackwell, Elizabeth; Dolley, Sarah Read Adamson; Fowler, Lydia Folger; Rutherford, Frances Armstrong

References

Circular of the Elmira Water Cure. April 1, 1882. [Elmira, N.Y.]: N.p.

Donegan, Jane B. 1999. "Gleason, Rachel Brooks." In *American National Biography*, edited by J.A. Garraty and M.C. Carnes. New York: Oxford University Press.

Gleason, Rachel Brooks. 1853. "Hints to Women." *Water-Cure Journal* 15 (1):7–8.

Gleason, Rachel Brooks. 1856. "Communication from Mrs. Dr. R.B. Gleason." In *Letters to the People on Health and Happiness*, edited by C.E. Beecher. New York: Harper and Brothers.

Gleason, Rachel Brooks. 1870. *Talks to My Patients, Hints on Getting Well and Keeping Well*. New York: Wood and Holbrook.

Waite, Frederick C. 1932. "Dr. Lydia Folger Fowler: The Second Woman to Receive the Degree of Doctor of Medicine in the United States." *Annals of Medical History* 4 (new series) (3):290–297.

JSB

Goggans, Lalla Mary (1906–1987)
Nurse-midwife

Lalla Goggans was a public health nurse and nurse-midwife in Florida and New York, as well as an administrator for the U.S. Children's Bureau. She was born on February 24, 1906, in Live Oak, Florida, the daughter of Joseph and Juanita (Gardner) Goggans. Her early education was at an Episcopal girls' school in Orlando, Florida. She became interested in nursing when her father was ill. She trained at Orange General Hospital's nursing school in Orlando. An affiliation at two Chicago maternity hospitals stimulated her interest in maternal and child health.

After graduating in 1927, Goggans received a scholarship from the Florida Federation of Women's Clubs for a year's study in public health nursing at William and Mary College in Virginia. A condition of the scholarship was that she return to Florida to work for the state's Department of Health for two years. Thus, after earning her certificate in public health nursing in 1929, she became a staff public health nurse in Marianna, Florida. Her job was to assist other nurses who were implementing the Sheppard-Towner Act of 1921, legislation that funded maternity, infant, and child hygiene programs. Goggans worked with, and taught classes for, African American lay midwives in the area. She also conducted a survey of the midwives and disabled children in her 10-county area.

Goggans helped sponsor an Institute for

Lay Midwives in 1933 at Florida A&M College in Tallahassee. More than 200 midwives attended the institute, where they completed courses on preparing the midwifery bag, conduct and care during delivery, and prenatal and infant care. Goggans was made district supervisor of nurses for the Florida Board of Health in 1934 and was then the board's statewide consultant on maternal and child health (1939–1942).

In 1942, Goggans took an educational leave of absence to study at Columbia University's Teachers College in New York, where she earned a B.S. in nursing education. She also earned a certificate in nurse-midwifery from the New York Maternity Center Association (MCA) that year. When she finished the course, she became an instructor and staff member at the MCA. In 1944, she was appointed by the federal Children's Bureau to supervise an emergency program to serve mothers and infants in the southwest region of the United States. She also helped to form the Catholic Maternity Institute at Santa Fe, New Mexico, during this time.

In 1949, Goggans earned a master's degree from Teachers College and was made nursing consultant for the Children's Bureau, Region III, headquartered in Charlottesville, Virginia. In addition to her work in the United States, Goggans supported the growth of nurse-midwifery in Puerto Rico, where she established a school of maternity nursing and nurse-midwifery in 1966. She retired from the Children's Bureau in 1972. She died on July 30, 1987, in Augusta, Georgia.

Selected Additional Achievements

Lecturer, School of Nursing, University of Virginia. Fellow, American Public Health Association. Member, American Association for Maternal and Infant Health, American College of Nurse-Midwifery, American Nurses Association, International Confederation Midwives, National League for Nursing.

References

Goggans, Lalla Mary. 1934. "Florida's First Institute for Midwives." *Public Health Nursing* (March):133–136.

"Miss Lalla Goggans." 1987. *The Augusta Chronicle* (August 1):14A.

Tom, Sally Austen. 1978. "With Loving Hands: The Life Stories of Four Nurse-Midwives." Master's thesis, University of Utah.

Who's Who of American Women with World Notables. 1969. 6th ed. Chicago: A.N. Marquis.

                                    LS

Goldman, Emma (1869–1940)
Nurse, Midwife

Emma Goldman is best known as a radical anarchist, but she was also an early advocate of birth control, a nurse, and a midwife. Goldman was born on June 27, 1869, in Kovno, Lithuania, the first of three children of Abraham and Taube (Bienowitch) Goldman. Her early education was at a *Realschule* in Königsberg, Prussia, and at a high school in St. Petersburg, Russia. In order to escape an arranged marriage, Goldman emigrated to the United States with her sister in 1885, and they settled in Rochester, New York.

Goldman found a job in a clothing factory but quickly became disillusioned by the exploitation of workers there and in other factories. The trial, conviction, and ultimate execution of prominent anarchists involved in the Haymarket Square riot in Chicago (1886–1887) made her further dissatisfied with democracy and capitalism and turned her toward the philosophy of anarchism, the belief that the hierarchical, political state should be replaced by a decentralized society rooted in cooperation. In 1887, Goldman married a fellow factory worker, Jacob Kersner, but divorced him after only two years. She moved to New York City in 1889 and became involved with members of the anarchist movement, including Alexander Berkman, with whom she had a lifelong love affair. She began giving public lectures on anarchism, and in 1893, after telling a crowd of unemployed men that they had a right to steal bread, she was sentenced to a year in prison on Blackwell's Island, New York.

Goldman was assigned to work in the prison hospital and learned practical nursing skills there. After her release from prison, she worked as a nurse and then studied nursing and midwifery at the Allgemeines Krankenhaus in Vienna, Austria (1895–1896). She earned diplomas in both fields and then returned to New York City. Her experience as a nurse and midwife put her in close contact with the very people whom she strove to help through her radical efforts. She was especially troubled by the plight of women who endured one unwanted pregnancy after another; however, she had no knowledge of effective methods of birth control to share with them. The Comstock Act of 1873 severely hindered efforts to distribute information on birth control, as it defined such information as obscene. Even when she asked physicians for help in advising her patients, none could, legally, help her.

Meanwhile, Goldman was becoming a well-known lecturer as she traveled across the country speaking on anarchism, women's equality, free speech, and labor rights. During a trip to Paris in 1900, she attended a secret conference and acquired information on methods of contraception. When she returned to New York, she resumed her work as a nurse and also continued her lectures, adding to them the subject of birth control. Fearing arrest, she gave specific information on methods of preventing conception only when privately asked. After Margaret Sanger's 1914 arrest for the publication of information about birth control, however, Goldman decided that she must also speak out on the issue. She began giving frank lectures on methods of birth control and was arrested for one such speech in February 1916. Rather than pay the $100 fine, Goldman chose to publicize the cause by spending 15 days in jail.

In 1919, after serving two years in prison for opposing the World War I draft, she was deported to Russia. In 1925, she married a British national to obtain citizenship. She supported herself through lectures and from royalties on her autobiography, *Living My Life* (originally published in 1931). She suffered a stroke while in Toronto and died there on May 14, 1940.

See also Sanger, Margaret Louise Higgins

Selected Additional Achievements

Editor, with Berkman, of the anarchist periodical *Mother Earth* (1906–1917). *Anarchism and Other Essays* (1911); *Marriage and Love* (1914); *The Social Significance of the Modern Drama* (1914); *My Disillusionment in Russia* (1923).

References

Drinnon, Richard. 1971. "Goldman, Emma." In *Notable American Women, 1607–1950: A Biographical Dictionary*, edited by E.T. James, J.W. James, and P.S. Boyer. Cambridge: Belknap Press of Harvard University Press.
Goldman, Emma. 1934. *Living My Life*. One volume ed. New York: Alfred A. Knopf.
Wexler, Alice. 1999. "Goldman, Emma." In *American National Biography*, edited by J.A. Garraty and M.C. Carnes. New York: Oxford University Press.

LS

Goodrich, Annie Warburton (1866–1954)
Nurse

Annie Goodrich was a leader in the reform of nursing education. She was born on February 6, 1866, in New Brunswick, New Jersey, the second of seven children of Samuel Griswold Goodrich, an insurance executive, and Annie Williams Butler Goodrich. She was educated by a governess and attended private schools in Connecticut, England, and

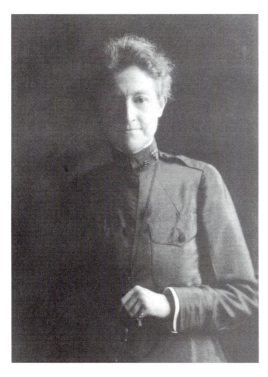

Annie Warburton Goodrich. National Library of Medicine.

France. Her grandfather, pioneering psychiatrist Dr. John Butler, fell ill in the late 1880s and was cared for by a poorly trained nurse, stimulating Goodrich's interest in nursing. At the same time, her family suffered financial reverses, and she felt it necessary to be self-supporting.

Consequently, Goodrich entered New York Hospital's Training School for Nurses in the fall of 1890. At the time, hospital apprenticeship was the standard method of training nurses; student nurses were overworked, underpaid, inadequately trained, and subject to strict discipline. An incident during her school years demonstrates Goodrich's early resolve to improve nursing education. One day during her rotation at Sloane Hospital's maternity ward, she found herself trying to perform the duties of attending all deliveries and feeding, bathing, weighing, and changing all babies, while also caring for all mothers. Because she was not at dinner as scheduled, a doctor demanded that she immediately go. That night, an angry, but determined, Goodrich carried out a time study that proved that 17 hours were actually required to do the tasks expected of nurses in 11 hours.

After she graduated in 1892, Goodrich became head nurse of New York Hospital's men's surgical ward. She then held a succession of jobs as superintendent of nursing at New York Post-Graduate Hospital (1893–1900), St. Luke's Hospital (1900–1902), New York Hospital (1902–1907), and Bellevue and Allied Hospitals (1907–1910), all in New York City. At New York Post-Graduate, she held weekly "class nights" for her students, who otherwise had very little classroom instruction, and in all these positions, she campaigned for better-qualified students, reorganized nursing curricula, and demanded better working conditions for the nurses whom she trained and supervised. She was said to be a born teacher; students spoke fondly of her ability to inspire them. About this ability, Goodrich said, "If you believe a thing deeply enough yourself, you can always get others to believe. And when people believe, they are able to think and to see" (quoted in Werminghaus, p. 17).

In addition to her other responsibilities, Goodrich taught hospital economics part-time at Columbia University's Teachers College (1904–1913) and was inspector of nurse training schools for the state of New York (1910–1914). In 1914, she accepted a full-time position as assistant professor of nursing and health at Columbia, teaching the administration of nursing schools. In 1917, while still working full-time at Columbia, she accepted Lillian Wald's call to become director of nurses at the Henry Street Visiting Nurse Service. Henry Street was founded by Wald to provide health care for the poor of New York City.

In her book *The Social and Ethical Significance of Nursing* (1932), Goodrich described her philosophy of nursing and social responsibility. She had a strong sense of community welfare and believed in using knowledge to produce a better world. She believed that no job had greater social significance than nursing. To her, the importance of the profession to society meant that nurses needed a liberal education as well as thorough professional preparation. She also believed that nursing should be taught at the university level and that nurses should be licensed.

At the outbreak of World War I, the U.S. government called upon Goodrich to serve as chief inspector of army hospitals. She thought that the best way to meet the demand for nurses was to establish an army nursing school. Opposing her was Jane Delano of the American Red Cross, who was convinced that the urgency of the war required the use of trained aides. The nursing profession and the War Department sided with Goodrich, and she was appointed dean (1918–1919) of the Army School of Nursing.

Following her term as dean of the army's school, Goodrich returned to her position at Henry Street in 1919. The year before, the Rockefeller Foundation had formed a committee to study nursing and nurse education in the United States. In 1923, the committee's summary, the Winslow-Goldmark report (published as *Nursing and Nursing Education in the United States*), led to the establishment of an experimental university school of nursing. Goodrich was selected as dean and professor (1923–1934) of the school chosen to host the experiment, Yale University. As dean of the School of Nursing, she was the first woman dean in the history of Yale University. Innovations brought about by Goodrich included requiring candidates for admission to have a high school education and, later, two years of college. Under her direction, Yale became the first school in the country to grant a bachelor's degree in nursing.

In 1934, Goodrich retired to a farmhouse in Colchester, Connecticut, but she continued to be an active member of the nursing community by giving speeches, serving on committees, and advising medical institutions. She died of a stroke on December 31, 1954, in Cobalt, Connecticut.

See also Delano, Jane Arminda; Wald, Lillian D.

Selected Additional Achievements

Distinguished Service Medal (1923); National Institute of Social Science Medal (1920); Médaille d'Honneur d'Hygène Publique, France (1928); Walter Burns Saunders Medal (1932); Bronze Medal, Belgium (1933); Medal of the Ministry of Social Welfare, France (1933); Mary Adelaide Nutting Award (1948); Yale Medal (1953); American Nurses Association Hall of Fame (1976). President, American Federation of Nurses (1909), International Council of Nurses (1912–1915), American Nurses Association (1915–1918), and Association of Collegiate Schools of Nursing (1933); vice president, Florence Nightingale International Foundation (1934). Honorary degrees from Mount Holyoke College (doctor of science, 1921), Yale University (master of arts, 1923), and Russell Sage University (doctor of laws, 1936).

References

Goodrich, Annie Warburton. 1932. *The Social and Ethical Significance of Nursing.* New York: Macmillan.

Gurney, Cindy. 1988. "Annie Warburton Goodrich." In *American Nursing: A Biographical Dictionary*, edited by V.L. Bullough, O.M. Church, and A.P. Stein. New York: Garland.

Henderson, Virginia. 1955. "Annie Warburton Goodrich." *The American Journal of Nursing* 55:1488–1492.

Koch, Harriett Berger. 1951. *Militant Angel.* New York: Macmillan.

Tomes, Nancy. 1980. "Goodrich, Annie Warburton." In *Notable American Women: The Modern Period: A Biographical Dictionary*, edited by B. Sicherman and C.H. Green. Cambridge: Belknap Press of Harvard University Press.

Werminghaus, Esther A. 1950. *Annie W. Goodrich: Her Journey to Yale.* New York: Macmillan.

LS

Greene, Cordelia Agnes (1831–1905)
Physician

Cordelia Greene was one of the first women to graduate from medical school in the United States. She was born on July 5, 1831, in Lyons, New York, the first of five children of Jabez and Phila (Cooke) Greene. In 1849, the family moved to Castile, New York, where Jabez Greene established a sanitarium, the Water-Cure. Based on the belief that water was the natural sustainer of life, water cure, or hydropathy, was a popular alternative to regular medical practice of the time. While assisting her father at the sanitarium, Greene read about Elizabeth Blackwell's graduation from medical school and decided to attend medical school herself. Greene earned the money for her medical school expenses by working as a nurse in several water cure facilities.

From 1854 to 1855, she attended Female (later, Woman's) Medical College of Pennsylvania in Philadelphia. For the 1855–1856 term, she transferred to Western Reserve University in Cleveland, where Greene and Marie Zakrzewska were two of four women in the class. After graduating in 1856, Greene was her father's chief assistant at the Water-Cure. She then returned to Female Medical for postgraduate study during the 1857–1858 school year. In 1859, she began practicing with Dr. Henry Foster at Clifton Springs Sanitarium in New York and remained there until 1865.

When her father died, Greene returned to Castile and took over management of the Water-Cure, renaming it the Castile Sanitarium. She was director of the institution until her death. Although Greene began in March 1865 with one patient, the Castile Sanitarium eventually became the place where many prominent women went to restore themselves mentally, physically, and spiritually. Greene's approach to medical care at the sanitarium was a combination of conventional medical care, spiritual guidance, and alternative methods, such as hydropathy. Greene often said that "health, like character, must be developed from within, not rubbed on from without" (quoted in Gordon, p. 25). She was a firm believer in proper diet, deep breathing of fresh air, and exercise. She also deplored alcohol and helped her alcoholic patients at the sanitarium overcome their addictions.

Greene never married, but she did adopt six children, one of whom, Edward Greene, also became a physician. Greene died as a result of complications from surgery on January 28, 1905, in New York City. After her death, Greene's niece, Dr. Mary T. Greene, took over management of the sanitarium; it remained open until 1954.

See also Blackwell, Elizabeth; Zakrzewska, Marie Elizabeth

Selected Additional Achievements

Greene's publications include *Build Well: The Basis of Individual, Home, and National Elevation: Plain Truths Relating to the Obligations of Marriage and Parentage* (1885) and *The Art of Keeping Well; or Common Sense Hygiene for Adults and Children* (published posthumously in 1906). Member, American Medical Association, New York State Medical Association, Wyoming County Medical Society, and Physician's League of Buffalo.

References

"Dr. Mary T. Greene Sanitarium 100 Year Celebration." 1949. *Medical Woman's Journal* 56 (6):21–25.

Female Medical College of Pennsylvania. 1857. *Eighth Annual Announcement of the Female Medical College of Pennsylvania.* Philadelphia: Deacon and Peterson, Printers.

Goldstein, Linda Lehmann. 1997. "Cordelia Agnes Greene." In *Doctors, Nurses, and Medical Practitioners: A Bio-Bibliographical Sourcebook*, edited by L. Magner. Westport, Conn.: Greenwood Press.

Gordon, Elizabeth Putnam. 1925. *The Story of the Life and Work of Cordelia A. Greene M.D.* Castile, N.Y.: Castilian.

"Obituary, Cordelia Agnes Greene, M.D." 1905. *Woman's Medical Journal* 15 (4):80–81.

LS

Guion, Connie Myers (1882–1971)
Physician

Connie Guion was the first female professor of clinical medicine in the United States. She was born on August 9, 1882, in Lincolnton, North Carolina, the 9th of 12 children of Benjamin Simmons and Catherine Coatesworth Caldwell Guion. She received her early education at home and in grade school in Charlotte, North Carolina. She attended Miss Kate Shipp's School in Lincolnton (1898–1900) and Northfield Seminary in Massachusetts.

After graduating from Wellesley College in Massachusetts in 1906, Guion was instructor of chemistry at Vassar College in Poughkeepsie, New York. She was then chemistry professor (1908–1910) and professor and head of the department of chemistry (1910–1913) at Sweet Briar College in Virginia. Concurrently, she studied biochemistry at Cornell University in New York. After earning an M.A. in 1913, she matriculated at Cornell's school of medicine. During her third year, she completed obstetrical requirements at New York Infirmary for Women and Children, founded by Dr. Elizabeth Blackwell in 1857.

Guion earned a medical degree in 1917 and then completed an internship at Bellevue Hospital in New York (1917–1920). At Bellevue, Guion was required to complete 24-hour ambulance shifts, sleeping only between emergency calls. When she rebelled against this practice, she was told that such shifts were a 100-year tradition. Her reply, that "the century's up!" led to the implementation of 12-hour shifts (Campion, p. 278). Over the course of her internship, Guion was promoted from intern to house physician and was responsible for teaching fourth-year medical students.

In 1919, Guion began teaching at Cornell University Medical School, where in 1922, she organized the Cornell Pay Clinic. The purpose of the Pay Clinic was twofold: to peak doctors' interest in clinical medicine and to provide fixed-fee treatment for working-class patients. She established a policy committing doctors to spend one hour with a patient for a first visit, 45 minutes for an annual visit, 30 minutes for a six-month revisit, and 15 minutes for a follow-up revisit. She taught physical diagnosis and general medicine at the clinic until 1929, when she was promoted to chief. After Cornell Medical School joined New York Hospital in 1932, she served as chief of the General Medical Clinic, New York Hospital-Cornell Medical Center.

Concurrently, Guion served as Cornell's assistant professor (1929–1936), then associate professor of clinical medicine (1936–1946). As professor of clinical medicine (1946–1951), she was the first female professor of clinical medicine in the country. At New York Hospital, she was assistant attending physician (1932–1942), associate attending physician (1942–1943), attending physician (1943–1949), and later, consulting physician. Her pioneering clinical work was honored by the hospital with the dedication of its new outpatient building, the Doctor Connie Guion Building, in May 1963.

Guion's other positions included assistant attending physician at New York Infirmary for Women and Children and attending physician at Booth Memorial Hospital (1920–1926). She then served as attending physician and director of the medical department of New York Infirmary (1926–1929) and afterward as consulting physician at the infirmary and at Booth (1926–1950). From 1926, she also maintained a private practice with her niece, Dr. Parks McComb.

Guion died on April 29, 1971.

See also Blackwell, Elizabeth

Selected Additional Achievements

First woman member (1946) and first female honorary member (1950), Medical Board, New York Hospital; first woman recipient, annual award of distinction, Cornell University Medical College Alumni Association (1951). Honorary doctor of science degrees from Wellesley College (1950), Woman's Medical College of Pennsylvania (1953), and Queen's College, Charlotte, North Carolina (1957). Elizabeth Blackwell Citation, New York Infirmary (1949); Medical Woman of the Year,

American Medical Women's Association (1954). Member, New York Academy of Medicine, New York State Medical Association, Women's Medical Association of New York City, County Medical Society, Cornell University Medical Council, Cornell Medical College Alumni Association (president 1946–1947). A scholarship in her name was established at Wellesley College.

References

Campion, Nardi Reeder, and Rosamond Wiffley Stanton. 1965. *Look to This Day! The Lively Education of a Great Woman Doctor, Connie Guion, M.D.* Boston: Little, Brown.

Gregory, Evelyn. 1992. "Works of Connie Guion, M.D." Unpublished paper written by a Sweet Briar College alumna at New York University.

"Guion, Connie Myers." Vertical file. Special Collections on Women in Medicine, Archives and Special Collections, MCP Hahnemann University, Philadelphia.

Moritz, C., ed. 1963. *Current Biography Yearbook 1962.* New York: H.W. Wilson.

JSB

Gullen, Augusta Stowe (1857–1943)
Physician

Augusta Stowe Gullen was the first woman physician to graduate from a Canadian university. She was the daughter of Emily Stowe, the first Canadian woman to practice medicine in Canada. Gullen was born on July 27, 1857, at Mount Pleasant, Ontario, the eldest of John and Emily (Jennings) Stowe's three children.

As Gullen was growing up, she was witness to Emily's frustration and anger as she attempted to become a licensed physician in Canada. Watching her mother practice medicine in an era where modesty prevented many women from seeking a physician's help, Gullen realized the great need for female doctors to serve women patients. Gullen therefore chose to follow her mother's path and become a physician.

In 1879, only two schools in Canada, Queen's College at Kingston and Victoria College in Coburg, both in the province of Ontario, were accepting women students. Since the medical course at Queen's met only in the summer and was for women only, Gullen's mother believed that a medical degree from Queen's would not be respected. Her mother therefore encouraged Gullen to apply to the coeducational Victoria College, where medical students took their classes at the more prestigious Toronto Faculty of Medicine. Gullen was accepted at Victoria and found herself to be the only woman in her class. Like her mother, she was subjected to rude behavior and pranks from the male students. After publicly intimidating a man who was the instigator of one particular disturbance, however, the abuse became less frequent.

In 1883, Gullen completed her training and married John Benjamin Gullen, a graduate of Trinity Medical College. Forgoing a typical honeymoon, the couple traveled to New York to take a postgraduate course in children's disease. Upon her return, Gullen was appointed demonstrator of anatomy at the newly formed Woman's Medical College in Toronto, with the distinction of being the only woman on the staff. Seven years later (1900), she became professor of pediatrics, a position that she held until 1906, when the college was absorbed by the University of Toronto. With the amalgamation of the colleges in 1906, the University of Toronto began to accept women medical students.

While teaching at the college, Gullen also ran a medical practice out of her home in Toronto. Additionally, she was actively involved in Western Hospital, which her husband had cofounded in Toronto. In 1896, she delivered the first child born at the new hospital. Recognizing a lack of linens and equipment at Western, she organized the doctors' wives to form the Women's Board of Western Hospital. The board provided the hospital with the much needed supplies. In 1910, Gullen was appointed the medical professional representative to the University of Toronto Senate.

In addition to practicing medicine, Gullen was active in the Canadian suffragist movement. In 1896, she, her mother, and the Dominion Women's Enfranchisement Association staged a mock parliament to raise public awareness of the cause of women's rights. Like her mother, Gullen served as president of the Dominion Women's Enfranchisement Association (1903–1907) and then its successor organization, the Canadian Suffrage Association (1907–1911).

Gullen died on September 25, 1943, in Toronto.

See also Stowe, Emily Jennings

Selected Additional Achievements

Founding member, National Council of Women (1893); chairwoman, National Council of Women's Standing Committee on Suffrage and Rights of Citizenship (1904–1921); Toronto School Board; Ontario Social Service Council; University Women's Club; Order of the British Empire (1935).

References

Hacker, Carlotta. 1974. *The Indomitable Lady Doctors.* Toronto: Clarke, Irwin.

Morgan, Henry J., ed. 1912. *The Canadian Men and Women of the Time: A Handbook of Canadian Biography of Living Characters.* 2nd ed. Toronto: W. Briggs.

National Library of Canada. *Women's Exhibition—Emily Jennings Stowe and Augusta Stowe Gullen.* Online. http://www.nlc-bnc.ca/digiproj/women/ewomen1f.htm. 15 December 1997.

Ray, Janet. 1978. *Emily Stowe.* Don Mills, Ont.: Fitzhenry and Whiteside.

CMB

Gunn, Jean Isabel (1882–1941)
Nurse

Jean Gunn was superintendent of nurses at Toronto General Hospital in Canada for more than 25 years and a leader in nursing in that country. She was born on February 11, 1882, in Belleville, Ontario, the fifth of eight surviving children of Donald and Ellen (Coons) Gunn. Because her father disapproved of her plans to become a nurse, she enrolled at Albert College in Belleville and studied to be a teacher. While a student there, a doctor encouraged her interest in nursing after she helped him treat a woman with a scalp wound. Gunn graduated second in her class around 1901.

In 1902, Gunn was accepted at the nurse training school of Presbyterian Hospital in New York City. After graduating in 1905, she remained in the United States for the next eight years, working at Presbyterian Hospital, at Morristown Hospital in New Jersey, and in a social service capacity for the city of New York. In September 1913, she accepted a position as the superintendent of nurses at Toronto General Hospital, a job that she would hold until her death. As su-perintendent, she was responsible for managing the nursing service of the hospital as well as running the nursing school.

Soon after she started, World War I erupted, and Gunn offered to coordinate the recruitment of trained nurses for Canada's war effort. The Dominion government accepted her offer; however, when she compiled a list of available nurses, the government ignored her recommendation. She was able to work with the Canadian Red Cross by supplying bandages and arranging for the sterilization and inspection of Red Cross supplies at Toronto General Hospital. She created instructions that volunteers could understand on how to make surgical dressings, and, because cotton was increasingly in short supply, she aided in the construction of sphagnum moss dressings. After the war, she chaired a committee to memorialize the 47 Canadian nurses killed. The monument was unveiled in August 1926 at the Parliament Buildings in Ottawa.

When Gunn began at Toronto General Hospital, more than 70 percent of the nursing staff was students, and most nurse training was on-the-job. She realized that nurse education must change, and among her innovations were arranging for students to hear lectures by the University of Toronto Social Services Department, expanding the curriculum to include such classes as chemistry, anatomy, and bacteriology, offering field experience with the city health department, and offering centralized lectures. Gunn also created a student government in the nursing school and provided in-service education for staff nurses. In 1926, the hospital and the University of Toronto collaborated on offering a four-year diploma to students.

As an officer and member in various national nursing organizations, Gunn was involved in at least 60 major nursing issues in her lifetime. Among these were helping to restructure the organizations, ensuring sufficient numbers of nurses in the workforce, raising education standards, developing national health policy, and fighting for the registration of nurses.

Gunn died of cancer on June 28, 1941, at Toronto General Hospital.

See also Snively, Mary Agnes

Selected Additional Achievements

Numerous articles in the *Canadian Nurse* and other nursing publications. Member (1914–1924), secretary (1914–1917), president (1917–1920), Canadian National Association of Trained Nurses; Canadian Society of Superintendents of Training Schools (1915–1917); Canadian Nurses Association (1924–1941); International Council of Nurses (1920–1941). Silver Medal, France (1933); Order of the British Empire (1935); King's Jubilee Medal (1935); Florence Nightingale Medal, International Red Cross (1935); Mary Agnes Snively Medal (1936); honorary doctor of laws, University of Toronto (1938).

References

Cosbie, W.G. 1975. *The Toronto General Hospital, 1819–1965: A Chronicle*. Toronto: Macmillan.
Riegler, Natalie Nitia. 1992. "The Work and Networks of Jean I. Gunn, Superintendent of Nurses, Toronto General Hospital 1913–1941: A Presentation of Some Issues in Nursing during Her Lifetime 1882–1941." Doctoral diss., University of Toronto.
Riegler, Natalie. 1997. *Jean I. Gunn: Nursing Leader*. Markham, Ont.: Fitzhenry and Whiteside.

LS

H

Hale, Mamie Odessa (1911–ca. 1968)
Nurse-midwife

Mamie Odessa Hale was a public health nurse whose innovative training program for lay midwives led to drastic declines in maternal mortality among African Americans in rural Arkansas. Born in Pennsylvania in 1911, she later worked as a public health nurse in Pittsburgh and attended the Tuskegee School of Nurse-Midwifery for Colored Nurses in Alabama.

From 1942 to 1945, Hale worked for the Arkansas State Board of Health as a public health nurse for the Crittendon County Health Department. In 1945, she was appointed as midwife consultant for the Maternal and Child Health Division of the Arkansas Health Department. In this position, she was responsible for developing educational programs for granny midwives in rural Arkansas. Granny midwives are elderly women who are experienced midwives but who have no formal training. Their role in rural Arkansas was crucial, as most African American women faced racial and financial barriers to finding professional obstetrical care.

By 1946, Hale was conducting midwifery education classes in four Arkansas counties. Her curriculum consisted of seven sessions, including "the fundamental principles concerning the equipment and care of the mid-wife bag; the filing of birth certificates; the conditions upon which the midwife accepts a case; prenatal care, including diet; the actual delivery; and post partum and newborn care" (Hale, 1946, p. 66). Developing effective programs was a daunting task since 75 percent of the midwives were illiterate. Hale compensated by using methods of instruction that included songs, pictures, and demonstrations. She also faced resistance by many midwives who believed that their talents came directly from God. Therefore, Hale began her sessions with prayers or hymns encouraging many of the students to accept the instruction as "extra enlightenment sent by God" (Hale, 1946, p. 68). By the end of the program, midwives were required to have a medical examination, a pledge card, a properly equipped midwife bag, and an application for a midwife permit. During the last session, she awarded permits to practice and gave certificates to retiring midwives.

By the time that Hale left her position in 1950, at least 600 granny midwives held permits, and the number of pregnancy- and childbirth-related deaths dropped dramatically. The success of the midwife training program can be partly attributed to her for helping the lay midwife accept such education as important and useful. Hale, who died

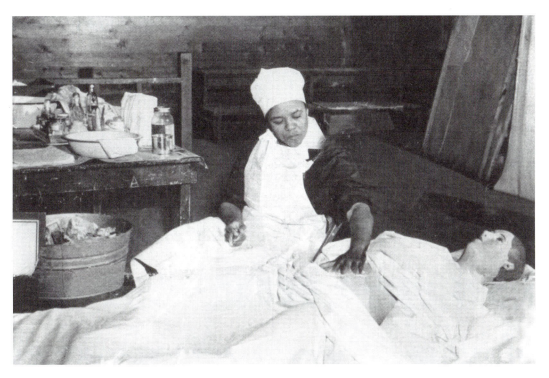

Mamie Odessa Hale. National Library of Medicine.

around 1968, believed that the public should "[s]tand by the midwife and help her as much as possible, since she is still a much needed person in her community" (Hale, 1946, p. 66).

References

Bell, Pegge. 1993. " 'Making Do' with the Midwife: Arkansas's Mamie O. Hale in the 1940s." *Nursing History Review* 1:155–169.

Bell, Pegge L. 2000. "Hale, Mamie Odessa." In *Arkansas Biography: A Collection of Notable Lives,* edited by N.A. Williams and J.M. Whayne. Fayetteville: University of Arkansas Press.

Hale, Mamie O. 1946. "Arkansas Teaches Her Midwives." *The Child* 2 (4):66–69.

Hale, Mamie O. 1948. "Arkansas Midwives Have All-Day Graduation Exercises." *The Child* 13 (4):53–54.

JSB

Hall, Lydia Eloise (1906–1969)
Nurse

Lydia Hall was a pioneer in the development of nurse-led care, demonstrating that professional and personalized nursing care is a necessary part of the healing process. She was born on September 21, 1906, the first of at least two children of Louis U. Williams, a surgeon, and Anna Ketterman Williams. Although born in New York City, she grew up in York, Pennsylvania.

Hall took liberal arts courses at Gettysburg College in Pennsylvania, and in 1927 she graduated from the New York Hospital School of Nursing. Ten years later, she earned a B.S. degree in public health nursing from Teachers College, Columbia University. From the same institution, she earned an M.A. in the teaching of natural life sciences (1942) and completed all but her dissertation for a doctoral degree. In 1945, she married Reginald A. Hall.

During her early career, Hall was a nurse in Pennsylvania and New York, worked for the Life Extension Institute of the New York Metropolitan Life Insurance Company (1930–1935), and was on the research staff of the New York Heart Association (1935–1940). Afterward, she accepted a position as staff nurse at the Visiting Nurse Association of New York, where she soon achieved the role of supervisor (1941–1947). She was then appointed to the faculty of Fordham School of Nursing but eventually returned to the New York Heart Association. In 1950, she was back at Teachers College, where she assisted in developing a new academic program designed to teach nurses to be medical consultants. This was a radical break from tradition, as physicians normally filled the role of adviser in a medical case.

While at Teachers College, Hall also served as research analyst in cardiovascular disease and as director of chronic diseases and tuberculosis studies for the U.S. Public Health Service. She was also visiting professor at the University of North Carolina School of Nursing and at Marquette University College of Nursing.

Hall's most important work began with the closing of the Solomon and Betty Loeb Memorial Home (a convalescent institution). The director of the Montefiore Medical Center asked her to assist him in converting the home into the Loeb Center for Nursing and Rehabilitation in Bronx, New York. She accepted and served as project director for the five-year construction phase and then as administrative director. The center began accepting patients in January 1963. As a nurse-led, inpatient institution, the center was the first of its kind. Patients came to Loeb after they passed through the critical stage of illness. Hall staffed the clinic with registered nurses, a senior staff nurse who held a bachelor's degree, and a chief nurse who held a master's degree. Messenger-attendants and ward secretaries kept nurses free from administrative tasks that interfered with nursing duties.

The care that patients received reflected Hall's philosophy that the intimate nature of nursing fostered a therapeutic environment, leading to a patient's full recovery. Most notably, nurses were in charge of the center, not doctors. Hall wrote the doctors' job descriptions and hired and fired them as necessary. Physicians saw the patient through the immediate crisis, after which nurses eased the patient through a process of self-awareness. Hall believed that sickness was based in psychology. She wrote, "From psychiatry, we learn that people can do three things with their feelings: Express them verbally, thus learning to know self as well as to grow and develop toward emotional maturity; repress verbal expression, in which case, the body communicates the feelings through sickness and *dis*-ease; [or] become psychotic" (Hall, 1964, p. 153). The success of her theory was supported by statistics that indicated that Loeb patients recovered in one-third to one-half the normal recovery time and were readmitted less frequently. The Loeb Center continued under its original mission until 1984, when it became a nursing home.

Hall died on February 27, 1969, at Queens Hospital.

Selected Additional Achievements

Hall wrote numerous professional articles. Member, American Nurses Association, National League for Nursing, National Organization for Public Health Nursing, and New York State Nurses Association. Honors include the Teachers College Alumni Award for Distinguished Achievement in Nursing Practice (1967), American Nurses Association Hall of Fame (1984), and the naming of Doctor's Hospital in Freeport, New York, the Lydia E. Hall Hospital (1974).

References

Birnbach, Nettie. 1988. "Lydia Eloise Hall." In *American Nursing: A Biographical Dictionary*, edited by V.L. Bullough, O.M. Church, and A.P. Stein. New York: Garland.

Griffiths, Peter. 1997. "In Search of the Pioneers of Nurse-Led Care." *Nursing Times* 93 (21): 46–48.

Hall, Lydia E. 1963. "A Center for Nursing." *Nursing Outlook* 11 (11): 805–806.

Hall, Lydia E. 1964. "Nursing—What Is It?" *The Canadian Nurse* 60 (2): 150–154.

"Hall, Lydia E." 1969. *American Journal of Nursing* 69 (4): 830, 832.

Wiggins, Lois Reeves. 1980. "Lydia Hall's Place in the Development of Theory in Nursing." *Image* 12 (1): 10–12.

JSB

Hamilton, Alice (1869–1970)
Physician

Alice Hamilton introduced the field of occupational medicine to the United States and was the first female professor at Harvard Medical School. She was born in New York City on February 17, 1869, the second of five children of Montgomery and Gertrude Hamilton, and raised in Fort Wayne, Indiana. Her sister, Edith Hamilton, became a world-renowned classicist, whose book *Mythology* is still used in classrooms today. After beginning her education at home, Alice Hamilton received her formal education at Miss Porter's School in Farmington, Connecticut (1886–1888). Around this time, her father's business ventures began failing, and Hamilton realized that she would need to support herself. She chose to study medicine, not because she "was scientifically minded" but because she "could go anywhere [she] pleased—to far-off lands or to city slums—and be quite sure that [she] could be of use anywhere" (Hamilton, p. 38).

Hamilton took preparatory courses at the Fort Wayne College of Medicine and then entered medical school at the University of Michigan in Ann Arbor in 1892. She graduated in 1893 and subsequently held internships at Northwestern Hospital of Women and Children in Minneapolis (1893) and New England Hospital for Women and Children in Boston (1893–1894). She returned to the University of Michigan in 1895 to study bacteriology and in the fall of that year traveled with her sister Edith to Germany to study at the Universities of Leipzig and Munich. She returned to the United States in the fall of 1896, where she studied pathology at Johns Hopkins Medical School in Baltimore.

In the summer of 1897, Hamilton accepted a position as instructor of pathology at the Woman's Medical School of Northwestern University in Chicago. She revolutionized the course of study at the school. She gave the all-female student body, previously schooled only through lectures and readings, hands-on experience with diseased tissues and autopsy specimens. Gaining the position in Chicago enabled Hamilton to realize her long-held dream of living in Jane Addams' Hull House settlement, which was dedicated to uplifting the living conditions of the poor of Chicago. At Hull House she established Chicago's first well-baby clinic.

In 1902, the Woman's Medical School at Northwestern closed, and Hamilton became a scientist at the Memorial Institute for In-

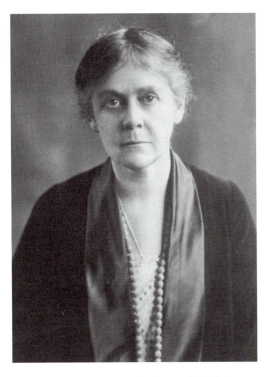

Alice Hamilton. National Library of Medicine.

fectious Diseases in Chicago. There she identified the source of a typhoid epidemic—flies that were infesting homes in the area surrounding Hull House. Serendipitously, she also learned of the extraordinarily large numbers of illnesses and deaths among male factory workers. Stockyard workers complained of pneumonia and rheumatism, while steel mill workers spoke of men falling unconscious while working. This information compelled her to learn as much as possible about occupational diseases, a relatively unknown branch of medicine in the United States. Her newfound expertise led her to be appointed director and chief medical investigator of a survey of industrial diseases in Illinois in 1910. The survey highlighted the toxicity of lead and stimulated the state of Illinois to enact the first worker's compensation law. In 1911, as a special investigator for the U.S. Bureau of Labor, Hamilton launched a study of the diseases associated with working in the lead, rubber, and munitions industries across the United States. As a result of her work many protective legislative acts for factory workers became law.

In the fall of 1919, Hamilton became the first female professor at Harvard Medical School. Despite this achievement, she was denied admission to the Harvard Club, was refused permission to take part in the commencement exercises, and was not allowed football tickets. While at Harvard, she continued to investigate the effects of noxious chemicals on U.S. factory workers and in 1924 published the first American textbook on industrial medicine, *Industrial Poisons in the United States*. In 1935, having never been promoted, she was asked to retire.

In her early years of retirement Hamilton worked as a consultant for the Department of Labor and served as the president of the National Consumer's League (1944–1949). After suffering a series of strokes, she died at her home in Hadlyme, Connecticut, on September 22, 1970.

Selected Additional Achievements

Hamilton was the first and only woman member of the Health Committee of the League of Nations, the predecessor of the World Health Organization (1924–1930). Honorary doctorate, University of Michigan (1948); Elizabeth Blackwell Citation, New York Infirmary (1954); New England Medical Woman of the Year (1956); 55-cent stamp in her honor, U.S. Post Office (1995).

References

Bendiner, Elmer. 1995. "Alice Hamilton's War on Occupational Disease." *Hospital Practice* (May 15):80–88.

Grant, Madeleine P. 1967. *Alice Hamilton: Pioneer Doctor in Industrial Medicine*. London: Abelard-Schuman.

Hamilton, Alice. 1985. *Exploring Dangerous Trades*. Boston: Northeastern University Press.

Sergeant, Elizabeth Shepley. 1929. "Alice Hamilton, M.D.: Crusader for Health in Industry." *Harper's* (May):763–771.

Sichermann, Barbara. 1984. *Alice Hamilton: A Life in Letters*. Cambridge.: Harvard University Press.

CMB

Hamilton, Elizabeth Jane Soley (1805–1897)
Midwife

Elizabeth Jane Hamilton was a Candian midwife whose long and honorable career spanned the middle of the nineteenth century. Known as Aunt Jenny, she was one of the most respected women in her community. She was born in 1805 to William and Mary Soley of Lower Truro, Nova Scotia. She married Robert Hamilton of Brookfield in 1825 and eventually had seven children, although two died in infancy.

Hamilton began her midwifery career in July 1851, when she was called on to assist at the birth of a woman who was probably a relative. It is unknown why she became a midwife at age 46, but by this time, she had already earned a reputation among her neighbors as a skilled and caring nurse. Hamilton's career spanned 42 years and covered the communities of Hilden, Pleasant Valley, Brookfield, Brentwood, Forest Glen, Alton, and Middle Stewiacke. She traveled on horseback, sometimes up to 10 miles, to get to her patients. During the winter, she often walked when deep snow made riding impossible. In a small notebook, she recorded that she attended 776 births, noting in each entry the mother's name, date, and sex of the newborn. She also listed when the baby was stillborn, but there is no record of her ever having lost a mother.

Hamilton continued to deliver babies after her husband's death in 1875. Her practice diminished during her 80s, when she mainly assisted at family births. Altogether she delivered 54 relatives; one of the last babies whom she delivered was her great-granddaughter. Hamilton retired at the age of 88 in 1893. She died in Brookfield, Nova Scotia, in October 1897.

References

Kennedy, Joan E. 1982. "Jane Soley Hamilton, Midwife." *Nova Scotia Historical Review* 2 (1): 6–29.

Kennedy, Joan. 1984. "Aunt Jenny." In *Fragments of the Past: History Notes of Brookfield and Area*, edited by A.J. Lindsay. Brookfield, Nova Scotia: Brookfield Bicentennial Committee.

"A Record of Children Delivered by Mrs. Jane (Soley) Hamilton, Midwife." [1980]. *Genealogical Newsletter of the Nova Scotia Historical Society* (31):321–336.

JSB

Hastings, Caroline Eliza (1841–1922)
Physician

Caroline Hastings was an eminent Boston physician and educator. She was born in Barre, Massachusetts, in 1841, the daughter of Emery and Mary (Bassett) Hastings. Hastings received her education in local schools, including two years at Mt. Holyoke College. It was probably while at Mt. Holyoke that she decided to become a physician, although her father opposed such a career for his daughter. At the age of 18, she learned of the New England Female Medical College in Boston. She eventually entered the college, graduated in 1868, and then established a local practice.

By 1873, the New England Female Medical College had been absorbed by Boston University Medical School as a coeducational homeopathic school of medicine. That year, despite opposition from many of the male faculty, Hastings began a 14-year teaching career at the Medical School. She held the positions of assistant demonstrator and special lecturer on anatomy (1873), assistant demonstrator and lecturer on embryology (1874–1877), lecturer and demonstrator of anatomy (1878–1879), and professor of anatomy (1880–1886). One of her students described her as "the idol of the strong-minded women, and for the same reason was the target, for some of the male students" (Alumni Medical Library Archives, Boston University School of Medicine). Hastings also spent a number of years as resident physician at Talitha Cumi, a home for unwed mothers.

Mary Jane Safford, a Civil War nurse and physician, joined the Boston University medical school the same year as Hastings. The two women participated in a lecture series promoting women's dress reform. Hastings opposed the then-fashionable corset, which inhibited the normal functions of women's vital organs. She urged women to ignore the dictates of fashion and to "adopt a style which allows the full and free use of all [her] powers, both physical and mental" (quoted in Woolson, p. 64).

In 1887, Hastings retired from Boston University but continued private practice. Aside from her regular medical duties, she founded and was first president of the Twentieth Century Club, Boston's first women's medical society. She also was a member of the Boston School Committee, through which she was successful in implementing one of the country's first free school lunch programs for poor children.

Hastings retired to Sharon, Massachusetts. She died at Massachusetts Homeopathic Hospital on July 19, 1922.

See also Safford, Mary Jane

References

Alumni Medical Library Archives, Boston University School of Medicine, Boston.
Archives and Special Collections, Mount Holyoke College, South Hadley, Mass.
Cameron, Mabel Ward, ed. 1974. *The Biographical Cyclopaedia of American Women.* Reprint ed. Vol. 1. Detroit: Gale Research. Original ed., New York: Halvord, 1924.
Kelly, Howard A., and Walter L. Burrage, eds. 1978. *Dictionary of American Medical Biography: Lives of Eminent Physicians of the United States and Canada, from the Earliest Times.* Reprint ed. West Newfield, Maine: Longwood Press. Original ed., New York: Appleton, 1928.
Woolson, Abba Goold, ed. 1874. *Dress-reform: A Series of Lectures, Delivered in Boston, on Dress as It Affects the Health of Women.* Boston: Roberts Brothers. (Five lectures given in the spring of 1874 by Mary J. Safford-Blake, Caroline E. Hastings, Mercy B. Jackson, Arvilla B. Haynes, and Abba Goold Woolson.)

JSB

Hegan, Eliza Parks (1861–1917)
Nurse

Eliza Hegan was a pioneer nurse in New Brunswick, Canada. She was born in 1861, probably in Saint John, New Brunswick, and was the daughter of John and Eliza (Black) Hegan. She received her early education at Miss Magstaff's private school in Saint John and in 1888 was one of 10 women chosen to study nursing at Saint John General Public Hospital.

Hegan graduated in 1890, becoming the sixth graduate of the school. She then became matron at Victoria Public Hospital in Fredericton, New Brunswick. In 1892, she accepted the same position at Saint John General Public, her alma mater. The following year, she refused to sign the diplomas of four students who had broken hospital rules. The Hospital Board did not support Hegan's actions, and she left in frustration in 1895. She afterward served as night supervisor at the New York Polyclinic Hospital, but a bout with typhoid fever compelled her to return to Saint John in 1898. At the suggestion of local physicians, she established one of the city's three private hospitals, which she ran until her death.

Hegan is credited with playing a role in the formation (1903) of the Graduate Nurses' Society of Saint John General Public Hospital, the first local nursing organization. By 1909, the society became the Saint John Graduate Nurses Association. She served as the association's fifth president and also served as registrar. In 1916, she helped establish the bylaws of the newly formed provincial organization, the New Brunswick Association of Graduate Nurses.

Hegan died of cirrhosis of the liver at General Public Hospital on February 18, 1917. After her death, she was recognized by both the New Brunswick and Canadian Nurses Associations for her contribution to the profession.

References

McGee, Arlee Hoyt. 1998. "Hegan, Eliza Parks." In *Dictionary of Canadian Biography: Volume 14, 1911–1920,* edited by R. Cook. Toronto: University of Toronto Press.
Slattery, Anne. 1929. *Pioneers of Nursing in Canada.* Montreal: Gazette Printing.

JSB

Henderson, Virginia Avenel (1897–1996)
Nurse

Virginia Henderson was often called the first lady of nursing for her contributions to the profession through writing and research. In her long career as a nurse, she produced noted textbooks, a standard definition of nursing, and an index to the nursing literature. She was born on November 30, 1897, in Kansas City, Missouri, the fifth of eight children of Lucy Minor Abbot and Daniel Brosius Henderson, an attorney. At a young age, Henderson and her family moved to northern Virginia. Her early education was primarily with relatives in the home. In 1918, out of a desire to assist in the nation's World War I effort, Henderson applied to, and was accepted at, the Army School of Nursing in Washington, D.C., headed by nurse Annie Goodrich.

After four months of classroom work, Henderson studied at several hospitals in New York and in Washington, D.C. In 1921, she graduated and joined Lillian Wald's Henry Street Visiting Nurse Service in New York City. She left the position after six months to direct a summer camp for underprivileged children. She next worked for the Visiting Nurse Association in Washington, D.C. Although she loved being a practitioner, in 1924 she accepted a position as a nursing instructor at Norfolk Protestant Hospital School in Virginia. She was both the school's and the state's first full-time nursing teacher. Among her innovations at Norfolk were bringing the school's admission policy up to the standard developed by the National League of Nursing Education, replacing physician instructors with nurses, and founding a nursing library and laboratory.

In 1929, Henderson attended Columbia University's Teachers College to further her education in the sciences. Financial constraints led her back to nursing practice, however, until she was awarded a Rockefeller Foundation grant in 1931. She earned a B.S. in 1932 and an M.A. in 1934, both in nursing education. She remained at Teachers College as an instructor and an associate professor of nursing education until 1948. During her time there, she taught research methods and medical and surgical nursing and began clinics that allowed patients to critique their nursing care. While at Teachers College, she revised a popular nursing text, *Textbook of the Principles and Practice of Nursing* (1939). After leaving the college in 1948, she devoted her attention to a fifth edition of the book, which was published in 1955. She condensed the work into *Basic Principles of Nursing Care* for the International Council of Nurses in 1960, and it was eventually translated into 25 languages.

In 1953 Yale University sociologist Leo Simmons asked Henderson to assist him in a survey and assessment of nursing research. Simmons had been charged by the National Committee for the Improvement of Nursing Service to develop a bibliography of nursing research. With funding from the U.S. Public Health Service, Henderson did much of the field research, visiting nursing schools and practicing nurses to determine what research had been done or might be done by nurses if resources were available. In 1959, she became director of the Nursing Studies Index Project. Assisted by Dean Florence Wald at the Yale School of Nursing, Henderson undertook the task of creating an index to the nursing literature. The first volume, *Nursing Studies Index, 1957–1959*, was published in 1963, and the final volume, containing retrospective coverage of the literature to 1900, was published in 1972.

While working on the *Index*, Henderson published an 84-page work, *The Nature of Nursing* (1966), which detailed her definition of nursing. She stated, "The unique function of the nurse is to assist the individual, sick or well, in the performance of those activities contributing to health or its recovery (or to peaceful death) that he would perform unaided if he had the necessary strength, will or knowledge" (quoted in Safier, p. 116). She further noted that the nurse's job is to deal with 14 fundamental human needs such as breathing, sleeping, expressing emotion, and participating in recreation. Henderson's definition has been adopted internationally.

In 1972, after completing the *Nursing Studies Index,* Henderson became a research associate emerita at Yale and began an international speaking tour. She died in Branford, Connecticut, on March 19, 1996. Sigma Theta Tau, the nursing honor society, named its library the Virginia Henderson International Nursing Library in her honor.

See also Goodrich, Annie Warburton; Wald, Florence Schorske; Wald, Lillian D.

Selected Additional Achievements

Nursing Research: A Survey and Assessment (1964, with Leo Simmons); *The Principles and Practice of Nursing* (1978); *The Nature of Nursing: A Definition and Its Implications for Practice, Research, and Education: Reflections after 25 Years* (1991); *A Virginia Henderson Reader: Excellence in Nursing* (1995, edited by Edward J. Halloran). Award for distinguished and exemplary service, American Nurses Association (1974); Mary Adelaide Nutting Award, National League for Nursing (1977); Christianne Reimann Prize, International Council of Nurses (1985); Merit Award, National Association of Nurses of Colombia, South America (1985); Excellence in Education Award (now the Virginia Henderson Award, National Association for Home Care, 1985); American Nurses Association Hall of Fame (1996); 12 honorary doctorates.

References

Hays, Judith C. 1992. "Virginia Henderson." In *American Nursing: A Biographical Dictionary,* edited by V.L. Bullough, L. Sentz, and A.P. Stein. New York: Garland.

McBride, Angela Barron. "Virginia Henderson (1897–1996)." *Sigma Theta Tau International, Honor Society of Nursing, Virginia Henderson International Library.* Online. http://www.stti.iupui.edu/library/vh_tribute.html. 25 February 2001. Original ed., *Reflections* (Spring 1996): 22–23.

Safier, Gwendolyn. 1977. *Contemporary American Leaders in Nursing: An Oral History.* New York: McGraw-Hill.

LS

Hogan, Aileen I. (1899–1981)
Nurse-midwife

Aileen Hogan was a leader in nurse-midwifery and in childbirth education in the United States and Canada. She was born on November 10, 1899, in Ottawa, Ontario, one of five children of James and Christina (McMaster) Hogan. She earned a high school diploma at age 16 and during World War I worked for the Canadian Federal War Department. Both of her parents died during the influenza epidemic of 1918–1919.

In 1920, Hogan emigrated to New York City, where she worked as a medical secretary. In the late 1930s she enrolled in the Columbia Presbyterian School of Nursing. During her studies, she also spent two years rotating as staff nurse at Sloane Hospital of the Presbyterian Medical Center. By 1942, she was head nurse of the hospital's labor and delivery service. In July 1942, with the nation at war, she sailed to Europe with the Presbyterian Hospital Unit. She served as a nurse in Ireland, England, and France and also provided informal parent education to the young soldiers with new babies at home.

After returning to the United States, Hogan attended Teachers College, Columbia University. She earned a B.S. in 1947 and then a certification in nurse-midwifery from the Maternity Center Association (MCA) in New York. After receiving an M.A. from Teachers College in 1948, she assumed the chair of the Maternity Nursing Department at Case Western Reserve University in Cleveland, Ohio. In 1951, she returned to the MCA and spent the next 15 years establishing childbirth education programs with nurses in the United States and Canada. The workshops taught the "principles of nurse-midwifery . . . the health approach for the family, continuity of care, [and a] cooperative team approach" (quoted in Tom, p. 9).

Hogan was also involved in the formation of the American College of Nurse-Midwifery (ACNM), the first national organization devoted solely to the professional needs and concerns of nurse-midwives. The college was incorporated in 1955 and continues to exist today as the American College of Nurse-Midwives. She retired from the MCA in 1965 and spent a short time in Santa Fe, New Mexico, at the Catholic Maternity Institute. She returned to New York to become the first executive secretary of the ACNM and in 1970 chaired the committee that established and administered the ACNM's archives. The following year, she helped organize the convention of the International Conference of Midwives in Washington, D.C.

Hogan retired in 1976. She died of a cardiopulmonary disorder on January 7, 1981, at her home in Whiting, New Jersey.

Selected Additional Achievements

Hogan's publications include "Bomb-Born Babies," *Public Health Nurse* 43 (1951): 383–385; "The Premature Baby," *American Journal of Nursing* 54 (1954): 575–577; and "A Tribute to the Pioneers," *Journal of Nurse-Midwifery* (Summer 1975): 6–11.

References

Stein, Alice P. 1992. "Aileen I. Hogan." In *American Nursing: A Biographical Dictionary*, edited by V.L. Bullough, L. Sentz, and A.P. Stein. New York: Garland.

Tom, Sally Austen. 1981. "Spokeswoman for Midwifery: Aileen Hogan." *Journal of Nurse-Midwifery* 26 (3):7–11.

JSB

Howell, Mary Catherine Raugust (1932–1998)
Physician

Mary Howell was a feminist physician who supported better health care for women and a woman's right to a career in medicine. She was born on September 2, 1932, in Grand Forks, North Dakota. She earned an A.B. from Radcliffe College in 1954 and an M.A. from the University of Minnesota in 1958. Around this time, she married Robert Jordan and had a son. When the marriage failed, she decided to become a pediatrician.

Before being admitted to the University of Minnesota medical school, Howell endured a lecture from an admissions officer who told her that women in medicine were a waste of taxpayers' money. She ignored the officer and went on to earn a medical degree as well as a Ph.D. in psychology in 1962. After graduating, she was an instructor in child development at Minnesota and then joined the Harvard Medical School faculty in 1969 as an instructor in pediatrics. She was also involved in the women's health movement and contributed to the Boston Women's Health

Book Collective's groundbreaking health information book *Our Bodies, Ourselves* (1st ed. 1971).

In 1972, Howell was made an associate dean for student affairs at Harvard, making her the highest-ranking woman there. She later said that she felt that her appointment was a token to the women's movement. While serving as dean, Howell surveyed women medical students across the country about their status as women in medicine. The surveys were the basis for her book, *Why Would a Girl Go into Medicine? Medical Education in the United States: A Guide for Women* (1973, as Margaret Campbell), which detailed discrimination against women in medical schools. In 1975, she helped to organize a national women's health conference at Harvard that contributed to the formation of the National Women's Health Network, a lobbying group for women's health care.

Howell left Harvard in 1975 for York,

Maine, where she practiced pediatrics for a year. Based on her experiences there, she wrote *Healing at Home: A Guide to Health Care for Children* (1978). While in Maine, she was divorced from her second husband, Dr. A. Ervin Howell. Howell returned to Boston and continued to practice pediatrics, as well as psychotherapy. She was also a columnist for *Working Mother* magazine (1977–1987). In 1991, she earned a law degree from Harvard and was a member of the Division of Medical Ethics at Harvard Medical School from 1992 to 1994. In 1995 she worked as executive director of a private adoption agency in Watertown, Massachusetts.

Howell died of breast cancer on February 5, 1998, at her home in Watertown.

References

Benjamin, Beth Cooper. "Mary Howell: Breaking Ground for Women in Medicine." *The National Women's Health Network.* Online. http:// www.womenshealthnetwork.org/nnartic.les/ howell.htm. 4 February 2001. Original ed., *The Network News* (September–October 1995).

Long, Tom. 1998. "Dr. Mary C. Raugust Howell, 65." *Boston Globe* (February 6):C17.

Saxon, Wolfgang. 1998. "Mary Howell, a Leader in Medicine, Dies at 65." *New York Times* (February 6):D19.

LS

Hunt, Harriot Kezia (1805–1875)
Physician

Harriot Hunt is considered to be the first American woman to practice medicine. She practiced with her younger sister, Sarah, for five years, until the latter left the profession.

Harriot was born in Boston on November 9, 1805, to Joab and Kezia (Wentworth) Hunt. Sarah, the second and last child, was born in 1808. During the late 1820s, the sisters ran a school that helped support the family after Joab's death in 1827. The course of their lives changed in 1830, when Sarah developed a prolonged and debilitating illness. The doctors called to the case were unable to cure her. Reading medical texts to educate themselves on disease and its cures sparked the sisters' interest in medicine. However, the unsuccessful and painful treatments prescribed by Sarah's physicians left the greatest impression. Harriot wrote of these treatments in her autobiography, *Glances and Glimpses* (1856): "Blisters and mercurials were tried; they were of no use. Leeches were resorted to; but without success. I marveled—all this agony—all these remedies—and no benefit!" (p. 81). In 1833, Harriot consulted a medical couple, the Motts, who offered alternative and apparently milder treatments. While it is unclear what the Motts prescribed, the results were favorable, and Sarah's health returned. The Hunt family moved in with the Motts while the sisters studied medicine with them.

In 1835, the Hunts established their own medical practice, championing prevention over the harsh cures that Sarah had endured. Harriot wrote, "That word—preventive—seemed a great word to me; curative, was small beside it" (Hunt, p. 122). In addition to curing illness, the Hunts taught women the importance of prevention through proper hygienic practices. While many mainstream physicians believed it unwise for women to have knowledge of their own physiology, Harriot was convinced that women's self-ignorance was the direct cause of many health problems. In 1843, she organized a local Ladies' Physiological Society to lecture on hygiene and preventive health. The society gave women a place to "meet together for the purpose of obtaining a knowledge of physical laws . . . [to] put them on their own responsibilities, and be a blessing to themselves and their children" (Hunt, pp. 170–171).

The Hunts became interested in the relationship between women's physical and mental health after observing many cases of "physical maladies growing out of concealed sorrows" (Hunt, p. 139). In 1838, Harriot attended a series of lectures on mental health, and in their own practice, the Hunts were "frequently surprised by the successful termination of many . . . cases through prescriptions for mental states" (Hunt, p. 139). Sarah left the profession to marry Edmund Wright in 1840. Harriot, who never married, continued her mission.

In 1847, Harriot learned that Geneva Medical College (New York) had accepted Elizabeth Blackwell, the first woman ever admitted into a mainstream medical school. The same year, Hunt applied to Harvard Medical School. She wrote to Dean Oliver Wendell Holmes, "I seek for that *scientific light*, which shall not only place my mind in more harmony with my professional duties, but enable me to become more worthy of the trust committed to me" (Hunt, p. 217). Despite years of successful practice, Hunt was rejected because of her sex. In 1850, she applied again to Harvard. She sent a letter to the faculty arguing that the growing demand for female physicians was forcing women to practice uneducated and unprepared. This time, her application was accepted. The senior class, however, protested the admission, and Hunt chose not to attend under such conditions. The Female (later, Woman's) Medical College of Pennsylvania in Philadelphia, the first conventional women's medical school, compensated Hunt with an honorary medical degree in 1853.

For the rest of her life, Hunt continued her practice and was active in women's rights issues. She attended a women's rights convention 1850 and expanded her lecture circuit beyond Boston. She traveled throughout New England, speaking on "Woman as Physician to Her Sex," calling "attention both publicly and privately, to the importance and propriety of her entering the medical profession" (Hunt, p. 311). Hunt was outspoken on other women's rights issues. Every year for 20 years, she included a letter of protest with her tax payment, arguing against taxation without representation. In 1853, she petitioned the Massachusetts constitutional convention for equal educational opportunities for women.

Hunt died of Bright's disease on January 2, 1875. She willed an endowment of $1,000 to be used to purchase textbooks for New England female medical students. The date and cause of Sarah's death are unknown.

See also Blackwell, Elizabeth

References

Elliot, H. B. 1868. "Miss Harriot K. Hunt, M. D." In *Eminent Women of the Age: Being Narratives of the Lives and Deeds of the Most Prominent Women of the Present Generation*, edited by J. Parton. Hartford, Conn.: S.M. Betts.

Hobson, Roberta, and Susan E. Cayleff. 1999. "Hunt, Harriot Kezia." In *American National Biography*, edited by J.A. Garraty and M.C. Carnes. New York: Oxford University Press.

Hunt, Harriot K. 1856. *Glances and Glimpses: Or, Fifty Years Social, including Twenty Years Professional Life*. Boston: John J. Jewett.

"Hunt, Harriot Kezia." 1899. In *The National Cyclopaedia of American Biography*. Vol. 9. New York: James T. White.

"Hunt, Harriot Kezia." 1978. In *Dictionary of American Medical Biography: Lives of Eminent Physicians of the United States and Canada, from the Earliest Times*, edited by H.A. Kelly and W.L. Burrage. West Newfield, Maine: Longwood Press. Original ed., New York: Appleton, 1928.

Tyler, Alice Felt. 1971. "Hunt, Harriot Kezia." In *Notable American Women, 1607–1950: A Biographical Dictionary*, edited by E.T. James, J.W. James, and P.S. Boyer. Cambridge: Belknap Press of Harvard University Press.

Viets, Henry R. 1932. "Hunt, Harriot Kezia." In *The Dictionary of American Biography*, edited by D. Malone. New York: Charles Scribner's Sons.

Warner, John Harley. 1984. "Hunt, Harriot Kezia." In *Dictionary of American Medical Biography*, edited by M. Kaufman, S. Galishoff, and T.L. Savitt. Westport, Conn.: Greenwood Press.

JSB

Hurd-Mead, Kate Campbell (1867–1941)
Physician

Kate Campbell Hurd-Mead was a practicing gynecologist but is probably best known for her historical research on women in medicine. She was born on April 6, 1867, in Danville, Quebec, the oldest of three children of Dr. Edward Payson Hurd and Sarah Elizabeth (Campbell) Hurd. When she was three, her family moved to Newburyport, Massachusetts, where she graduated from high school in 1883. She wanted to be a physician like her father; so, on the advice of pioneering woman physician Mary Putnam Jacobi, she studied medicine privately for two years before matriculating at the Woman's Medical College of Pennsylvania in Philadelphia at the age of 18.

After graduating in 1888, Hurd-Mead interned at Boston's New England Hospital for Women and Children, founded by Dr. Marie Zakrzewska in 1862. She then went to Europe to do postgraduate work (1889–1890) and in 1890 moved to Baltimore. There she became medical director of the Bryn Mawr School for Girls and set up a private practice with Dr. Alice Hall. The two women also established the Evening Dispensary for Working Women and Girls in 1891, which, in addition to providing medical care for women, offered women physicians a place to practice medicine.

On June 21, 1893, Kate Campbell Hurd married William Edward Mead, a professor of English at Wesleyan University in Middletown, Connecticut. Shortly after her marriage, Hurd-Mead opened a private gynecological practice in Middletown, which she operated for 37 years. In 1895, she helped establish Middlesex County Hospital; she was later secretary of the hospital. She also helped organize the Middletown District Nurses Association in 1900. In 1904, she went to Vienna for further medical training and upon her return became the consulting gynecologist to Middlesex Hospital (1907–1925). She retired from medical practice in 1925 and traveled to Britain, the European continent, Asia, and Africa to research the history of women in medicine.

Hurd-Mead had originally been inspired to study the topic during her Baltimore days, when she attended Johns Hopkins Hospital Historical Club meetings. She wrote that "as a class, women seem always to have been too busy to say much about themselves," and she was determined to record the missing history of women healers (1977, p. vi). In 1929, she and her husband settled in Haddam, Connecticut, where she continued her research and writing. She published her research in the journal literature and wrote two books, *Medical Women of America* (1933) and *A History of Women in Medicine from the Earliest Times to the Beginning of the Nineteenth Century* (1938). She had hoped to bring the latter work up-to-date in two more volumes but died before she could finish it.

Hurd-Mead died of a heart attack on January 1, 1941, at her home in Haddam. She left $10,000 to the Woman's Medical College of Pennsylvania, as well as her library of books.

See also Jacobi, Mary Corinna Putnam; Zakrzewska, Marie Elizabeth

Selected Additional Achievements

Vice president, State Medical Society of Connecticut (1913–1914); president, Women's Medical Society of Connecticut (1922–1925); president, American Medical Women's Association (1923–1924). Manuscripts of the second and third volumes of *A History of Women in Medicine* are at the Schlesinger Library, Radcliffe College (Vol. 2, *Medical Women in the Eastern Hemisphere*) and at the Special Collections on Women in Medicine, MCP Hahnemann University, formerly Woman's Medical College of Pennsylvania (Vol. 3, *Medical Women in England*).

References

Hurd-Mead, Kate Campbell. 1925. "Forty Years of Medical Progress: Reminiscences and Comparisons." In *Seventy-fifth Anniversary Volume of the Woman's Medical College of Pennsylvania*. Philadelphia: Woman's Medical College of Pennsylvania.

Hurd-Mead, Kate Campbell. 1977. *A History of Women in Medicine from the Earliest Times to the Beginning of the Nineteenth Century*. Reprint ed. New York: AMS Press. Original ed., Haddam, Conn.: Haddam Press, 1938.

Lovejoy, Esther P. 1941. "Kate Campbell Hurd-Mead (1867–1941)." *Bulletin of the History of Medicine* (July):314–317.

Miller, Genevieve. 1971. "Hurd-Mead, Kate Campbell." In *Notable American Women, 1607–1950: A Biographical Dictionary*, edited by E.T. James, J.W. James, and P.S. Boyer. Cambridge: Belknap Press of Harvard University Press.

LS

Hurdon, Elizabeth (1868–1941)
Physician

Elizabeth Hurdon was the first woman physician appointed to the staff of Johns Hopkins University Hospital. She is also known for developing a uterine cancer treatment utilizing radium and X-rays. She was born in Exeter, England, on January 28, 1868, one of two daughters of John Hurdon, a linen and woolen manufacturer, and Ann (Coom) Hurdon. When she was very young, her family emigrated to Ontario, Canada. At the age of 13, Hurdon entered the Wesleyan Ladies' College in Hamilton, Ontario, from which she graduated in 1886 with the degree of mistress of English literature. She received her medical degree from Trinity College at the University of Toronto in 1895.

When she graduated, Hurdon took a position at the Evening Dispensary for Working Women and Girls in Baltimore, founded in part by physician Kate Campbell Hurd-Mead. This position was ideal for her as it paid her living expenses and left her free during the day to pursue her primary interest, gynecological pathology research at Johns Hopkins University School of Medicine. With Dr. Howard A. Kelly, Hurdon studied the efficacy of radium for the treatment of gynecological diseases.

In 1897, Hurdon was appointed assistant gynecologist at the dispensary of Johns Hopkins Hospital. This marked the first appointment of a woman physician to the staff of the Hospital. In February 1898, she achieved another first when she became the first woman member of the medical faculty at Johns Hopkins University Medical School. For the next 18 years, she taught gynecological pathology to the students of Johns Hopkins University Medical School and worked in her private practice. During this time she coauthored several articles and book chapters on gynecological pathology with Howard Kelly. In 1913, she was one of approximately 12 women who qualified for election into the newly formed American College of Surgeons.

In 1915 she requested a leave of absence from Johns Hopkins to volunteer for service in the Royal Army Medical Corps of her native England. She was given the rank of captain and was assigned to active duty in army hospitals in Malta and Salonika. After the war she continued working in military hospitals in England until 1921. Family obligations detained her in London and prevented her planned return to Johns Hopkins.

Hurdon did not practice medicine again until 1925, when she was to assist in the founding of a hospital in London for clinical research and treatment of cancer in women. The first studies took place at the four women's hospitals in London, but the success of the treatment led to the founding of a separate institution, Marie Curie Hospital, in 1929. Originally, Hurdon was concerned with treating cancer of the cervix with radium and X-rays but eventually extended her work to include the treatment of cancer of the uterus, vagina, vulva, breast, and rectum. Hurdon's research significantly advanced the treatment of cancer in women, especially for cases that were poor surgical risks or inoperable.

In 1938, Hurdon retired from her position as director of the hospital. She died on January 29, 1941, from cancer of the liver.

See also Hurd-Mead, Kate Campbell

Selected Additional Achievements

The Variform Appendix and Its Diseases (1905, with H. A. Kelly); chapters in *Gynecology and Ab-*

dominal *Surgery* (2 vols., 1907–1908, edited by H. A. Kelly and C.P. Noble); *Cancer of the Uterus* (1942, published posthumously). Order of Commander of the British Empire (1938).

References

Chesney, Alan Mason. 1958. *The Johns Hopkins Hospital and the Johns Hopkins University School of Medicine: A Chronicle, Volume 2, 1893–1905.* Baltimore: Johns Hopkins Press.

Hurdon, Elizabeth. 1936. "The Marie Curie Hospital of London." *Medical Woman's Journal* 43: 233–235.

Koudelka, Janet Brock. 1971. "Hurdon, Elizabeth." In *Notable American Women, 1607–1950: A Biographical Dictionary*, edited by E.T. James, J.W. James, and P.S. Boyer. Cambridge: Belknap Press of Harvard University Press.

"Obituary." 1941. *Lancet* (February 8):199.

CMB

Huson, Florence (1857–1915)
Physician

Florence Huson's success as an early female physician in Michigan helped open the doors for future women to practice in that state. She was born in Ann Arbor, Michigan, on June 17, 1857, to Frederick C. and Mary L. (Bradley) Huson. After receiving her early education in local schools, she graduated from the University of Michigan College of Medicine in 1885. Following a year of study at Massachusetts Hospital in Boston, she returned to Michigan to become assistant to Donald McLean, her former instructor of surgery.

After McLean's resignation in 1889, Huson began a successful 25-year surgical and obstetrical practice in Detroit. Additionally, she founded and was first president of the Woman's Hospital Free Dispensary (1893), where she administered health care to many of Detroit's women and children. She also served as vice chief of staff at Detroit Woman's Hospital, the first woman to be on staff at that institution.

In 1905, Huson established and presided over the Elizabeth Blackwell Medical Society for Women Physicians, Detroit's first woman's medical society. She was also vice president of the Michigan Medical Society. Outside of her medical work, Huson supported causes and associations devoted to assisting wayward young women and was director of the local Young Women's Christian Association. She died in Detroit on August 12, 1915.

See also Blackwell, Elizabeth

References

The National Cyclopaedia of American Biography. 1921. Vol. 17. New York: James T. White.

Pernick, M. 1984. "Huson, Florence." In *Dictionary of American Medical Biography*, edited by M. Kaufman, S. Galishoff, and T.L. Savitt. Westport, Conn.: Greenwood Press.

JSB

Hutchinson, Anne Marbury (ca. 1591–1643)
Midwife

Anne Hutchinson is best remembered as a religious leader in colonial Massachusetts, but she was also a midwife and healer. She was born around 1591 in Alford, Lincolnshire, England, the second of 13 children of Francis and Bridget (Dryden) Marbury. Her father was a minister in the Church of Eng-

land who had been imprisoned for his nonconformist views. Presumably, he taught Hutchinson to read and write using Scripture and theological writings as her textbooks. In 1612, she married William Hutchinson, a merchant, and the couple eventually had 14 children. Her own experience in giving birth and in assisting other women in childbirth helped Hutchinson develop her skills as a midwife and as a lay nurse.

The Hutchinsons were followers of Puritan preacher John Cotton. Cotton sailed to the Massachusetts Bay Colony in 1633 to avoid arrest, and the Hutchinsons sailed the next year, arriving in Boston in September 1634. William Hutchinson prospered in the cloth trade, while Anne continued her work as a midwife. There is little direct evidence of Hutchinson's midwifery methods or healing techniques, but she was most likely skilled in herbal medicine. As a midwife, she probably prepared and administered herbs and supervised the entire ritual of childbirth. Certain midwifery practices, such as the gathering of female relatives and neighbors and the designation of the room in which the birth would take place, were most likely brought with her from England.

Much of a midwife's duty in Puritan Massachusetts was to help women be spiritually prepared to face the very real possibility of death in childbirth. Hutchinson's knowledge of the physiology of birth and her understanding of Puritan theology made her ideally suited to be a midwife. She was confident in her own religious beliefs and shared them with pregnant and laboring women. In the process of performing her duties as a midwife and healer, she learned that many women in the community believed in the Covenant of Works—that personal good deeds would provide salvation. This was inconsistent with her own commitment to the Covenant of Grace, the belief that salvation comes only through reliance on the grace of God, which she stressed in prayer meetings held in her home. Hutchinson came to be seen as a threat by Boston's religious leaders, who emphasized the Covenant of Works; she and her followers were called "Antinomians," because they were seen as being in opposition to customary law.

In August 1637 a synod was held to denounce Hutchinson; she was brought to trial in November. She was accused of failing to honor the ministers of the colony and of presuming to teach men who attended her meetings. Hutchinson claimed the spirit of God as an authorization to teach, leading the court to declare her a heretic. During this difficult time, a woman whose labor Hutchinson attended gave birth to a premature and severely deformed infant who was born dead. The religious community took the deformed child as a sign of God's wrath at Hutchinson's heretical doctrine.

Hutchinson spent the winter exiled from her family and appeared, pregnant and exhausted, before the Church of Boston in March 1638, where she attempted to defend herself and her beliefs. Hutchinson was exiled from the colony and excommunicated from the church. She moved to Rhode Island and shortly thereafter, instead of bearing a child, gave birth to a hydatidiform mole, a rare tumor of placental tissue that may occur when an embryo fails to develop. After her husband's death in 1642, she and the rest of her family left for Dutch territory on Long Island, New York. In 1643, Hutchinson and all but one of her daughters were killed in an Indian raid.

References

Huber, Elaine C. 1999. "Hutchinson, Anne." In *American National Biography*, edited by J.A. Garraty and M.C. Carnes. New York: Oxford University Press.

McGregor, Deborah Kuhn. 1989. " 'Childbirth-Travells' and 'Spiritual Estates': Anne Hutchinson and Colonial Boston, 1634–1638." *Caduceus: A Museum Quarterly for the Health Sciences* 5 (4):1–33.

LS

J

Jackson, Mary Percy (1904–2000)
Physician

Mary Percy Jackson was one of the first doctors recruited to provide medical care for the early settlers of northern Alberta, Canada. She was born in 1904 in the town of Dudley near Birmingham, England. Her father was the director of a woolen manufacturing company, and her mother was a teacher. At about age 10, she decided to become a doctor and was allowed to engage in serious study, rather than the more traditional domestic training of the day.

Jackson studied medicine at Birmingham University, where the professors assigned women students the most difficult tasks "on the grounds that if women wanted medical degrees, they should be forced to earn them" (McGinnis and Jackson, p. 11). Male students often asked Jackson to take their shifts, which she did willingly in order to gain the extra experience. Jackson graduated in 1927, winning the Queen's Prize as the best all-round student.

For two years following graduation, Jackson interned in medicine, obstetrics, and anesthetics and worked as a house surgeon at Children's Hospital in Birmingham. She was interested in finding adventure, however, and intended to take a post in obstetrics at Women's Hospital in Calcutta. Her plans changed when she saw an advertisement in the February 1929 issue of the *British Medical Journal* calling for "strong energetic medical women with post-graduate experience in midwifery for country work in western Canada" (Jackson and Lehn, p. 11). At the time, the government of Alberta was promoting the establishment of communities in northern Alberta and had come to realize that their success depended on the survival of the homesteading families. In fact, women were refusing to follow their husbands to this remote region unless proper medical care was made available. The government chose to recruit female doctors to provide the necessary health care primarily because the patients would be mostly women and children. Women were also favored because Canada's minister of public health believed that they could be relied upon to perform the jobs of both nurse and doctor, would be less likely to "turn to drink," and could be paid less since they did not need to support a wife (McGinnis and Jackson, p. 19).

Jackson was accepted for a position, along with two other women, and sailed for Canada in June 1929. After gaining a minimum of experience in frontier medicine with a traveling clinic in late June, Jackson took her post as district medical officer in Battle River Prairie, 100 miles from the nearest hospital at Peace River. She was provided with a small shack that was to serve as both her home and surgery. The area lacked all modern conveniences including roads, bridges, telegraphs, and telephones. Jackson fought long battles with typhoid and tuberculosis that plagued the white settlers and the native Metis. She also worked endlessly to improve the public health of the region through education. Although she often found herself house-bound by snow for days or was so busy that she went without sleep for three or fours days in a row, she flourished in the lifestyle. She enjoyed the freedom of being both an independent woman and an independent physician, opportunities that she believed would not have been available to her in England.

In 1931, she married a settler, Frank Jackson, and moved to his ranch 100 miles north of Battle River, in the Keg River area. The financially deficient Alberta government was unwilling to transfer Jackson's appointment as district medical officer to Keg River, yet she elected to practice there without the benefit of a salary. Despite daily hard work and her valiant campaign against a rabies epidemic, she was not paid again for her efforts until health insurance was instituted in 1969. She retired in 1974 and continued to live in the log house that her husband had built before their marriage. Jackson died in May 2000 in Edmonton, Alberta.

Selected Additional Achievements

Centennial Medal of Canada (1967); senior life membership, Alberta Medical Association (1969); senior membership, Canadian Medical Association (1971); life membership, College of Family Physicians (1974); Woman of the Year, Voice of Native Women (1975); honorary doctor of laws, University of Alberta (1976); Alberta Order of Excellence (1983); honorary life membership, Geriatric Medical Society of Alberta (1985); Order of Canada (1990).

References

Andrews, P. J., ed. 1933. *On the Last Frontier; Pioneering in the Peace River Block; Letters of Mary Percy Jackson.* Toronto: General Board of Religious Education.

Hacker, Carlotta. 1974. *The Indomitable Lady Doctors.* Toronto: Clarke, Irwin.

Jackson, Mary Percy, and Cornelia Lehn. 1988. *The Homemade Brass Plate: The Story of Dr. Mary Percy Jackson as Told to Cornelia Lehn.* Sardis, Brit. Col.: H. Braun.

Keywan, Zonia. 1977. "Mary Percy Jackson: Pioneer Doctor." *The Beaver* 308:41–46.

McGinnis, Janice P. Dickin, and Mary Percy Jackson. 1995. *Suitable for the Wilds: Letters from Northern Alberta, 1929–1931.* Toronto: University of Toronto Press.

CMB

Jacobi, Mary Corinna Putnam (1842–1906)
Physician

Mary Putnam Jacobi, one of the most highly regarded pioneering American women physicians, believed that limited opportunities for quality medical education stood in women's way to full acceptance into the profession. Throughout her career, she strove to improve medical education available to women. Several of her essays and speeches on women in medicine are published in *Mary Putnam Jacobi, M.D.: A Pathfinder in Medicine* (1925).

Jacobi, the oldest of 11 children of American publisher George Putnam and Victorine (Haven) Putnam, was born in London, England, on August 31, 1842. The family returned to the United States around 1848, ultimately settling in Morrisania, New York. She received her early education at home and in New York public and private schools. When she was only 17, the *Atlantic Monthly* published her story "Found and Lost"; despite this indication of a future literary life, she decided on a career in medicine.

At the age of 19, Jacobi undertook private

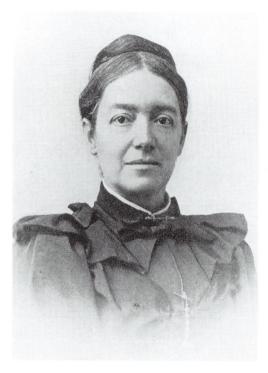

Mary Corinna Putnam Jacobi. Archives & Special Collections on Women in Medicine, MCP Hahnemann University.

studies in medicine with Elizabeth Blackwell and other physicians. Afterward, she earned the distinction of being the first woman enrolled at the New York College of Pharmacy. She graduated in 1863 and the following year received a medical degree from the Female (later, Woman's) Medical College of Pennsylvania (now MCP Hahnemann University) and was the only student at the college to write a thesis in Latin. After graduation, she studied clinical medicine with Marie Zakrzewska and Lucy Sewall at New England Hospital for Women and Children in Boston. In addition to her formal training, Jacobi volunteered at soldiers' hospitals in New York and studied chemistry privately. In the summer of 1863, she went to Louisiana to care for her brother, George, who was suffering from malaria, and in 1864, she went to South Carolina to treat a sister with typhoid.

Dissatisfied with the quality of medical education that she received in the United States, Jacobi went to Paris in 1866 for further training at the prestigious École de Médecine. The school, however, had not yet opened its doors to women, and she was unable to gain entry into the École for a year and a half. One professor agreed to allow her into his dissecting lectures if she would disguise herself as a man, a condition that she refused. Impressed by her determination, the professor admitted Jacobi into his lecture hall. In the meantime, she attended hospital and clinical lectures and visited laboratories. She continued her efforts to be fully accepted in the school, and in 1868, by order of the minister of public education, she became the school's first female matriculant. She graduated in 1871, receiving the highest possible grade on her examinations and a bronze medal for her thesis.

In Paris, Jacobi wrote for American journals. She contributed a series of 19 articles to the *Medical Record* titled "Medical Matters in Paris." She signed these essays P.C.M., fearing that a woman's signature would discredit them. She also wrote for *Putnam's Magazine* and *Scribner's Magazine* and for the *New York Evening Post.* Her accounts of French politics and the Franco-Prussian War were published in the *American Historical Review.* Over the course of her career, she published nearly 150 medical articles.

In 1871, Jacobi returned to New York with a medical education surpassing that of many men and was soon considered one of the leading women physicians in the United States. In addition to her practice, she had a long career (1871–1888) as lecturer and physician at the Woman's Medical College of the New York Infirmary, founded by Elizabeth Blackwell in 1857. In 1873, she and Dr. Anna Angel, a graduate of the infirmary, launched a dispensary service for children at Mount Sinai Hospital in New York, the hospital's first outpatient service. Later the same year, she initiated a separate children's ward at the New York Infirmary. On July 22, 1873, she married Dr. Abraham Jacobi, the father of modern pediatrics. The couple had three children, but only one, Marjorie (b. 1878), survived to adulthood.

During her career, Jacobi was active in medical societies open to women. Shortly after her return from Paris, she was accepted into the Medical Library and Journal Association. A paper that she presented to the association was one of the first given by a woman to a medical society. In 1873, she became the second woman member admitted to the New York County Medical Society. She also joined the state's pathological, neurological, and therapeutic societies but was, ironically, excluded from the obstetrical society. In 1880, she became the first woman accepted into the New York Academy of Medicine and eventually chaired the neurology section.

Like many of the pioneering women physicians, Jacobi blamed the state of the medical education available to American women for their difficulty in gaining full and equal acceptance in the medical profession. In her essay "Shall Women Study Medicine?" she concluded that the "only possible excuse for this wide-spread assumption that women physicians must be inferior to men . . . may be found in the conditions under which women have hitherto been obliged to study medicine" (1925, p. 374). In an 1880 speech, she argued that "since society is . . . already supplied with quite enough doctors, the only way in which women can possibly gain footing is by displacing a certain number of men," an impossible goal as long as the "preparation afforded to the mass of women students is still inferior to that which is attainable . . . by men" (1925, p. 351).

To raise standards in women's medical education, Jacobi organized and served as president (1874–1903) of the Association for the Advancement of the Medical Education of Women (later, the Women's Medical Association). In the same vein, she was interested in improving the clinical training available to graduate women physicians who were unable to receive such training in the more advanced European hospitals. In 1880, the faculty of the infirmary appointed her to organize postgraduate instruction for the college. This plan became unnecessary when the New York Post-Graduate Medical School began admit-

ting women in 1882. When this institution appointed Jacobi as clinical lecturer of childhood diseases (1882–1885), she became the first woman to lecture at a formerly all-male school. Between 1893 and 1902, she was also visiting physician at St. Mark's Hospital in New York.

Jacobi was also a strong proponent of woman suffrage and was instrumental in the establishment of the Working Women's Society. In her essay "The Question of Rest for Women during Menstruation," (1876) she challenged the idea that menstruation required physical and mental rest, a belief that impeded women's entrance into any profession. She won Harvard's Boylston Prize for her essay in 1876, the first woman to be awarded this distinguished award.

In 1896, Jacobi began experiencing the first symptoms of the brain tumor that eventually led to her death. She died in New York City on June 10, 1906. To continue her efforts to further the medical advancement of women, the Women's Medical Association of New York City established the Mary Putnam Jacobi Fellowship to fund postgraduate study for women physicians.

See also Blackwell, Elizabeth; Sewall, Lucy Ellen; Zakrzewska, Marie Elizabeth

Selected Additional Achievements

Infant Diet (1874); *The Value of Life* (1879); *Essays on Hysteria, Brain-Tumor, and some Other Cases of Nervous Disease* (1888); *Physiological Notes on Primary Education and the Study of Language* (1889, based on her experiences educating her daughter); *"Common Sense" Applied to Women Suffrage* (1894); and *Stories and Sketches* (1907). Her last essay, "Description of the Early Symptoms of the Meningeal Tumor Compressing the Cerebellum," is an unemotional account of the symptoms of the brain tumor from which she died (see Jacobi, *Pathfinder in Medicine*, p. 501).

References

Gartner, Carol B. 1999. "Jacobi, Mary Corinna Putnam." In *American National Biography*, edited by J.A. Garraty and M.C. Carnes. New York: Oxford University Press.

Hartt, Mary Bronson. 1932. "Jacobi, Mary Corinna Putnam." In *The Dictionary of American*

Biography, edited by D. Malone. New York: Charles Scribner's Sons.

Jacobi, Mary Putnam. Memorial Pamphlet. Deceased Alumnae Files, Special Collections on Women in Medicine, Archives and Special Collections, MCP Hahnemann University, Philadelphia.

Jacobi, Mary Putnam, and Women's Medical Association of New York City. 1925. *Mary Putnam Jacobi, M.D., A Pathfinder in Medicine, with Selections from her Writings and a Complete Biography*. New York: G.P. Putnam's Sons.

Lubove, Roy. 1971. "Jacobi, Mary Corinna Putnam." In *Notable American Women, 1607–1950: A Biographical Dictionary*, edited by E.T. James, J.W. James, and P.S. Boyer. Cambridge: Belknap Press of Harvard University Press.

The National Cyclopaedia of American Biography. 1898. Vol. 8. New York: James T. White.

Withington, Alfreda B. 1978. "Jacobi, Mary Putnam." In *Dictionary of American Medical Biography: Lives of Eminent Physicians of the United States and Canada, from the Earliest Times*, edited by H.A. Kelly and W.L. Burrage. West Newfield, Maine: Longwood Press. Original ed., New York: Appleton, 1928.

JSB

James, Susan Gail (1953–   )
Nurse, Midwife

Susan James is a leader in the profession of midwifery in Canada. She was born on June 21, 1953, in Toronto, Ontario, the eldest of four children of Barbara Joan (Bagsley) and Alan Leslie James. After graduating from high school in Toronto, she entered the Women's College Hospital School of Nursing there and earned an R.N. diploma in 1973.

James then accepted a position as a staff nurse in labor and delivery at Women's College Hospital (1973–1982) and earned a bachelor's degree in nursing from the University of Toronto (1979). From 1983 to 1987, she held obstetrical nursing positions in Toronto and taught part-time continuing education courses in advanced obstetrics at Humber College. She enjoyed working with childbearing women but did not enjoy being a nurse. Moreover, although the hospital where she worked was initially supportive of natural childbirth, it gradually changed; she disliked the "distinct shift to treating all women as though they were about to die in labor" (James, interview with author).

Around this time, James began to take notice of midwives who brought their clients into the hospital. She came to see that midwifery offered a special relationship between midwife and client, a relationship of relaxed communication, trust, humor, and love that was not available in the hospital nursing environment. She decided to become a midwife but was unable to find training in Toronto. In 1987, she moved to Edmonton, Alberta, and was one of three students admitted to the first dual midwifery certification and nursing master's degree program at the University of Alberta. During her second year of study, James was allowed to train with two practicing midwives in Edmonton, Sandy Pullin and Noreen Walker. This experience, her attendance at a home birth on her own, and six weeks at a hospital where she was required to attend 30 deliveries, solidified her decision to become a midwife and not go back into obstetrical nursing. She earned her midwifery certificate in 1989 and master's degree in 1990.

In 1989, James joined Pullin's practice, With Woman Midwifery Care. The practice offered clients continuity of care, choice of birthplace, prenatal classes, postnatal support groups, and informal drop-in sessions. The midwives assisted women in the large geographical area surrounding Edmonton and had a diverse clientele, including stereotypical hippies, academics, artists, and fundamentalist Christians. With Woman Midwifery Care averaged from 50 to 60 home births and 23 to 35 hospital births per year. In addition to practicing midwifery, James supervised apprentice midwives and student midwives from the University of Alberta and taught maternal and child nursing at the university (1989–1990).

In 1990, James returned home to Toronto, where she was on the faculty of the University of Toronto's nursing school (1990–1992), as well as a coordinator for the Homecare Program of Metropolitan Toronto (1991–1992) and a prenatal educator for the Public Health Department (1990–1992). In 1992, she returned to Edmonton and the With Woman Midwifery Care practice and began working on her doctorate in nursing at the University of Alberta, which she earned in 1997. At the university, she became a research associate with the John Dossetor Health Ethics Centre (1992–present) and was a guest lecturer for a variety of undergraduate and graduate courses (1994–1999).

In 1999, James left her practice in Edmonton to accept a position as director of the Midwifery Education Programme at Laurentian University in Sudbury, Ontario. In this position she teaches theoretical and clinical midwifery courses and is involved in the administration and design of the program.

Selected Additional Achievements

Two chapters in *Reconceiving Midwifery: The "New" Canadian Model of Care* (forthcoming); "Regulation: Changing the Face of Midwifery?" in *The New Midwifery* (1997); articles in the nursing, midwifery, and health care literature. Midwifery Implementation Committee, Midwifery Regulation Advisory Committee, government of Alberta (1993–1998); assessment consultant, College of Midwives of Ontario (1994–1998), College of Midwives of British Columbia (1998–present). Midwives' Alliance of North America; president, Alberta Association of Midwives (1994–1996); coordinator, Canadian Confederation of Midwives (1997–1999). Midwifery Certificate Programme Book Prize; Ph.D. Dissertation Fellowship.

References

James, Susan. (2001). Curriculum Vitae.
James, Susan. Interview with author via E-mail. May 1, 2001.

LS

Jean, Sally Lucas (1878–1971)
Nurse

Sally Lucas Jean was a nurse and health educator who coined the term "health education" and received acclaim for her work teaching better hygiene and health habits to children. She was born in Towson, Maryland, on June 18, 1878, the youngest of three children of George and Emilie Watkins (Selby) Jean. As a child, Jean played Florence Nightingale in a school play. She was inspired by the life story of Nightingale and chose nursing as her career. However, after Jean's father died when she was 15, her family convinced her to enter his profession, teaching.

Jean completed teacher's training at Maryland State Normal School in 1896 but then entered the Maryland Homeopathic Training School for Nurses, from which she graduated in 1898. She became an army nurse, serving in hospitals in Lexington, Kentucky, and Chikamauga, Georgia, during the Spanish-American War. Following the war, she returned to Maryland, first working in a hospital, then as a private-duty nurse. She later worked for the Baltimore Department of Health as a school nurse in the Baltimore public school system. She worked with teachers and students in the classroom, teaching basic hygiene. She also opened a public bathing facility for children and began a program that lent children dry shoes and socks. In 1914, she was appointed director of the Maryland Social Health Service.

Jean moved to New York in 1917 to organize the department of health service for the People's Institute. As a member of the Committee on Wartime Problems of Childhood created by the New York Academy of Medicine, she learned that one in five children in New York City suffered from malnutrition. The findings of the committee led to the creation of the Child Health Organization (CHO) in 1918. Jean was named the organization's first director.

Jean emphasized the role of teachers in health education and encouraged teacher-training institutions to include health information in their curricula. Her work led to the formation of a separate health education section within the American Public Health Association. In 1923, the American Child Health Association was formed as a result of a merger of the CHO and the American Child Hygiene Association. Jean was named director of health education but left the association the following year.

Jean continued developing health education programs, working in the Panama Canal Zone, the Philippines, Japan, China, and the Virgin Islands. She worked for the Navajo division of the U.S. Indian Service as a health education coordinator from 1933 to 1936. She also worked as a health consultant to companies such as the National Dairy Council and Quaker Oats. In 1944, she directed health education work for the National Foundation for Infantile Paralysis.

Jean shared a home with her secretary and close friend, Dorothy Goodwin. Jean died on July 5, 1971, in New York City.

Selected Additional Achievements

Spending the Day in China, Japan, and the Philippines (1932, with Grace T. Hallock). State Service Award, New York State Association for Health, Physical Education and Recreation (1948); William Howe Award, American School Health Association (1948); honorary M.A., Bates College (1924). President, Association of Women in Public Health (1937–1940); fellow, American Public Health Association.

References

Bullough, Vern L. 1988. "Sally Lucas Jean." In *American Nursing: A Biographical Dictionary*, edited by V.L. Bullough, O.M. Church, and A.P. Stein. New York: Garland.

Gevitz, N. 1984. "Jean, Sally Lucas." In *Dictionary of American Medical Biography*, edited by M. Kaufman, S. Galishoff, and T.L. Savitt. Westport, Conn.: Greenwood Press.

Rudavsky, Shari. 1999. "Jean, Sally Lucas." In *American National Biography*, edited by J.A. Garraty and M.C. Carnes. New York: Oxford University Press.

Who Was Who in America with World Notables: Volume V, 1969–1973. 1973. Chicago: Marquis-Who's Who.

DTW

Johns, Ethel Mary Incledon (1879–1968)
Nurse

Ethel Johns was the first director of the University of British Columbia's School of Nursing and a leader in the field of nursing in Canada as well as internationally. She was born on May 13, 1879, in Meonstoke, Southampton, England, the oldest of three children of Henry Incledon and Amy (Robinson) Johns. Her early education was at a boarding school in Denbigh, Wales, and at a school on the Wabigoon Indian Reserve in Ontario, Canada, where her father had accepted a teaching position.

In 1899, Johns entered the Winnipeg (Manitoba) Hospital Training School for Nurses. She graduated in 1902 and then held various nursing positions in Canada and in the United States. In 1905, she was an instructor and a head nurse at Winnipeg General Hospital, and in 1907 she was placed in charge of the hospital's newly created X-ray department. Also in 1907, she helped to found and was named editor of the *Nurses' Alumnae Journal* of the Winnipeg General Hospital. In 1909, she was elected president of the Alumnae Association and in 1911 was elected president of the Manitoba Association of Graduate Nurses. She became superintendent and director of nurses at McKellar General Hospital in Fort William, Ontario, in 1911 but resigned after only a year in order to care for her ailing mother.

In 1914 Johns took courses in science,

public health, teaching methods, and nursing school administration at Teachers College, Columbia University in New York City. In 1915, she returned to Manitoba as superintendent and principal of the nursing school at Children's Hospital of Winnipeg, where she taught anatomy and physiology, practical nursing, and history of nursing. She was also active in the Manitoba Association of Registered Nurses and the Canadian Society of Superintendents of Training Schools, for which she served on a committee to study nursing education. In October 1917, she was appointed to the Public Welfare Commission of Manitoba.

In 1919, Johns resigned from Children's Hospital and became director of nursing service and education at Vancouver General Hospital as well as coordinator of the nursing program at the University of British Columbia in Vancouver. She helped to transform the hospital from a small, specialized institution into a 1,000-bed multifunction hospital. Johns designed a two-track program for the nursing school, where students could receive either a nursing diploma after studying at the hospital or a diploma and a degree if they combined hospital study with university courses. She resigned as director of nursing in 1921 but remained director of education until May 1922, when she became a full-time member of the university's faculty.

In 1925, Johns accepted a job with the Rockefeller Foundation in Europe as a special member of the Field Staff in Nursing Education. She served there in an advisory capacity and was responsible for the management of a nursing fellows program. She was also instrumental in the reorganization of the

nursing school in Debrecen, Hungary. After her service in Europe, she served on two nursing committees in the United States before returning to Canada in 1933 to become editor and business manager of the Canadian Nurses Association official journal, *Canadian Nurse*. She enhanced the journal by ensuring that it reflected provincial, national, and international nursing concerns, and within three years, circulation increased by 1,000.

After her retirement in 1944, Johns continued to be active in nursing organizations and wrote a series of pamphlets called *Just Plain Nursing*, as well as two histories of nursing schools. She died on September 2, 1968, in Vancouver.

Selected Additional Achievements

The Johns Hopkins Hospital School of Nursing 1889–1929 (with Blanche Pfefferkorn, 1954); *The Winnipeg General Hospital School of Nursing, 1887–1953* (1957). Mary Agnes Snively Medal (1940); honorary doctor of laws, Mount Allison University (1948); honorary life membership, Canadian Nurses Association (1958).

References

Davis, Althea T. 1992. "Ethel Mary Incledon Johns." In *American Nursing: A Biographical Dictionary*, edited by V.L. Bullough, L. Sentz, and A.P. Stein. New York: Garland.

Street, Margaret M. 1973. *Watch-fires on the Mountains: The Life and Writings of Ethel Johns.* Toronto: University of Toronto Press.

University of British Columbia Archives. *Ethel Johns Fonds.* Online. http://www.library.ubc.ca/spcoll/ubc_arch/u_arch/johns.html. 29 April 2001.

LS

Johnson, Halle Tanner Dillon (1864–1901)
Physician

Halle Dillon Johnson was an early African American physician who became the first woman licensed to practice medicine in Alabama. She was born on October 17, 1864,

in Pittsburgh, the daughter of Benjamin Tucker Tanner, a leader in the African Methodist Episcopal Church, and Sarah Elizabeth (Miller) Tanner and the sister of Henry Ossawa Tanner, a famous artist. In 1886, she married Charles E. Dillon, of Trenton, New Jersey, and a child was born to the couple the next year. Dillon soon died, and Halle returned to her family home in Philadelphia. In 1888, she enrolled at the city's Woman's Medical College of Pennsylvania (now MCP Hahnemann University), the only black student in her class. She graduated on May 7, 1891, with high honors.

Around the same time, Booker T. Washington, president of the African American Tuskegee Institute in Alabama, wrote to the dean of the Woman's Medical College in search of a black woman physician for the institute. Johnson's name was mentioned, and she accepted Washington's offer. She arrived in Tuskegee on August 3, 1891. All physicians in Alabama were required to pass a difficult examination before practicing, so she soon traveled to the state capital at Montgomery to sit for the 10-day exam. The local press watched the black woman physician's comings and goings with great curiosity, ridiculing the idea that she would even dare to appear. She held up well to the scrutiny and passed the examinations, thus becoming the first woman, of any race, to legally practice medicine in Alabama.

As resident physician at the Tuskegee In-

stitute (1891–1894), Johnson taught two classes a day, headed the Institute's health department, and compounded medicine as needed. She also established the Lafayette Dispensary to help care for the local people of Tuskegee and a training school for nurses.

In 1894, Johnson married an African Methodist Episcopal minister and Tuskegee math instructor, John Quincy Johnson. The next year, the couple moved to Columbia, South Carolina, and later to Princeton, New Jersey, before settling in Nashville, Tennessee. Nothing is known about Johnson's medical career after she moved from Tuskegee. She died in Nashville on April 26, 1901, from complications of childbirth. She had three sons with John Quincy Johnson.

References

Dillon, Halle Tanner. Deceased Alumnae Files, Special Collections on Women in Medicine, Archives and Special Collections, MCP Hahnemann University, Philadelphia.

Smith, Jessie Carney. 1992. "Halle Tanner Dillon Johnson." In *Notable Black American Women*, edited by J.C. Smith. Detroit: Gale.

Smith, Jessie Carney. 1999. "Johnson, Halle Tanner Dillon." In *American National Biography*, edited by J.A. Garraty and M.C. Carnes. New York: Oxford University Press.

LS

Jumper, Betty Mae Tiger (1923–   )
Nurse

Betty Mae Jumper was the first Seminole Indian woman to become a nurse. She was born near Lake Okeechobee in the Florida Everglades on April 27, 1923, the daughter of Mae Tiger, a full-blooded Seminole, and Abe Partan, a white French trapper and cane cutter. Partan had little direct influence on Jumper's life, however, as he left the area while Jumper was still very young.

Jumper's maternal grandmother, Mary Tiger, was a midwife who assisted with Jumper's birth. At that time, the Seminoles did not accept multiracial children and often smothered or drowned them immediately af-

ter birth. Although her maternal grandfather protected Jumper and, later, her brother Howard, the family continued to live in fear until Mae Tiger moved her family to the Dania Indian Reservation near Fort Lauderdale when Jumper was five years old.

Jumper's mother followed family tradition and practiced midwifery and traditional Native American medicine. She watched her mother and soon recognized the limitations of Indian medicine. She witnessed the deaths of many newborns and children, including the death of her three-year-old sister from whooping cough. She realized that an education could help her learn to save children from dying, and she attended the day school on the reservation until it closed in 1936. She also persuaded her family to allow her and her brother to attend a government-funded Indian boarding school in Cherokee, North Carolina, over 1,000 miles from home. Four other Seminole children accompanied the Jumper children to North Carolina. Jumper and a cousin later became the first Seminoles to graduate from high school (1945).

After graduation, Jumper moved to Lawton, Oklahoma, to study nursing at the Kiowa Indian Hospital. She chose nursing partly because her ancestors had been healers but also because she realized the value of modern medicine and was driven by the desire to help her people. She completed a one-year course in public health nursing, becoming the first Seminole trained nurse. She returned to Florida in 1946 to work as a nurse for the Bureau of Indian Affairs on the Seminole reservations. Also in 1946, she married Moses Jumper, one of only two Seminoles to serve in World War II. Together they raised two sons and a daughter. In the 1950s, Jumper traveled between the reservations of Dania, Big Cypress, and Brighton in the Everglades, working tirelessly to improve the health of the Seminole people. Her work was met with prejudice and sometimes firearms by those who did not trust modern medicine. Gradually, she was able to gain the respect of tribal members by speaking with them in traditional languages and helping to improve their health. In recognition of her work, a health clinic on the Dania Reservation (now the Hollywood Reservation) is named in her honor.

During the late 1950s the status of the Seminoles as a recognized Indian nation was threatened by the termination policy of the Bureau of Indian Affairs. During this turbulent time, Jumper acted as an interpreter of the new ways for the older members of the tribes. For the next decade, she was active in the administration of the Seminole tribe, culminating with her election as the first and only female tribal council chair (1967–1971). Although she became less involved in nursing as her political career advanced, she continued to emphasize the importance of public health. During her tenure with the Seminole Tribal Council, she improved the health care as well as the education, social, economic, and housing conditions of the Seminoles.

Since leaving political life in 1971, Jumper has served as the director of operations for Seminole Communications. In 1979, she founded the *Seminole Tribune*, the official newspaper of the Seminole Nation, and is editor in chief.

Selected Additional Achievements

. . . *and with the Wagon Came God's Word* (her memoirs, 1980); *Legends of the Seminoles* (1994). National Congress of Indian Opportunity Council (1970); Florida Women's Hall of Fame (1995); Top 50 Indian Women in the United States, North American Indian Woman's Association (1971); Woman of the Year, Jewish Women's Defense League (1990); Folklife Heritage Award, Florida Department of State (1994); honorary doctorate of humane letters, Florida State University (1994); Lifetime Achievement Award, Native American Journalists Association (1997).

References

Kasee, Cynthia R. 1995. "Betty Mae Tiger Jumper." In *Notable Native Americans*, edited by S. Malinowski and G.H.J. Abrams. New York: Gale Research.

Kersey, Harry A. 1993. "Jumper, Betty Mae." In *Native American Women: A Biographical Dictionary*, edited by G.M. Bataille. New York: Garland.

McDonald, Dan. 1997. "Betty Mae Jumper." *The Seminole Tribune*. Online. http://seminole tribe.com/tribune/40anniversary/interview_bjumper.shtml. 7 May 1998.

CMB

K

Kinney, Dita Hopkins (1854–1921)
Nurse

Dita Kinney was the first superintendent of the United States Army Nurse Corps. She was born in New York City on September 13, 1854, to C.T. and Myra (Burtnett) Hopkins. After graduating from Mills Seminary in California, she married Mark Kinney in 1874 and had one son. Following her husband's death in 1878, Kinney moved to Boston, where she graduated from the Massachusetts General Hospital Training School for Nurses (1892). Afterward, Kinney taught nursing for the Young Women's Christian Association and trained women to be nursing assistants. She was then superintendent of the Long Island Almshouse (1892–1896) in Boston Harbor and superintendent for the City and County Hospital in St. Paul, Minnesota (1897).

In September 1898, Kinney joined the United States Army as a contract nurse to care for veterans of the Spanish-American War. During the next two years, she worked at the General Hospital and the French Hospital, both in San Francisco, the convalescent home of the Oakland, California, Red Cross Society, and the Army Hospital at Fort Bayard, New Mexico. In August 1900, she was transferred to the Office of the Surgeon General of the Army

in Washington, D.C. She was assigned as one of the chief nurses on the staff of acting assistant surgeon general Anita McGee. That year, McGee wrote the section of the Army Reorganization Act that established a permanent Army Nurse Corps. McGee then resigned from her position and appointed Kinney to direct the corps.

On March 15, 1901, Kinney began her duties as the first superintendent of the Army Nurse Corps. Army nurses received low pay and did not enjoy high professional or social status, and her efforts to raise the nurses' standing were thwarted by the fact that she had very little authoritative power. Although she was able to secure some improvements for the nurses, her most important recommendations—those regarding the education, evaluation, supervision, and promotion of nurses—were rejected by army surgeon general George Torney. In 1904, he announced a plan to establish an army nurse reserve to be used in times of national emergency. However, the status of army nurses made it difficult for Kinney to attract a sufficient number of applicants, and in July 1906 she resigned at Torney's request. She was succeeded by Jane Delano, whose association with the American Red Cross allowed her to transfer the members of the Red Cross Nursing Corps into the Army Nurse Reserve.

Following her resignation, Kinney completed a course in hospital management at Massachusetts General Hospital and took a position as superintendent of Addison Gilbert Hospital in Gloucester, Massachusetts. A heart problem forced her resignation in 1912. Despite her ailment, she taught home nursing during World War I for the Penobscott, Maine, Red Cross and at the Eastern Maine General Hospital. She died in Bangor, Maine, on April 16, 1921.

See also Delano, Jane Arminda; McGee, Anita Newcomb

References

Danis, Eileen M., and Rosemary T. McCarthy. 1988. "Dita Hopkins Kinney." In *American Nursing: A Biographical Dictionary*, edited by V.L. Bullough, O.M. Church, and A.P. Stein. New York: Garland.

Dock, Lavinia L., Sarah Elizabeth Pickett, Clara D. Noyes, Fannie F. Clement, Elizabeth G. Fox, and Ann R. Van Meter. 1922. *History of American Red Cross Nursing*. New York: Macmillan.

Surgeon General, Department of the Army. 1958. *Highlights in the History of the Army Nurse Corps*. Washington, D.C.: Government Printing Office.

JSB

L

Lang, Raven (1942–   )
Midwife

Raven Lang helped reestablish and legitimate the practice of lay midwifery in the United States in the 1970s. Her Santa Cruz [California] Birth Center demonstrated the safety and efficacy of home birth and natural childbirth methods and made them more acceptable to American women. She was born to Emma Parenti Lang on December 17, 1942, in San Francisco and was given the name Patricia, which she later changed to Raven. Lang attended San Francisco City College and graduated with an associate's degree in premedical studies in 1962. She also pursued art studies at San Francisco State College (1964) and at the San Francisco Art Institute (1965–1966).

While attending the institute, she met and fell in love with Ken Kinzie; the couple married in 1966. When she was 25, Lang became pregnant. She was interested in experiencing a natural childbirth, rather than being sedated, so she began reading on the topic. Despite her determination and self-education, her obstetrician rushed the birth along by performing an unnecessarily extensive episiotomy, which resulted in a painful recovery for Lang. This experience led her to question the medicalization of childbirth, a process that she believed should be normal and natural. She began to attend home births as a witness and continued her studies on natural childbirth. She became a childbirth educator and accompanied laboring women to the hospital, where she coached them through the birthing process and encouraged them to remain conscious.

An experience attending a woman named Kathy in a hospital in 1970 caused Lang to lose faith in the hospital as the ideal location for having a baby. Kathy's labor progressed normally until a doctor, who wished to keep a lunch appointment, ordered a drug to slow her progress. Later, when it was convenient for the physician, Kathy was given the powerful hormone pitocin to speed up the labor. The rapid progress put the baby in distress and forced the physician to use forceps to extract it quickly, giving the baby a concussion. Lang later said, "Seeing Kathy there like that after having worked with her and knowing her expectations and dreams for herself and her baby made my heart scream. It was then that I vowed to help the next pregnant woman seeking an alternative method of birth" (quoted in Arms, p. 267).

Lang continued to teach childbirth classes, emphasizing the rights of pregnant women in the hospital, and began collecting data on hospital versus home birth. Before long, expectant mothers and their mates started asking her to act as their midwife. Believing that she and others like her must begin to take responsibility for reclaiming the birth process, she agreed to become a midwife and helped women give birth in their own homes. In 1971, physicians called a meeting to discuss the increasing incidence of midwife-attended home births in the Santa Cruz area. Lang and a physician friend, the primary people who were attending these births, were not allowed to attend the meeting or to speak on behalf of the Santa Cruz women. The meeting concluded with the physicians declaring their intention to refuse prenatal care to pregnant women who chose to have their babies at home or who chose to seek the help of midwives.

Lang and other local midwives responded by offering prenatal care themselves at the Santa Cruz Birth Center, which opened in March 1971. It was a place for them to learn from one another, as well as a clinic for prenatal care and for other care related to pregnancy and childbirth. Lang's efforts with the center inspired women in other communities to take similar action. On March 25, 1972, she invited the medical community, parents, midwives, and supporters to a symposium to show that the Santa Cruz midwives were competent birth attendants. The meeting room was decorated with large black and white photographs of actual home births, and statistics were presented by the midwives showing the safety of home birth. Later that year, Lang published the *Birth Book*, which contained photographs of home births and personal narratives of women who had given birth at home. The book was an instant success and was published in Germany and Italy and in braille in the United States.

In 1973 Lang went to Canada to begin work at a clinic funded by the government of British Columbia and the federal government of Canada. From 1973 to 1976, she was a midwife in Vancouver, British Columbia, and in 1974 she began to work on Vancouver Island and acted as a midwife to women of the Gulf Islands. She cowrote and codirected a Canadian federal grant that allowed women to be educated for direct entry to the midwifery profession and funded pre-, intra-, and postpartum care. In the spring of 1976, she returned to California to give birth to her second child and in the fall moved back to California with her family.

From 1978 to 1984, Lang was director of the Institute of Feminine Arts, a California state-certified college dedicated to the study of midwifery. From 1982 to 1984, she studied at the American College of Traditional Chinese Medicine in San Francisco and earned the doctor of Oriental medicine degree from the Tokyo College of Oriental Medicine in 1985. She is currently a practitioner of traditional Chinese medicine and a licensed acupuncturist in Santa Cruz, California. She has lectured across North America and in Canada on women's health, childbirth, and women's studies.

Selected Additional Achievements

Mother Roasting: The Use of Traditional Chinese Medicine in Postpartum Care (1985); *Blessingway into Birth: A Rite of Passage* (1993); *The History and Politics of Women's Health Care* (1996). Woman of the Year Award, Santa Cruz County (1985); Brazen Women's Award, California Association of Midwives (1999).

References

Arms, Suzanne. 1975. *Immaculate Deception: A New Look at Women and Childbirth in America.* Boston: Houghton Mifflin.

Edwards, Margot, and Mary Waldorf. 1984. *Reclaiming Birth: History and Heroines of American Childbirth Reform.* Trumansberg, N.Y.: Crossing Press.

Lang, Raven. N.d. Curriculum Vitae.

Mitchell, Selena. 2001. "An Interview with Raven Lang, OMD, LAc." *California Journal of Oriental Medicine* 12(1):38–41.

LS

La Roe, Else Kienle (1900–1970)
Physician

Else La Roe, a German-born physician, re-located to New York during World War II. There, she became a pioneer in cosmetic surgery and was most noted for her work in breast reconstructive surgery. She was born in Heidenheim, Germany, on June 26, 1900, the eldest daughter of Otto and Elisabeth Kienle. During World War I she volunteered at a Red Cross Hospital. After observing an operation on the mutilated face of a soldier, she decided to become a plastic surgeon. In 1918, she graduated from a high school in Esslingen and in 1923 graduated from the University of Heidelberg Medical School. Afterward, she was accepted for clinical training in reconstructive surgery at the Lexer Clinic in Freiburg.

La Roe's first position was at Catherine's Hospital in Stuttgart, where she worked as a dermatologist in the venereal disease department. She was especially moved by the plight of her female patients, whose infections led to the loss of their respectability and often their chance at motherhood. Around 1928, she borrowed money from her fiancé to purchase a small surgical hospital (according to her autobiography, her fiancé was named Stephan Arnold; however, Riepl-Schmidt refers to him as Stephan Jacobowitz).

During the early 1930s, La Roe was actively involved in the German movement for accessible birth control and legal abortion. She performed many abortions and was placed under arrest until her release following a well-publicized hunger strike. In the meantime, she and her husband divorced. When the Nazis seized power, many members of the sex reform movement were forced into exile. La Roe was found guilty of high treason but was rescued from Germany when she married American George Henry La Roe. In 1932, they moved to New York, where she could practice safely. The couple eventually divorced, and she was later married for a short time to a dentist.

According to historian Atina Grossmann, in New York La Roe "quickly transferred her passionate commitment to the betterment of women from the struggle for birth control . . . to women's right to bodily self-improvement" (p. 173). At the time, the breast was not considered integral to women's physical health, and surgical improvements to the breast were often seen as vain and unnecessary. To counteract this belief, La Roe published two books: *The Breast Beautiful* (1940) and *Care of the Breast* (1947). These books were instrumental in legitimating the importance of the breast to women's physiological and psychological health. She wrote *The Breast Beautiful* to help "every woman to preserve . . . the health and beauty of so important an organ of her body" (1947 reprint, p. 17). She criticized fads that encouraged women to wear stiff undergarments that affected blood circulation and caused deformities. In the preface of *Care of the Breast*, she wrote: "I hope that my detailed advice based on vast experience in this particular field . . . will be of benefit to the practicing physician and to women in their quest for a better physical and emotional outlook on life." She prescribed surgery as a legitimate treatment for women with overly large breasts, a condition that led to back pain and pressure on the diaphragm, heart, lungs, and spine.

La Roe instructed women on the latest methods of breast examination to alert them to potential cancer. For women who were forced to have one cancerous breast removed, La Roe devised an operation by which the remaining breast was grafted onto the amputated one and eventually divided to form two breasts. Around 1952, she founded the American Society for the Reduction of Cancer Casualties, formed to encourage patients to seek early treatment when they or their doctors suspected that cancer was present.

In 1951, La Roe married her fourth husband, Wesley Le Roy Robertson, a Native American musician. She died in 1970.

References

Grossmann, Atina. 1995. *Reforming Sex: The German Movement for Birth Control and Abortion Reform, 1920–1950.* New York: Oxford University Press.

La Roe, Else K. 1947a. *Care of the Breast.* New York: Froben Press.

La Roe, Else K. 1947b. Table of contents and introduction from *The Breast Beautiful.* Reprint ed. New York: Froben Press. Original ed., New York: House of Field, 1940.

La Roe, Else K. 1957. *Woman Surgeon.* New York: Dial Press.

"News of Women in Medicine." 1952. *Journal of the American Medical Women's Association* 7 (9):357–358.

Riepl-Schmidt, Maja. 1993. "Else Kienle (1900–1970)." In *Frauen im Deutschen Südwesten*, edited by B. Knorr and R. Wehling. Stuttgart: Verlag W. Kohlhammer.

"Science Notes." 1940. *Newsweek* (September 23):46.

JSB

Leete, Harriet L. (ca. 1875–1927)
Nurse

Harriet Leete was an early leader in the effort to promote child health care in the United States. She was born around 1875 in Cleveland, Ohio, where she received her nursing education at the Lakeside Training School for Nurses. She graduated on March 23, 1901, and was then a private-duty nurse in various New York cities and served as head of the men's surgical ward at Lakeside Hospital in Cleveland (1902–1906). In 1906, she became a nurse at the Infant's Clinic of the Babies Dispensary, also in Cleveland, where she developed well-baby programs until 1917.

During World War I, Leete sailed for Europe (1917). She worked for the Red Cross Bureau of Tuberculosis and then for the Rockefeller Commission for the Prevention of Tuberculosis in conjunction with French hospitals. In September the same year, she became chief nurse of the Children's Bureau of the Department of Civil Affairs for the Red Cross Commission for France. In this capacity, she trained Frenchwomen to make home visits in Paris. After being transferred to military duty, she was appointed chief nurse of the American Red Cross Military Hospital, Number 5, Auteuil Tent Hospital. Beginning in early 1919, she became chief nurse in northern Siberia for the Balkan Commission. She received government recognition for the work there but was forced to return home in July after contracting typhus.

Back in the United States, Leete accepted a position with the American Child Hygiene Association. As field director for the association, she oversaw adoption and child-care standards for young children. Her duties were expanded to include older children when the association joined the American Child Health Association. During the early 1920s, as director of the Maternity Center Association (New York), she organized a Mothercraft Club to provide prenatal care and instruction. The recurring effects of typhus forced her to obtain a less demanding career as director of Wavecrest, a convalescent home for children in Far Rockaway, New York.

Leete died of an acute mastoid infection on November 9, 1927, in Brooklyn. She was buried near Jamestown, New York, with full military honors.

References

Bullough, Vern L. "Harriet L. Leete." 1992. In *American Nursing: A Biographical Dictionary*, edited by V.L. Bullough, L. Sentz, and A.P. Stein. New York: Garland.

Hawkins, Joellen Watson. 1988. "Leete, Harriet L." In *Dictionary of American Nursing Biography*, edited by M. Kaufman. New York: Greenwood Press.

Noyes, Clara D. 1928. "The Passing of Harriet L. Leete." *American Journal of Nursing* 28(1):71–72.

JSB

Leonard, Carol L. (1950–   )
Midwife

Carol Leonard is a New Hampshire midwife who was instrumental in seeing the passage of midwifery legislation enabling the legal certification of midwives practicing in that state. She was born in Bangor, Maine, on June 10, 1950, the oldest of four children of Parker and Louis Leonard. She attended West Side High School in Manchester, New Hampshire, and then received a biology degree from New England College in Henniker, New Hampshire (1974). In 1981, she married Dr. Kenneth McKinney, an obstetrician.

After the birth of her son, Milan Mc-Alevey, in 1975, Leonard decided to become a midwife. During her labor, the hospital staff left her alone in the bathroom, discouraged her from pushing or making noises, and tied her hands down when her son's head began to crown. After the delivery, Leonard was ignored when she asked to hold her son. This experience sparked a desire to "help women know about sane childbirth" (quoted in Chester, p. 183). Later the same year, she began training with a local physician in rural New Hampshire (1975–1977) and co-founded the Concord Midwifery Service. During her twelve-year practice with the service, she attended over 1,000 healthy births.

Leonard was very active in promoting midwifery in New Hampshire. She spearheaded a successful campaign for the passage of legislation that allowed for the legal certification of midwives in 1982. Hundreds of women who had midwife-attended births came to state hearings to attest to the safety of such births. Leonard also served on the Advisory Committee to the New Hampshire Director of Health and Welfare to develop rules and regulations for midwives (1981–1984). She then worked on a review committee to oversee the implementation of the certification program, and in 1985, she became the state's first certified independent midwife. In 1999, the governor appointed her as the first chairperson of the Midwifery Council. The council is the country's first independent midwife regulatory agency.

Leonard has also worked on behalf of her profession outside her home state. She was a charter member (1982) of the Midwives' Alliance of North American (MANA), a national organization representing midwives in the United States, Canada, and Mexico. In 1984, she was elected vice president of MANA and then president in 1986. In 1984, she went to Sydney, Australia, to represent MANA in its successful bid for membership in the International Confederation of Midwives. In 1991, she traveled to Moscow to improve maternity care in Russia and was the first American midwife to teach midwifery there. The following year she spoke to the U.S. Congress about the deplorable birth practices in Russia, and her testimony appeared in the *Congressional Record*.

After the death of her husband in 1987, Leonard limited her practice. She presents workshops to women's groups around the country on "Women's Ordinary Magic" and "Witches, Midwives and Other Healers." She also teaches alternative medicine and therapies to women going through menopause and those with chronic illnesses. In September 2000, she opened the Longmeadow Farm Midwifery Service and Birthing Home, central New Hampshire's only freestanding birth center and the second out-of-hospital center in the state. The center offers a safe alternative to hospital births and serves as a teaching facility for student midwives.

Selected Additional Achievements

"Hearts and Bones: The Baby Boomer's Survival Guide to Menopause," in *WomenWise* (1997); *Lady's Hands, Lion's Heart: Memoirs of a Radical Midwife* (unpublished autobiography, 1998). President, New Hampshire Midwives Association (1976–1985); original board member, Concord Feminist Health Center (1976–1978); member, New Hampshire Homebirth Committee (1978–1979); Bronze Medal for Bravery, Australian government (1984).

References

Chester, Penfield. 1997. *Sisters on a Journey: Portraits of American Midwives*. New Brunswick, N.J.: Rutgers University Press.

Davis, Elizabeth, and Carol Leonard. 1996. *The Women's Wheel of Life, Thirteen Archetypes of Woman at Her Fullest Power*. New York: Viking Arkana.

Leonard, Carol. 1999. Curriculum Vitae.

Leonard, Carol. May 17, 2001. Interview with author via E-mail.

Leonard, Carol. N.d. Biographical Sketch.

Longmeadow Farm Midwifery Service & Birthing Home. Online. http://www.longmeadowfarm midwifery.com. 12 May 2001.

JSB

Leone, Lucile Petry (1902–1999)
Nurse

Lucile Petry Leone, an American nursing leader, was the first female assistant surgeon general of the U.S. Public Health Service. She was born in Lewiston, Ohio, on January 23, 1902, the only child of David Petry, a high school principal, and Dora (Murray) Petry. She chose nursing because the field combined her love of science with her desire to contribute to the public good.

Leone earned a B.A. degree in chemistry from the University of Delaware (1924) and then entered the Johns Hopkins School of Nursing. She graduated from Johns Hopkins in 1928 and continued there doing postgraduate work in psychiatric nursing while also working as head nurse in several Johns Hopkins hospital wards. In 1929, she earned an M.A. degree from Teachers College, Columbia University and then began work at the University of Minnesota School of Nursing, where she advanced from clinical instructor, to associate professor, to assistant director. At Minnesota, she was involved in early efforts to encourage students to become involved in other university departments and thus broaden their educational experiences.

In 1940, Leone was asked to complete a study for the North Central Accrediting Association on local baccalaureate nursing programs. According to Leone, the report that she wrote as a result of the study "helped place nursing programs in universities in the region as credible and valuable university offerings and . . . supported other universities that were considering the development of nursing programs" (Leone, p. 209). After two years with the association, Leone was appointed as dean of the New York Hospital School of Nursing at Cornell University. However, the military and civilian nursing demands created by World War II called her out of this position after only one month.

In 1943, Leone was recruited by U.S. surgeon general, Dr. Thomas Parran, to serve as director of the Cadet Nurse Corps in the Division of Nurse Education of the U.S. Public Health Service (USPHS). Over a three-year period, Leone recruited 179,000 cadets into the corps. To meet heightened demands for training military nurses, she oversaw improved nurse education in 1,150 nursing schools. Despite these impressive achievements, she believed that the most beneficial effect of the corps was elevated public awareness of the importance of nursing and increased efforts by school administrators to improve educational standards. At the close of the Cadet Nurse Corps program, in 1949, Leone was appointed as chief nurse officer of the USPHS. With this appointment, she was given the rank of assistant surgeon general of the Public Health Service Commissioned Officer Corps and thus earned the distinction of being the first woman to earn this rank.

Leone was also a member of the U.S. Delegation to the first World Health Organization assembly held in Geneva, Switzerland, in 1948. She was later a member of the organization's Expert Committee on Nursing and worked with member nations to improve health conditions in those countries. In 1952, she married USPHS researcher Dr.

Nicholas C. Leone. She retired from the Public Health Service in February 1966, and that year, the service awarded her its Distinguished Service Medal and established the Lucile Petry Leone Award in her honor. She and her husband relocated to Dallas, Texas, where she served as associate dean of Texas Woman's University until 1971. She died on November 25, 1999.

Selected Additional Achievements

President, National League for Nursing; fellow, American College of Hospital Administrators. Board member, National League of Nursing Education, National Academy of Sciences, Board of Medical Education and Research, American Journal of Nursing, and *American Journal of Public Health*; editorial adviser on nursing for McGraw-Hill Book Company. Her presentation "Today's Challenge to the College Women in the Professions" was entered into the *Congressional Record*. Awards include the American Legion Auxiliary Award (1955); the Lasker Award (1955), the Florence Nightingale Medal of the International Committee of the Red Cross; and at least six honorary degrees.

References

Haritos, Delores J. 1992. "Lucile Petry Leone." In *American Nursing: A Biographical Dictionary*, edited by V.L. Bullough, L. Sentz, and A.P. Stein. New York: Garland.

Leone, Lucile Petry. 1988. "Lucile Petry Leone." In *Making Choices, Taking Chances: Nurse Leaders Tell Their Stories*, edited by T.M. Schorr and A. Zimmerman. St. Louis: C.V. Mosby.

"Obituary." 1999. *Cleveland Plain Dealer* (December 6):5B.

Petry, Lucile. 1945. "The U.S. Cadet Nurse Corps: A Summing Up." *American Journal of Nursing* 45 (12):1027–1028.

Petry, Lucile. 1949. "We Hail an Important 'First.' " *American Journal of Nursing* 49 (10): 630.

Roberts, Mary. 1954. *American Nursing: History and Interpretation*. New York: Macmillan.

JSB

L'Esperance, Elise Depew Strang (ca. 1878–1959)
Physician

Elise L'Esperance, an American physician, founded the world's first clinic devoted to the detection and prevention of cancer. L'Esperance was born around 1878 in Yorktown, New York, the second daughter of Dr. Albert Strang and Kate (Depew) Strang. She received her early education at the St. Agnes Episcopal School in Albany, New York. In 1896, she entered the Woman's Medical College of the New York Infirmary for Women and Children, founded by Dr. Elizabeth Blackwell in 1868. Although the college closed in 1899, a bout with diphtheria kept her from receiving her diploma until 1900. That year, she also entered into a short marriage with David L'Esperance, a lawyer.

After graduation, L'Esperance began a one-year internship at New York Babies Hospital. She was then in private practice for two years in Detroit and in New York until 1908. She specialized in pediatrics, but an interest in tuberculosis led to her association with the Tuberculosis Research Commission of New York. With the commission, she studied bacteriology for the New York City Department of Health. This work led to her ultimate desire to specialize in pathology. She sought a position with James Ewing, a cancer specialist at Cornell University Medical College. Although Ewing had refused to employ women in the past, he accepted L'Esperance as his assistant in 1910. She studied with him until 1912, when she was appointed as an instructor at Cornell's Pathology Department. In 1914, she took a six-month leave from Cornell to study pathology in Munich, Germany, on a Mary Putnam Jacobi Fellowship. Her work there was published in the *Journal of Medical Research* (1915).

L'Esperance continued as instructor until she was appointed assistant professor in the Pathology Department (1920–1932), the first woman ever to obtain that status at Cornell. From 1942 to 1950, she held an appointment as assistant professor in Cornell's Department of Preventative Medicine. She earned status as a full professor in the same department in 1950, a post that she held until her death. In addition to her teaching duties at Cornell, L'Esperance served in other capacities at New York area hospitals. She was pathologist and director of laboratories at the New York Infirmary for Women and Children (1917–1927, 1929–1954). Between 1917 and 1920, she served as assistant pathologist at New York Hospital, as pathologist at Manhattan Maternity Hospital, and as assistant pathologist at Memorial Hospital for Cancer, and she was instructor of surgical pathology at Bellevue Hospital (1919–1932).

After their mother died of cancer in 1930, L'Esperance and her sister, May Strang, founded the Kate Depew Strang Tumor Clinic at the New York Infirmary for Women and Children in 1933. The clinic was dedicated to the diagnosis and treatment of cancer in women. Realizing that early detection was more important than cure, the clinic became the Kate Depew Strang Cancer Prevention Clinic in 1937. Staffed entirely by women, it was not only the first clinic established to prevent cancer in women through early diagnosis but also the first cancer detection facility in the world. In 1940, L'Esperance established the Strang Cancer Prevention Clinic at New York's Memorial Hospital for Cancer and Allied Diseases, later including care for men and children. By 1950, the two clinics had examined 35,000 patients, detecting precancerous conditions in 18 percent of them.

In a 1945 article, L'Esperance wrote that her facilities "differed from the diagnostic cancer clinics in that regular visits from normal . . . persons were encouraged believing that in this way the habit of periodic cancer health examinations may be formed" (p. 25). If no evidence of cancer was detected, the patient was instructed to return in six months to one year. If the examination revealed disease, the patient was referred to another doctor or hospital for treatment. Several

important developments in cancer detection were made at the clinics, such as the Pap smear for cervical cancer and the protoscope for colon or rectal cancers. The Strang Cancer Prevention Center exists today and is considered the foremost cancer prevention institute in the United States.

In her later years, L'Esperance was still active in many medical societies and served as consultant pathologist to the New York Infirmary (1954–1955). She lived with her sister in a home in Pelham Manor, New York. L'Esperance died on January 21, 1959.

See also Blackwell, Elizabeth; Jacobi, Mary Corinna Putnam

Selected Additional Achievements

President, New York State Women's Medical Society (1935–1936); editor, *Medical Woman's Journal* (1936–1941); first editor, *Journal of the American Medical Women's Association* (1946–1948); delegate, Fourth International Cancer Research Conference (1947); first woman recipient, Clement Cleveland Medal, New York City Cancer Committee (1942); president, American Medical Women's Association (1948–1949); Elizabeth Blackwell Citation, New York City Cancer Committee (1950); Lasker Award for Medical Research, American Public Health Association (1951).

References

Dwork, Deborah. 1980. "L'Esperance, Elise Strang." In *Notable American Women: The Modern Period: A Biographical Dictionary*, edited by B. Sicherman and C.H. Green. Cambridge: Belknap Press of Harvard University Press.

L'Esperance, Elise S. 1944. "Cancer Prevention Clinics." *Medical Woman's Journal* 51 (1):17–21.

L'Esperance, Elise S. 1945. "Progress in Cancer Prevention Clinics." *Medical Woman's Journal* 52 (4):25–31.

Perry, Marilyn Elizabeth. 1999. "L'Esperance, Elise Strang." In *American National Biography*, edited by J.A. Garraty and M.C. Carnes. New York: Oxford University Press.

Rothe, Anna, ed. 1951. *Current Biography Who's News and Why 1950*. New York: H.W. Wilson.

JSB

Livingston, Nora G.E. [Gertrude Elizabeth] (1848–1927)
Nurse

Nora Livingston, one of the pioneers of nursing education in Canada, helped to found and was a longtime superintendent of the nursing school at Montreal General Hospital in Quebec. She was born in Sault Ste. Marie, Michigan, on May 17, 1848, to English parents. At an early age, she and her family moved to Como, Quebec. She returned to the United States to study at New York Hospital Training School and graduated in 1889.

For a short time, Livingston was superintendent of nurses at New York Hospital. In February 1890, she was named superintendent of nurses at Montreal General Hospital. In April, the nurse training school opened, and she became director of the school. The course was originally two years, with three terms of eight months each, but was among the first nursing schools in Canada or the United States to expand to three years in 1895. Applicants were required to be between 25 and 35 years of age with a common school education and had to present certificates of good character and health. If accepted, students were on probation for two months and received free board and lodging. After the probationary period, they were paid a salary and were the hospital's primary nursing staff, as was common in nursing schools of the era.

In addition to Livingston, physicians of the hospital and head nurses on wards were the school's instructors. Students were required to attend 22 lectures on topics ranging from anatomy and materia medica to hygiene ventilation. They also received practical instruction in wound dressing, bed making, and the application of blisters, poultices, and leeches.

As with most nurse training of the time, strict rules governed the lives of nursing students, and Livingston, as superintendent, was a disciplinarian as well as a teacher. Students were to rise by 6:00 A.M. and be in bed with lights out by 10:00 P.M. At Livingston's discretion, nurses were allowed one afternoon off per week and were permitted one hour every day in the fresh air. In 1897, Livingston established a nurses' home at the school, and in 1906 she instituted the first preliminary class in Canada, with nurse Flora Shaw as instructor. The preliminary class allowed nursing students to have some training before beginning their work on the hospital's wards.

Livingston retired from Montreal General in 1919, due to illness. She died at her home in Val Morin, Quebec, on July 24, 1927.

See also Shaw, Flora Madeline

References

MacDermot, H.E. 1940. *History of the School for Nurses of the Montreal General Hospital.* Montreal: Alumnae Association.

Slattery, Anne. 1929. *Pioneers of Nursing in Canada.* Montreal: Gazette Printing.

Training School for Nurses in Connection with the Montreal General Hospital Formal Opening, Windsor Hall, Montreal, December 11th, 1890. 1890. Montreal: Gazette Printing.

LS

Lockrey, Sarah Hunt (1863–1929)
Physician

Sarah Lockrey was a Philadelphia surgeon who devoted her professional career to providing better health care for women, and who worked as a private citizen toward winning them the right to vote. She was born in Philadelphia on April 21, 1863, to Charles and Martha Jane (Wisner) Lockrey. She graduated from Girls' Normal School and then began teaching at age 17. She attended the Woman's Medical College of Pennsylvania in Philadelphia (now MCP Hahnemann University), teaching night school and tutoring in physiology while there. She graduated from Woman's Medical in 1888 and then interned at the college's Woman's Hospital.

In 1895, Lockery was appointed as assistant to Dr. Anna Broomall at the Woman's Hospital; later, Lockrey became chief of the gynecological staff at the hospital. Shortly afterward, she was also made a visiting chief on the surgical staff of West Philadelphia Hospital for Women; her specialty was abdominal surgery. She held the latter two positions until her death. In addition to her positions at the two hospitals, she was a consultant to the Elwyn School for the Feeble-Minded and was physician at the Methodist Deaconess Home for more than 25 years. At the home, she helped start a women's clinic. Lockrey was a member of many medical societies and associations, including the American College of Surgeons, the American Medical Association, the Pennsylvania State Medical Society, the Philadelphia County Medical Society, and the Broomall Medical Club.

Lockrey was also active in the woman suffrage movement. In 1918, she was given a jail sentence for taking part in a Lafayette Square meeting in Washington, D.C., and was one of 26 women who went on a hunger strike in protest of a fine for suffrage demonstration. She died in Philadelphia on November 8, 1929.

See also Broomall, Anna Elizabeth

References

Lingelbach, Anna Lane. 1933. "Lockrey, Sarah Hunt." In *The Dictionary of American Biography*, edited by D. Malone. New York: Charles Scribner's Sons.

Lockrey, Sarah Hunt. Deceased Alumnae Files, Special Collections on Women in Medicine, Archives and Special Collections, MCP Hahnemann University, Philadelphia.

"Obituary." 1929. *Pennsylvania Medical Journal* (December):201.

LS

Logan, Laura Rebekah (1879–1974)
Nurse

Laura Logan was a prominent leader in nursing education in the United States. She was born on September 15, 1879, at Amherst Point, Nova Scotia, Canada. Her early education was at the private Amherst Academy. In 1901 she earned a bachelor's degree in English from Acadia University in Wolfville, Nova Scotia. Three years later, she received a diploma in nursing from Mount Sinai Hospital School of Nursing in New York.

After graduating from nursing school, Logan spent several years as a private-duty nurse in New York City before earning a bachelor's degree in hospital economics from Columbia University (1908). She also worked at Mt. Sinai Hospital as an instructor and supervisor until about 1911. She was then superintendent of Hope Hospital in Fort Wayne, Indiana, and principal of the hospital's nursing school for three years. In 1914, she became director of the Cincinnati General Hospital School of Nursing and the hospital's nursing service. Two years later, she helped to establish the University of Cincinnati School of Nursing and Health and was the second nurse in the United States to be granted the title professor of nursing, after Adelaide Nutting. Additionally, she founded the nation's first five-year combined baccalaureate and diploma nursing program at the university.

During World War I, Logan was chair of the state and local branches of the nursing section of the women's committee of the Council of National Defense. She helped to recruit 600 women for wartime nursing service. In 1924, she was named dean of the Illinois Training School for Nurses in Chicago, which became the Cook County School of Nursing in 1929. She remained as dean of that school and became director of Cook

County Hospital's nursing service. She retired from Cook County in 1932 and then traveled to Europe to survey schools of nursing for the Rockefeller Foundation.

In 1936, Logan was named director of the nursing service and principal of the school of nursing at Flower-Fifth Avenue Hospital in New York City. From 1937 to 1940, she was director of nursing at Boston City Hospital and then was director of nursing services and the nursing school at St. Louis City Hospital. She retired from the position in 1953.

As director at the various schools of nursing, Logan was known for expanding curricula and recruiting first-rate instructors, including Alma Gault at Illinois. She required nursing students to write case studies of typical patients and expanded their clinical experience to include the care of neurological and mental patients and communicable disease cases. Logan also required basic courses in the social sciences and in anatomy, physiology, bacteriology, and pharmacology. To accommodate the expanded curricula she believed that nursing programs should be lengthened from 30 to 36 months.

Logan died on July 16, 1974, at a nursing home in Sackville, Nova Scotia.

See also Gault, Alma Elizabeth; Nutting, [Mary] Adelaide

Selected Additional Achievements

Taught summer sessions at Stanford University (1924), University of Chicago (1925), Marquette University (1927). Editor, department of nursing education, *American Journal of Nursing* (1920–1929). Education Committee, National Organization for Public Health Nursing; National Committee on Red Cross Nursing Service; secretary, first vice president, board member (1918–1935) and president (1922–1925), National League of Nursing Education. Honorary master of arts (1929) and doctor of civil law (1938), Acadia University; honorary doctor of science, University of Cincinnati (1954).

References

Densford, Katharine J. 1933. "Leaders in Nursing Education: Laura R. Logan, A.M., R.N." *Trained Nurse and Hospital Review* (July):23–24.

Friedman, Alice Howell. 1988. "Logan, Laura R." In *Dictionary of American Nursing Biography*, edited by M. Kaufman. New York: Greenwood Press.

Glass, Laurie K. 1988. "Laura Rebekah Logan." In *American Nursing: A Biographical Dictionary*, edited by V.L. Bullough, O.M. Church, and A.P. Stein. New York: Garland.

"Laura Logan Dies." 1974. *American Journal of Nursing* 74 (September):1722, 1724.

LS

Logan, Onnie Lee (ca. 1910–1995)
Midwife

Onnie Lee Logan was an African American "granny," or lay midwife, in Alabama who successfully delivered hundreds of infants in her lifetime. She estimated that she was born in Sweet Water, Marengo County, Alabama, about 1910. She was the 14th of 16 children and helped her family make a living by picking cotton and taking in laundry. She did not attend school and was only marginally literate. She was a remarkable optimist who dealt with adversity with the attitude, "If you get yo' mind set on that [adversity] you cain't go on to nothin else" (Clark, p. 43).

Descended from two generations of mid-wives, Logan came to her calling naturally. As a teenager, she assisted her mother with births around the Sweet Water area. In 1949, at the age of 39, she received her first midwife permit from the Alabama Board of Health. She first worked in the predominantly poor, black Mobile suburbs of Prichard and Crighton. Later, she assisted physicians in delivering infants in the homes where she worked as a maid. Consequently, her clientele expanded to include all classes of black and white women, including a Mobile physician's wife for whom she worked as a maid for over 40 years. The physician encouraged Logan to obtain her midwife permit and told her that she would have made a good doctor.

Logan was forward-thinking in her philosophy of childbirth. She believed that childbirth is not an illness and that a mother should be allowed to have her baby in the manner of her choice. She also believed that the mother and father should be alone together during the first stages of labor. As labor progressed, Logan would help the mother with kind words and a smile. She coaxed the laboring mother up from her bed and helped her walk through her contractions. After the birth, Logan would place the baby on the mother's stomach to let her enjoy the child whom she had carried for nine months. Logan did not learn these procedures, which are common practice today, from the Board of Health. She attributed them to her "motherwit," or God-given ability.

In the 1960s, Logan's attendance at births dramatically decreased as mothers began to favor the growing number of maternity clinics in rural Alabama. During this time, the majority of her patients were lower-middle-class, white women. In 1976, the state of Alabama outlawed lay midwifery. However, because Logan's record was exemplary and she was so respected by the local medical community, she was allowed to continue her practice.

This privilege came to an abrupt halt in 1984, when the Board of Health sent Logan a notice telling her that her services were no longer needed. Logan's candid reaction to the news that her permit was not to be renewed was that she did not "want no man stoppin these hands from doing what says the Lord. I don't need a permit to deliver no babies. If God tell me not to do it I won't do it" (Clark, p. 174). By 1984, Logan very much wanted to tell her story, so she was introduced to Katherine Clark, an English instructor at the University of South Alabama. Together they wrote Logan's memoir, *Motherwit: An Alabama Midwife's Story* (1989). At the close of her memoir in 1989, Logan was continuing to assist in home deliveries, without the knowledge of the Board of Health. She said that "they didn't say I was not supposed to deliver anymo'. They said they wasn't gonna issue me a permit" (Clark, p. 174).

Logan died on July 9, 1995, at the Mobile Infirmary in Mobile, Alabama. She was survived by her third husband, Roosevelt Logan, a son by her first husband, six grandchildren, and nine great-grandchildren.

References

Clark, Katherine. 1989. *Motherwit: An Alabama Midwife's Story.* New York: Dutton.

Lewis, Michael. 1993. "Driving Miss Onnie." *The New Republic* 209:11–12.

"Obituary." 1995. *Time* 146 (July 24):19.

Thomas, Robert McG. 1995. "Onnie Lee Logan, 85, Midwife Whose 'Motherwit' Drew Praise (Obituary)." *The New York Times Biographical Service* 26 (7):1007.

CMB

Longshore, Hannah E. Myers (1819–1901)
Physician

Hannah Longshore was one of the first women in the United States to earn a medical degree and the first woman to practice medicine in Philadelphia. She was born on May 30, 1819, in Sandy Spring, Maryland, the first of seven children of a Quaker couple, Samuel and Paulina (Iden) Myers. Two of Longshore's sisters, Mary Frame Myers (later, Thomas) and Jane Viola Myers, would also become physicians. Longshore's early education was at a Quaker school in Washington, D.C., and at the New Lisbon Academy in New Lisbon, Ohio.

Samuel Myers helped his daughter overcome her teenage shyness by encouraging her to give lectures on women's rights and

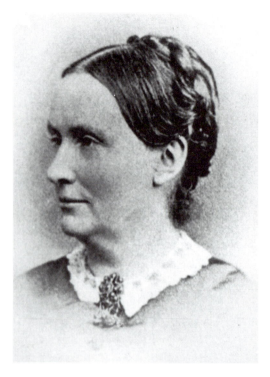

Hannah E. Myers Longshore. National Library of Medicine.

scientific subjects. Longshore soon decided that she wanted to be a doctor, and the family's physician was consulted around 1836 as to the best method to train her. The doctor could offer no useful suggestions for her, however, because no woman had yet been admitted to a medical school in the United States. Longshore also desired to attend Oberlin College in Ohio to further her general education, but a lack of funds prevented her from attending. Undaunted, she studied chemistry, physiology, and botany on her own.

In March 1841, Hannah Myers married Thomas Ellwood Longshore, a teacher at New Lisbon Academy who was a strong supporter of women's rights. The couple lived with her family for the next four years, and they had two children. In 1845, Thomas Longshore's antislavery views forced him and his family to move to his hometown of Attleboro, Pennsylvania. In Attleboro, Hannah Longshore and her husband's sister, Anna Mary Longshore, began studying medicine with Thomas' brother, Dr. Joseph Skelton

Longshore. Like Thomas, Joseph Longshore was a supporter of women's rights, particularly their right to medical education.

Soon Joseph helped establish the Female (later, Woman's) Medical College of Pennsylvania in Philadelphia (now MCP Hahnemann University). The state granted the college a charter in March 1850, and Joseph became the first professor of obstetrics and diseases of women and children there. In October of that year, Hannah Longshore enrolled in the college's first session; her classmates included Ann Preston, future dean of the college, and her sister-in-law Anna. Because of her previous medical study, Longshore also acted as demonstrator of anatomy for the school, making her one of the first women faculty members at an American medical school. When she and seven other women of the Female Medical College's first class graduated on December 31, 1851, Philadelphia police were present because local male medical students had threatened to disrupt the event.

Longshore became demonstrator of anatomy at the New England Female Medical College in Boston in February 1852 as a result of a faculty exchange program between the two women's schools. She was the first woman to teach at the school and was there until June 1852. From September 1852 to January 1853, she was again demonstrator of anatomy at the Female Medical College in Philadelphia. In 1853, when Joseph Longshore and other faculty members were asked to resign from the school because of their eclectic medical beliefs, Hannah Longshore also resigned. Joseph Longshore founded the sectarian school Penn Medical University, in Philadelphia, and Hannah joined him there. She taught at Penn's female department for the next four years, and her older sister, Mary Frame Myers Thomas, was one of her students.

In addition to her teaching duties, Longshore opened a private practice in her home in Philadelphia. She was the first woman to practice in the city, and as such she encountered a great deal of skepticism and hostility. Two incidents from her unpublished autobiography illustrate the obstacles that she faced and her resolve to overcome them. Soon after establishing her medical practice, she wrote a prescription for a woman patient. The patient took the prescription to a pharmacist, but he refused to fill it, cautioning the patient against women healers. For a time, she was forced to carry an emergency medical bag with her own supply of drugs. Later, Longshore herself encountered hostility from a local pharmacist when she went to his pharmacy to purchase some medications. In Longshore's words, "The proprietor . . . said, 'I will not sell the drugs to you! You are out of your sphere! Go home and darn your husband's stockings!' " (Longshore Family Papers, MCP Hahnemann University). Longshore proceeded to lay her emergency medical bag on the counter and tell the pharmacist that her bag had kept dollars out of his pocket and that it would keep out many more in the future if he refused her. Eventually, the man conceded and sold her the medications.

In addition to teaching and her medical practice, Longshore gave public lectures in Philadelphia. Her first lecture, in the spring of 1852, was on medical education for women. Later, she gave a series of five lectures to women on physiology and hygiene that included a frank discussion of sex. Although the content of her lectures may have shocked some, their popularity helped Longshore attract many patients to her medical practice. By 1855, her practice had grown such that she had no time for teaching or lecturing. Longshore devoted the remainder of her medical career to caring for the 300 families in Philadelphia that relied on her.

In 1892, Longshore retired after 40 years of medical practice. She died in Philadelphia on October 18, 1901, of uremia.

See also Preston, Ann; Thomas, Mary Frame Myers

References

Boyer, Ida Porter. 1901. "In Memoriam." *Woman's Journal* (November 9):357.
Elliot, H.B. 1868. "Mrs. Hannah E. Longshore, M.D." In *Eminent Women of the Age: Being Narratives of the Lives and Deeds of the Most Prominent Women of the Present Generation*, edited by J. Parton. Hartford, Conn.: S.M. Betts.
Longshore Family Papers, Several undated, handwritten drafts of an autobiography of Hannah Longshore, Manuscript Collection MS-75, Special Collections on Women in Medicine, Archives and Special Collections, MCP Hahnemann University, Philadelphia.
Waite, Frederick C. 1933. "The Three Myers Sisters—Pioneer Women Physicians." *Medical Review of Reviews* 39 (March):114–120.
Ward, Patricia Spain. 1971. "Longshore, Hannah E. Myers." In *Notable American Women, 1607–1950: A Biographical Dictionary*, edited by E.T. James, J.W. James, and P.S. Boyer. Cambridge: Belknap Press of Harvard University Press.

LS

Love, Susan M. (1948–   )
Physician

Susan Love, a conventionally trained breast surgeon, has revolutionized the treatment of breast cancer. She is skeptical of modern medicine because she believes that it perpetuates a condescending attitude toward women; consequently, she entreats women to become their bodies' own advocate. She was born in Long Branch, New Jersey, on February 9, 1948, the first of five children of James and Peggy Love. When Love was 13, her family relocated to Puerto Rico and within a year moved again to Mexico City, where Love finished high school. After two years of premedical studies at the College of Notre Dame of Maryland in Baltimore, she entered a convent in New York City. After four or five months, she left the convent and enrolled at Fordham University in the Bronx borough of New York City to continue her premedical education.

Beating the quota system that limited women medical students to 10 percent, Love attended the State University of New York Downstate Medical Center in Brooklyn. She graduated cum laude in 1974, ranked fourth in her class. She then began her surgical residency at Beth Israel Hospital in Boston and in 1979 opened a private practice there. After treating a variety of people for many different conditions, it became apparent that women patients preferred to go to her with breast problems because she was a woman. Realizing that she could make a contribution in this area, in 1981, she became a member of the staff of the Dana Farber Cancer Research Institute in Boston. Here she was part of a team of specialists, including radiologists and oncologists, who were among the first to challenge the use of radical mastectomies and to champion more conservative surgeries such as lumpectomies and partial mastectomies.

In 1987, Love accepted an appointment as an assistant clinical professor in surgery at Harvard Medical School, and in the next year she established the Faulkner Breast Center in Boston. This center was originally, and remains today, staffed with women surgeons who specialize in breast disease and breast reconstruction. In 1990 she cofounded the National Breast Cancer Coalition, an organization that was instrumental in increasing national breast cancer research funding from $90 million in 1990 to more than $420 million in 1994. Also in 1990, Love (with Karen Lindsey) published *Dr. Susan Love's Breast Book*, a comprehensive guide to breast health and disease. Her vision, to empower women with knowledge of their own breasts and thereby enable them to make their own decisions about the type of treatment that they receive, forms the basis of the book.

In 1992, Love was appointed director of the Revlon/UCLA [University of California, Los Angeles] Breast Center and became interested in hormone replacement therapy during menopause. Once again, Love challenged conventional wisdom by casting doubt on routine hormone replacement therapy during menopause because high hormonal levels at this stage in life are not normal. To help women make informed decisions, a second guide to women's health, *Dr. Susan Love's Hormone Book*, was published in 1997, again with Karen Lindsey. The subtitle, *Making Informed Choices about Menopause*, captures the essence of the book. It is a guide to the process of menopause and stresses Love's conviction that menopause is not a disease and should not be treated as one.

In 1996 Love became an adjunct professor of surgery at UCLA and the medical director of the Santa Barbara Breast Cancer Institute, a nonprofit organization. In 1998 she was appointed to the National Cancer Board, and in the fall of 1999, she launched SusanLoveMD.com, an interactive Web site for women's health information.

Love lives in Pacific Palisades, California, with her partner and their daughter.

Selected Additional Achievements

Woman of the Year, the Canadian Women's Cancer Foundation (1990); the Rose Kushner Award, American Medical Writers Association (1991); Women Who Have Made a Difference Award, International Women's Forum (1991); "The Muses" Women Making History Award, the California Museum of Science and Industry (1993); Community Role Model Award, Los Angeles Gay and Lesbian Center (1997).

References

Gover, Tzivia. 1997. "Dr. Love and the Politics of Disease." *The Advocate* (March 4):38–40.

O'Neill, Molly. 1994. "A Day with Dr. Susan M. Love: A Surgeon's War on Breast Cancer." *New York Times Biographical Service* 25 (6):958–959.

Seglin, Jeffrey. 1997. "Is There an M.B.A. in the House?" *Inc.* 19 (April):26.

Stabiner, Karen. 1997. *To Dance with the Devil: The New War on Breast Cancer.* New York: Delacorte Press.

SusanLoveMD.com, Dr. Susan Love's Website for Women. Online. http://susanlovemd.com. 14 April 2000.

CMB

Lovejoy, Esther Pohl (1869–1967)
Physician

Esther Pohl Lovejoy is most notable for her directorship of the American Women's Hospitals. She was born in a lumber camp near Seabeck, Washington Territory, on November 16, 1869, one of six children of Edward and Annie (Quinton) Clayson. She received her education in the lumber camp school and from a professor who boarded at the family-owned hotel.

Lovejoy's interest in medicine was sparked after watching a woman doctor deliver her youngest sister, and in 1894, she graduated from the Medical School at the University of Oregon. She was the school's second woman graduate but the first to practice medicine. Three weeks later, she married classmate Emil Pohl. The two set up practice in Portland, he as a surgeon and she as an obstetrician. In 1896, she went to Chicago for further training in gynecology and obstetrics at the West Side Post-Graduate School. The couple then became the first physicians in Skagway, Alaska, where they founded Union Hospital in 1898.

In 1905, after spending the previous year studying gynecology and obstetrics in Vienna, Lovejoy was appointed to the Portland Board of Health. She became the board's director in 1907 and earned the distinction of being the first woman to hold that position in a major American city. As a direct result of her work, Portland received recognition for its excellent sanitation standards. Tragedy struck in 1909, when her son died of septic peritonitis, and again in 1911, when Pohl died during an encephalitis epidemic. She married George A. Lovejoy in 1913 but divorced him seven years later.

Lovejoy returned to private practice in 1909 and took further medical training in Berlin (1910). At the outbreak of World War I, she focused her career on overseas medical relief efforts. In 1917, in France as a representative of the American Medical Women's Association (AMWA), she worked in a Red Cross center and volunteered at a charity hospital. Her experiences in France are described in her book *The House of the Good Neighbor* (1919).

Lovejoy returned to the United States in 1918 to secure funds for the American Women's Hospitals (AWH). The AWH was established by the AMWA in 1917 to provide medical aid in war-torn countries. As explained in her book *Certain Samaritans* (1927), the AWH was established for female physicians who, though not accepted by the military, wanted to contribute their skills to the war effort. As director of the AWH for 48 years, she led the establishment of hospitals, clinics, orphanages, and other public health services to provide medical and health care to those suffering from the effects of war. The organization also assisted during a Tokyo earthquake (1923) and a Florida hurricane (1926). During World War II, the AWH provided medical care in Britain, France, and Greece, moving into the Far East and Latin America during the postwar period. Lovejoy oversaw relief efforts in over 30 countries with American Women's Hospital Service (AWHS), as it was later called.

Lovejoy was involved in politics and also encouraged women to go into medicine. In 1920, she ran unsuccessfully for Congress on

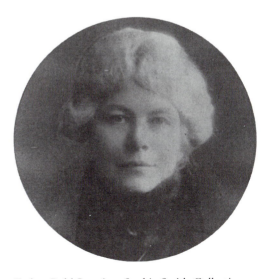

Esther Pohl Lovejoy. Sophia Smith Collection, © Underwood & Underwood.

the Democratic ticket, campaigning on behalf of women's rights, Prohibition, and the League of Nations. She endowed a scholarship for medical students at her alma mater and stipulated that one-third of the awards go to women students. She also wrote two books, *Women Physicians and Surgeons* (1939) and *Women Doctors of the World* (1957), chronicling the achievements of women physicians around the globe. Additionally, she was a founder and first president (1919–1924) of the Medical Women's International Association, created to increase status for women physicians and to provide medical aid worldwide.

Lovejoy died of pneumonia in New York City on August 17, 1967.

Selected Additional Achievements

President, American Medical Women's Association (1932–1933) and the only woman to have received the organization's Elizabeth Blackwell

Medal twice. Her overseas work earned her the Legion of Honor (France), the Gold Cross of Saint Sava (Yugoslavia), the Gold Cross of the Holy Sepulcher (Jerusalem), and the Gold Cross of the Order of George I (Greece).

References

"Esther Pohl Lovejoy, M.D." 1944. *Medical Woman's Journal* 55 (6):33–34.
Lovejoy, Esther Pohl. 1919. *The House of the Good Neighbor.* New York: Macmillan.
Lovejoy, Esther Pohl. 1927. *Certain Samaritans.* New York: Macmillan.
Perry Marilyn, Elizabeth. 1999. "Lovejoy, Esther Pohl." In *American National Biography*, edited by J.A. Garraty and M.C. Carnes. New York: Oxford University Press.
Thomson, Elizabeth H. 1980. "Lovejoy, Esther Pohl." In *Notable American Women: The Modern Period: A Biographical Dictionary*, edited by B. Sicherman and C.H. Green. Cambridge: Belknap Press of Harvard University Press.

JSB

Loveridge, Emily Lemoine (1860–1941)
Nurse

Emily Loveridge established the first nurse training school in the American Northwest. She was born on August 28, 1860, in Hammondsport, New York, the daughter of the Reverend Daniel Loveridge and Marie Lemoine (Wolfolk) Loveridge. She graduated from a Norwich, New York, high school in 1879 and then began teaching in Otsego County (New York) public schools.

Loveridge left teaching in 1887 to attend Bellevue Hospital Training School of Nursing in New York City. During her senior year, the superintendent of Good Samaritan Hospital in Portland, Oregon, asked Loveridge to establish a nurse training school at the hospital. After graduating from Bellevue in 1889, she went to Portland, where she organized the first school of nursing in the American Northwest. The School of Nursing at Good Samaritan Hospital opened in June 1890. Loveridge published a description of

her busy 12-to 16-hour days: "In addition to being superintendent of nurses, I was floor nurse and operating room supervisor, and in my leisure moments did any necessary work—sewing, cleaning, painting, etc.—that there was to be done" (p. 777).

Loveridge served as nursing superintendent until 1905, when she became superintendent of the entire hospital. In 1910, she played a role in the establishment of what is now the Oregon State Board of Nursing. Loveridge was also an active member of the American Hospital Association, president of the Northwest Hospital Association (1926–1927), and head of the Western Hospital Association (1928). Outside of nursing, she raised a niece, a nephew, and a girl orphaned by the influenza epidemic of 1919. She retired from Good Samaritan in 1930.

Loveridge died in Portland on April 26, 1941. In 1966, Loveridge Hall was dedicated to her memory at Good Samaritan Hospital.

References

Loveridge, Emily L. 1930. "Reminiscences of Forty Years in Hospital Work." *American Journal of Nursing* 30 (6):777–778.

Pennock, Meta Rutter, ed. 1940. *Makers of Nursing History; Portraits and Pen Sketches of One Hundred and Nine Prominent Women.* New York: Lakeside.

Sentz, Lilli. 1992. "Emily Lemoine Loveridge." In *American Nursing: A Biographical Dictionary,* edited by V.L. Bullough, L. Sentz, and A.P. Stein. New York: Garland.

JSB

Lozier, Clemence Sophia Harned (1813–1888)
Physician

Clemence Lozier founded New York Medical College and Hospital for Women (Homeopathic), the third women's medical college in the United States. She was born on December 11, 1813, in Plainfield, New Jersey, the youngest of 13 children of David and Hannah (Walker) Harned. In her youth, Lozier attended Plainfield Academy. She was orphaned at age 11, and five or six years later she married Abraham Witton Lozier, a carpenter from New York City. The couple settled in the city and had several children. Only the youngest, Abraham Witton Jr., survived infancy. Soon after their marriage, Lozier's husband's health began to fail, and she opened a girl's school in her home to help support her family. Each year, for the next 11 years, she taught an average of 60 girls physiology, anatomy, and hygiene, subjects not commonly taught to girls of that era.

While teaching school, Lozier began to study medicine with her brother, Dr. William Harned. She was also active in the New York Female Moral Reform Society, an organization founded to prevent prostitution. Her husband died in 1837, and in 1844, she moved to Albany, then Webster, New York, where she gave lectures at the local Presbyterian Church on physiology and hygiene. Around this time, she married John Baker. In 1853, she graduated from the sectarian medical school Syracuse Medical College with highest honors. After graduation, Clemence, as Dr. Baker, set up practice in New York City. She specialized in obstetrics and in the removal of tumors, and she quickly gained a wide following. By the mid-1860s, she was earning $25,000 a year from her practice.

Lozier's second marriage was an unhappy one, so she filed for divorce; it was granted on April 27, 1861, and she resumed using the surname Lozier. In 1860, she had begun offering lectures in her home to some of her women patients on anatomy, physiology, and hygiene. She also organized a Medical Library Association to encourage these women to read on their own. Women's enthusiasm for medical study, made clear by the popularity of her lectures, led her to found a medical college.

On April 14, 1863, with the help of suffragist Elizabeth Cady Stanton, Lozier secured a charter from the state of New York for the New York Medical College and Hospital for Women (Homeopathic). Homeopathic medicine is based on the use of minute doses of drugs administered according to the principle of "like cures like." The school, with Lozier as president and clinical professor of diseases of women and children, opened on November 1 of that year. Lozier's niece, Anna Comfort, was one of the college's first students. The New York Medical College and Hospital for Women (Homeopathic) was the state's first women's medical school and the third in the country. It was opened five years before Dr. Elizabeth Blackwell's Woman's Medical College of the New York Infirmary in the same city. Although the schools coexisted for nearly 30 years, the two women had an antagonistic relationship due, in part, to Blackwell's contempt for sectarian medicine.

In 1867, after a tour of European hospitals, Lozier reorganized the school. She served as dean and professor of gynecology and obstetrics there for the next 20 years, and she helped support the school with money from her private medical practice. Against her advice, in 1878 the college and hospital were moved to a new site. The expense of the move forced her into bankruptcy, but she was able to keep her private practice. The school also persisted; by the time of Lozier's death in 1888, it had graduated over 200 women.

In addition to practicing medicine, Lozier was active in reform movements, especially the campaign for woman suffrage. She was president of the New York City Woman Suffrage Society (1873–1886) and the National Woman Suffrage Association (1877–1878). Her medical practice helped support the *Revolution*, Susan B. Anthony's suffrage publication. Lozier also supported sanitary reform, international arbitration, better treatment of Native Americans, prison reform, and temperance.

Lozier died of heart disease on April 26, 1888, at her home in New York. Forty-eight women doctors, all graduates of her school, attended her funeral.

See also Blackwell, Elizabeth; Comfort, Anna Amelia Manning

Selected Additional Achievements

First woman to read a paper before New York state's homeopathic society; wrote *Child-Birth Made Easy* (1870) and *Dress* (n.d.); editor, *Moral Reform Gazette*; member, New York Sorosis club and National Working Women's League; president, Moral Education Society of New York; president, local Woman's Christian Temperance Union; secretary, American Female Guardian Society; vice president, Universal Peace Union.

References

Cantor, Milton. 1971. "Lozier, Clemence Sophia Harned." In *Notable American Women, 1607–1950: A Biographical Dictionary*, edited by E.T. James, J.W. James, and P.S. Boyer. Cambridge: Belknap Press of Harvard University Press.

Elliot, H. B. 1868. "Mrs. Clemence S. Lozier, M.D." In *Eminent Women of the Age: Being Narratives of the Lives and Deeds of the Most Prominent Women of the Present Generation*, edited by J. Parton. Hartford, Conn.: S. M. Betts.

"Funeral of Mrs. Lozier." 1888. *New York Times* (April 30):8.

Selmon, Bertha L. 1946. "The New York Medical College and Hospital for Women (Homeopathic): 1863–1918." *Medical Woman's Journal* 53 (4):43–46.

"Woman's Power to Invent: What She Has Accomplished in Business and the Professions: Some Prominent New-York Examples." 1895. *New York Times* (December 22):25.

LS

Lubic, Ruth Watson (1927–   )
Nurse-midwife

Ruth Lubic is a leader in the field of nurse-midwifery in the United States. She was born on January 18, 1927, in Bristol, Pennsylvania, the second of two daughters of John Russell and Lillian (Kraft) Watson. She was influenced to become a nurse by an aunt who was a nurse and by two local physicians. After graduating from Bristol High School in 1944, she went to work at her family's drugstore to earn money for nursing school.

In 1952, Lubic enrolled at the School of Nursing of the Hospital of the University of Pennsylvania in Philadelphia and earned a diploma three years later. Just before graduating, she married William James Lubic, an attorney. Lubic worked at the Memorial Center for Cancer and Allied Diseases in New York City from 1955 to 1958, working her way up from staff to head nurse. At the same time, she took courses toward a bachelor's degree in nursing at Hunter College. In 1958, she was awarded a full scholarship to Teachers College, Columbia University and completed her degree there in 1959. Two weeks after graduating, she gave birth to a son, Douglas Watson Lubic. She had begun working on a master's degree in medical-surgical nursing at Teacher's College, which she earned in 1961, but changed her mind about the specialty after becoming a mother. Lubic confided her doubts to her obstetrician, who suggested that she become a midwife. After speaking with Hazel Corbin, general director of the Maternity Center Association (MCA), she decided to enroll in the association's nurse-midwifery certificate program and earned a certificate in June 1962.

Lubic then worked as a clinical instructor at the MCA (1962) and as a clinical associate in nursing at the graduate nursing school at New York Medical College (1962–1963). In 1963, she became a parent educator and counselor at the MCA (1963–1967). To help her understand her multicultural clientele, Lubic enrolled in an applied anthropology doctoral program at Teachers College. She had finished most of her course work in 1970, when she was named general director of the MCA, delaying completion of her degree until 1979.

At the time she became director, many pregnant women were choosing to give birth at home. To offer an alternative, Lubic and nurse-midwife Kitty Ernst opened the MCA Childbearing Center in Manhattan in 1975. The birth center's success in the face of medical opposition inspired many other similar facilities across the country. Other achievements during Lubic's tenure as director include a 1978 self-help education program designed to allow expectant mothers to perform their own health checks and the 1988 opening of a birth center in the economically depressed Bronx area of New York. In 1995, she stepped down as general director of the MCA to become director of its clinical projects (1995–1997).

In addition to her work for the MCA, Lubic has done extensive consulting work, helped to found, and is active in, the National Association of Childbearing Centers, and has held nursing professorships at the Frances Payne Bolton School of Nursing at Case Western Reserve University (1991), New York University (1995–), and Georgetown University (1997–). In 1993, she was the first nurse to win the prestigious John D. and Catherine T. MacArthur Foundation Fellowship. Lubic decided to use the $375,000 grant money to address the high infant mortality rate in Washington, D.C. Thus, in 1998 she established the District of Columbia Developing Families Center (DCDFC). The DCDFC is a nonprofit collaborative corporation including the D.C. Birth Center, the Healthy Babies Project, and the National Child Day Care Association. Lubic is currently president and chief executive officer (CEO) of the DCDFC and the D.C. Birth Center.

See also Corbin, Hazel; Ernst, Eunice Katherine MacDonald [Kitty]

Selected Additional Achievements

Numerous articles and book chapters in the nursing and health care literature; *Childbearing: A Book of Choices* (with Gene R. Hawes, 1987). Fellow, American Academy of Nursing (1978); Rockefeller Public Service Award, Woodrow Wilson School of Public and International Affairs, Princeton University (1981); Hattie Hemschemeyer Award, American College of Nurse-Midwives (1983); Honorary Recognition, American Nurses Association (1994); Lillian D. Wald Spirit of Nursing Award, Visiting Nurse Service of New York (1994); Carola Warburg Rothschild Award for Distinguished Service to Women and Families, MCA (1997); at least five honorary doctorates.

References

Graham, Judith, ed. 1996. *Current Biography Yearbook 1996.* New York: H.W. Wilson.
Loose, Cindy. 1998. "A Battle Won, a Center Born; Nurse-Midwife to Open Birthing Facility for D.C.'s Poor." *Washington Post* (September 30):A01.
Lubic, Ruth Watson. 1988. "Ruth Watson Lu-

bic." In *Making Choices, Taking Chances: Nurse Leaders Tell Their Stories*, edited by T.M. Schorr and A. Zimmerman. St. Louis: C. V. Mosby.

Lubic, Ruth Watson. September 4, 1999. Curriculum Vitae.

LS

Lytle, Nancy A. (1924–1987)
Nurse

Nancy Lytle was a specialist in maternity nursing. She was born on October 14, 1924, in Fredericksburg, Ohio, one of three children of George B. and Bertha G. Lytle. In 1945, she graduated from Fairview Park Hospital School of Nursing in Cleveland, Ohio, and worked there for a year before accepting a nursing position at Elizabeth Steele McGee Hospital in Pittsburgh.

While in Pittsburgh, Lytle earned a bachelor's degree in nursing from the University of Pittsburgh (1948), after which she became teaching supervisor at St. Margaret's Memorial Hospital and then supervisor of obstetrics at Western Pennsylvania Hospital, both in Pittsburgh. From 1953 to 1957, she was an assistant professor of obstetrical nursing at Ohio State University. She earned a master's degree in maternity nursing from Columbia University's Teachers College in 1954 and was an instructor there until 1964. Next, she was professor and chair of maternal health nursing at the State University of New York at Buffalo.

In 1968, Lytle earned a doctorate in nursing education from Teachers College and was recruited by Rozella Schlotfeldt to be a professor of nursing at Case Western Reserve University's Frances Payne Bolton School of Nursing in Cleveland, Ohio, and the director of maternity nursing at the University Hospitals. Among her accomplishments were developing a graduate program in maternity nursing and introducing innovative methods of instruction, such as having new parents talk to nursing students about the birth experience. In 1969, she initiated a program at the University Hospitals to increase the father's role in the childbirth experience. In the 1970s, at the urging of the Ohio Department of Health, she conducted continuing education programs for nurses who provided prenatal health care.

Lytle was also a consultant to the Ohio and Virgin Islands Departments of Health and to several universities. In 1971 she was made professor and director (at University Hospitals) of maternity and gynecologic nursing at Case Western and was chair of the program from 1973. She held these positions until her death from cancer on August 24, 1987, in Cleveland.

See also Schlotfeldt, Rozella May

Selected Additional Achievements

Maternal Health Nursing: A Book of Readings (1967); *Nursing of Women in the Age of Liberation* (1977). Charter member, American Academy of Nursing; Sigma Theta Tau. Outstanding Service in Health Care Award, Ohio Senate (1980); March of Dimes Nurse of the Year, Ohio Nurses' Association (1984).

References

Brook, Marianne. 1992. "Nancy A. Lytle." In *American Nursing: A Biographical Dictionary*, edited by V.L. Bullough, L. Sentz, and A.P. Stein. New York: Garland.

Lytle, Nancy. 1986–1987. Curriculum Vitae. University Archives, Case Western Reserve University. Cleveland, Ohio.

"Nancy A. Lytle, Regarded as Expert in Nursing Field." 1987. *Cleveland Plain Dealer* (August 27):18D.

"Professor Was Leader in Health Care." 1987. (Case Western Reserve University) *Campus News* (September 16).

LS

M

Macleod, Charlotte (1852–1950)
Nurse

Charlotte Macleod was the first chief superintendent of the Victorian Order of Nurses in Canada. She was also responsible for the establishment of the earliest training programs for public health nurses in both Canada and the United States in the late 1890s. She was born on November 11, 1852, in New Brunswick, Canada. Orphaned as a young child, she was raised by an uncle who taught her to believe that, above all, her life should serve God and humankind. This conviction first led Macleod to become a teacher. She taught grammar school for 15 years until she decided to train for a nursing career.

Macleod graduated from the Waltham Training School for Nurses in Waltham, Massachusetts, in 1891 and went on to take additional courses at Long Island College Hospital in Brooklyn, New York, and at McLane Insane Hospital in Massachusetts. In 1892, Macleod returned to the Waltham School as the principal, and she soon left for Scotland and England (1896) to study the education of nurses in Britain. While abroad, she visited the slums of Liverpool and London and discussed nursing education with famed English nurse Florence Nightingale. Based on her observations in England, she established at the Waltham School the first

training program in the United States to offer a course in home nursing. Macleod's initial curriculum laid the foundation for what is now the discipline of public health nursing education.

In 1898, Lady Aberdeen of Canada entreated Macleod to leave the Waltham School and establish the first visiting nursing service in Canada, the Victorian Order of Nurses (VON). Originally, Macleod agreed to return to Canada for three months to help set up the visiting nursing service, but eventually she assumed a permanent position as chief superintendent. She designed a six-month course in district nursing that was required for nurses wishing to serve with the VON. She traveled extensively across Canada for six and a half years, establishing district offices for the VON until ill health forced her to step down.

After further travel abroad (1904–1905), Macleod returned to Massachusetts in 1906 to establish, and then direct, the Training School for Visiting Nurses of the Boston Instructive Visiting Nurses Association. Shortly thereafter, she acted in a similar capacity for the Training School for Attendants, which was formed by the Brattleboro Mutual Aid Association in Brattleboro, Vermont (1909–

1912). Over the next four years, she held a series of short-term positions, including superintendent of nursing services at Miradero Sanitarium in Santa Barbara, California (1913), superintendent of Waltham Hospital (1913), and acting matron of the Roxbury House of Mercy in Boston (1914). From 1915 to 1917 she turned her attention away from nursing education and devoted her time to parish and social service work at Christ Church in New York City.

Macleod retired to Winchendon, Massachusetts, in 1917, returning to the Waltham School temporarily in 1921 to give a course in home nursing. She died on October 21, 1950.

References

Dodd, Diane, and Deborah Gorham, eds. 1994. *Caring and Curing: Historical Perspectives on Women and Healing in Canada.* Ottawa: University of Ottawa Press.

Penney, Sheila M. 1996. *A Century of Caring: 1897–1997: The History of the Victorian Order of Nurses for Canada.* Ottawa: VON Canada.

Pennock, Meta Rutter, ed. 1940. *Makers of Nursing History; Portraits and Pen Sketches of One Hundred and Nine Prominent Women.* New York: Lakeside.

Stein, Alice P. 1992. "Charlotte Macleod." In *American Nursing: A Biographical Dictionary,* edited by V.L. Bullough, L. Sentz, and A.P. Stein. New York: Garland.

CMB

MacMurchy, Helen (1862–1953)
Physician

Helen MacMurchy was chief of the Division of Child Welfare for the Canadian Department of Health. In this role, she led a successful campaign to decrease maternal and infant mortality rates in Canada. She was born in Toronto on January 7, 1862, to Archibald and Marjorie Jardine (Ramsay) MacMurchy. After completing her preliminary education in Toronto, she taught at the Jarvis Collegiate Institute, also in Toronto (1880).

While teaching, MacMurchy took medical courses at the Ontario Medical College for Women. After receiving her M.D. in 1901, she became the first woman intern at Toronto General Hospital. Following postgraduate studies at Johns Hopkins Hospital in Baltimore, and at the Woman's Medical College of Pennsylvania in Philadelphia, she returned to Toronto in 1902 to start an obstetrics, gynecology, and pediatrics practice.

In 1905 MacMurchy was commissioned by the Ontario government to conduct a census of the "feeble-minded." The survey resulted in the Ontario Auxiliary Classes Act (1914), which provided special educational training for physically and mentally handicapped children. In 1914, she was appointed inspector of auxiliary classes in the province of Ontario. She also strove to improve the milk supply and to decrease the maternal and infant mortality rates by being the first to write special reports on these subjects for the Ontario government (1910–1912). During this time she also served as medical inspector of schools for the Toronto Board of Education (1910) and became an assistant demonstrator of obstetrics and gynecology at the University of Toronto (1911). In 1912, she wrote her first book, *A Little Talk about the Baby.* Additionally, she held close ties to the Canadian nursing community. She was the first editor in chief of *The Canadian Nurse* (1905–1911) and worked with the nurses of Opington War Hospital before they were deployed overseas during World War I.

In 1920, MacMurchy was appointed chief of the Division of Child Welfare for the Canadian Department of Health. In this post she examined approximately 11,000 reports of deaths occurring between 1925 and 1926 of women aged 15 to 50 and discovered a maternal mortality rate of approximately 6 per 1,000 live births. She believed that the keys to maternal and infant survival were the provision of proper prenatal care and contraception, to avoid overburdening the mother with too many children.

To pass on such practical information to women, MacMurchy wrote a series of books, the *Little Blue Books*, approximately 1 million copies of which were distributed throughout Canada by 1940. In these books, MacMurchy walked a fine line between advocating lay midwifery and the more conventional physician-attended hospital delivery that her colleagues supported. Prior to World War I, she advocated the training and licensing of midwives, but throughout the *Blue Books* MacMurchy was cautious not to endorse midwifery by appending her advice with the assertion that medical attendance was needed during childbirth. Nonetheless, her books provided minute detail of the birth process and the actions that were required in the case of unusual circumstances such as breech births.

MacMurchy retired as chief of child welfare in 1934. She died in Toronto on October 8, 1953.

Selected Additional Achievements

Organization and Management of Auxiliary Classes (1914); *The Almosts: A Study of the Feebleminded* (1920); *The Canadian Mother's Book* (1920). President, University Women's Club of Toronto (1904–1906); honorary M.D., University of Toronto (1923); Commander of the Most Excellent Order of the British Empire, King George V, England (1934); life fellow, Academy of Medicine of Toronto (1939); Elizabeth Blackwell Citation, Hobart and William Smith Colleges (1949).

References

Buckley, Suzann. 1988. "The Search for the Decline of Maternal Mortality: The Place of Hospital Records." In *Essays in the History of Canadian Medicine*, edited by W. Mitchinson and J.D. McGinnis. Toronto: McClelland and Stewart.

"Centennial of a Trailblazer." 1949. *Journal of the American Medical Women's Association* 4 (3): 125–128.

Dodd, Diane. 1991. "Advice to Parents: The Blue Books, Helen MacMurchy, M.D. and the Federal Department of Health, 1920–1934." *Canadian Bulletin of Medical History* 8 (2): 203–230.

Dodd, Diane, and Deborah Gorham, eds. 1994. *Caring and Curing: Historical Perspectives on Women and Healing in Canada*. Ottawa: University of Ottawa Press.

Hacker, Carlotta. 1974. *The Indomitable Lady Doctors*. Toronto: Clarke, Irwin.

MacLennan, David. 1987. "Beyond the Asylum: Professionalization and the Mental Hygiene Movement in Canada, 1914–1928." *Canadian Bulletin of Medical History* 4:7–23.

Snelgrove, Erle E. 1949. "The First Woman Doctor." *Hygeia* 27 (8): 534–535.

CMB

Magee, Joni Lahr (1941–   )
Physician

Joni Magee is an obstetrician and gynecologist known for her insistence that physicians must understand the needs and perspectives of their female patients. She was born in Philadelphia in 1941. She decided in childhood to become a doctor; however, someone convinced the young Magee that female physicians were unfeminine. She changed her plans to nursing, only to discover that her parents did not support her new career choice. At her father's request, she entered the University of Pennsylvania liberal arts program. It was near her graduation when she realized that her true calling had always been medicine.

After graduation, Magee returned to the University of Pennsylvania for one year of premedical course work. In 1963, she began her medical education at New York University (NYU), one of only 10 women in a class of 120. After completing her second year at NYU, newly married and pregnant, she joined her husband in Philadelphia and transferred to the Medical College of Pennsylvania. She decided to specialize in obstetrics and gynecology after her terrible experience during the birth of her first child. She had looked forward to natural childbirth. However, her doctor and husband persuaded her to use painkillers, which left her weak and incoherent. She ended up with a "forceps delivery, a depressed baby, a sphincter tear and a great deal of blood loss" (quoted in Morantz-Sanchez et al., p. 216). The hospital staff also refused to allow the baby to room-in with her and discouraged her from breast-feeding. The day after giving birth, she thought to herself that "there's got to be somebody who will treat people the way I want to be treated, so I think I'll go into OB-GYN" (quoted in Morantz-Sanchez et al., p. 217).

After receiving her medical degree in 1968, Magee completed a one-year internship in pediatrics at Philadelphia's Presbyterian Hospital. This was followed by another year as resident in internal medicine at the Medical College of Pennsylvania and a second year as house physician at Haverford General Hospital. In 1971, she began a residency in obstetrics and gynecology at Philadelphia's Jefferson Hospital. When she began the residency program, she was three months pregnant, and the hospital agreed to a maternity leave. However, she became pregnant with her third child soon after her return from leave. Neither the hospital staff nor her husband supported the third pregnancy. Although the hospital administration was originally against a second leave, she was able to convince them otherwise. She was not able to salvage the situation with her husband, however, and the two divorced. After completing her residency in 1976, she began a full-time position at Booth Maternity Cen-

ter, a unique institution that encouraged childbirth with minimal institutional interference. She also opened a small private gynecological practice.

Magee's published articles are aimed at educating physicians to the needs and experiences of the female patient. In "Labor: What the Doctor Learns as a Patient," she reminds physicians that, while they are treating the baby, they are also treating the mother, who "has a fully developed brain which harbors hopes and fears, as well as a grown body with unaccustomed aches and pains and strange sensations" (p. 27). In a similar article on the pelvic examination, she discusses ways to make the examination more comfortable for women. In both articles, she explains certain manual techniques but stresses that the most important technique is to communicate continually with the patient. Magee encourages communication because "[n]ot only does the patient have a right to know what you are doing to, and finding out about, her body, but being treated as worthy of this knowledge makes her more cooperative" (Magee, 1994, p. 34).

Today, Magee continues to maintain her practice in Merion Station, Pennsylvania.

References

Magee, Joni. 1976. "Labor: What the Doctor Learns as a Patient." *The Female Patient* 1 (December):27–29.

Magee, Joni. 1994. "The Pelvic Examination: A View from the Other End of the Table." *Minnesota Medicine* 77 (5):8–9, 34.

Morantz-Sanchez, Regina Markell, Cynthia Stodola Pomerleau, and Carol Fenichel, eds. 1982. *In Her Own Words: Oral Histories of Women Physicians.* Westport, Conn.: Greenwood Press.

JSB

Mageras, Georgia Lathouris (1867–1950)
Midwife

The career of Georgia Mageras exemplifies the central importance of midwifery among immigrant communities in America at a time when the medical community was waging a

campaign against it. She was born in 1867 in Achladokambos, Greece. At the age of 14, while taking lunch to her father and brothers tending goats on a mountainside, she heard a woman crying in pain. The cries frightened her; but, after initially running away, she returned to help the woman deliver her baby. After this successful first case, she was increasingly called on to assist pregnant women in the village and became known as the *Mamí*, or midwife.

She met and married Niko Mageras, an Austrian who was in Greece to do construction work. The couple had four children before Niko left to find work in the United States in 1902. He was in the United States for seven years before his family was able to join him in Snaketown, Utah, where they settled near three other Greek families. In 1912, Mageras gave birth to another child and eventually had seven children. She used her healing knowledge to care for immigrant male workers in the area who distrusted company doctors, and she was particularly known for her ability to set broken bones. As the men in the area married, she again took on the role of midwife. She continued as midwife even after physicians were used for other illnesses and injuries because modesty prevented immigrant women from accepting a male attendant at birth.

Throughout the time that Mageras practiced, the family moved to different areas of Utah before finally settling in the town of Magna. No matter where she lived, she was a busy midwife and was most active in the 1920s. She never lost a mother or child in her years of practice and was careful to bring abnormal pregnancies to the attention of local physicians. Part of her success was likely due to her insistence on cleanliness. She kept her fingernails cut short and neat and thoroughly scrubbed her hands and arms before a birth. In time, she also began using alcohol and rubber gloves. Her responsibility for a mother and baby lasted though the postnatal period until the baby was baptized. Toward the end of her career, which lasted until she was in her late 70s, she increasingly assisted physicians at births rather than delivering babies herself.

Mageras died of leukemia in 1950.

References

Edwards, Jane. "Midwife Delivered, Cared for Generation of Greeks in Utah." *Salt Lake Tribune Centennial Collection Series.* Online. http://www.sltrib/com/archive/centennial/cent1233.html. 3 March 2001.

Papanikolas, Helen Z. 1996. "Georgia Lathouris Mageras, Magerou, the Greek Midwife." In *Worth Their Salt: Notable but Often Unnoted Women of Utah*, edited by C. Whitley. Logan: Utah State University Press.

LS

Mahoney, Mary Eliza (1845–1926)
Nurse

Mary Mahoney was the first African American woman to become a professional nurse. She was born on May 7, 1845, in Dorchester, Massachusetts, the eldest of three children of Charles and Mary Jane (Stewart) Mahoney. Little is known of Mahoney's life before March 23, 1878, when she enrolled in the nursing school of New England Hospital for Women and Children.

The hospital, founded by physician Marie Zakrzewska in 1862, graduated one of the country's first trained nurses, Linda Richards, in 1873. By the time that Mahoney entered the school, the training period included 12 months of study in the hospital's maternity, surgical, and medical wards and four months of private-duty nursing. Standards for graduation were rigorous; of the 40 students in the 1878 class, only 4, including Mahoney, received the diploma. Her graduation helped pave the way for future African American nurses at a time when few nursing schools accepted black students. After receiving her diploma on August 1, 1879, she registered with the Massachusetts Medical Library Nurses' Directory as a private-duty nurse. She developed a reputation as a skilled nurse and was often called to work outside Massachusetts.

In 1896, Mahoney joined the Nurses Associated Alumnae of the United States and Canada. She continued her membership after the alumnae became the American Nurses Association. She was one of the association's few black members, as membership required registration in a state nursing association, a prerequisite that few African American nurses could achieve since many state associations would not admit black women. Throughout her career, she worked to alleviate the continuing racial bias in her profession. She supported Martha Franklin's establishment of the National Association of Colored Graduate Nurses (NACGN) in 1908. At the association's first annual meeting in 1909, Mahoney presented the welcoming address and was elected chaplain. She attended the association's yearly meetings and actively recruited new members until 1921. In 1911, she was honored with life membership in the NACGN. The same year, she became head of the Howard Orphan Asylum for African American children in Kings Park, Long Island, a position that she held for only one year.

Mahoney was a longtime supporter of woman suffrage, and after ratification of the Nineteenth Amendment in 1920, she was one of Boston's first women to register and vote. She became ill with breast cancer in 1923 and died at New England Hospital on January 4, 1926. In 1936, the NACGN established the Mary Mahoney Medal to honor distinguished service to nursing. When the association merged with the American Nurses Association in 1951, the award was continued. Many local chapters of the NACGN were named after her, as are various health care clinics around the country. She was inducted into the American Nurses Association Hall of Fame on the 75th anniversary of her graduation from nursing school.

See also Franklin, Martha Minerva; Richards, Linda Ann Judson; Zakrzewska, Marie Elizabeth

References

Chayer, Mary Ella. 1954. "Mary Eliza Mahoney." *American Journal of Nursing* 54 (4):429–431.
Chayer, Mary Ella. 1971. "Mary Eliza Mahoney." In *Notable American Women, 1607–1950: A Biographical Dictionary*, edited by E.T. James, J.W. James, and P.S. Boyer. Cambridge: Belknap Press of Harvard University Press.
Doona, Mary Ellen. 1986. "Glimpses of Mary Eliza Mahoney (7 May 1845–4 January 1929)." *Journal of Nursing History* 1 (2):20–34.

JSB

Mance, Jeanne (1606–1673)
Nurse

Jeanne Mance was the founder of Montreal's Hôtel-Dieu, one of the first hospitals in North America. She is also celebrated as the first lay nurse in Canada. She was born in Langres, Champagne, France, in November 1606, the 2nd of 12 children of Catherine Émonnot and Charles Mance. As a child, Mance most likely studied with Ursuline nuns, who emphasized Christian principles and skills such as handwriting, reading, and arithmetic. Her mother died when she was about 20, leaving Mance and an older sister to care for their younger siblings.

Mance probably first practiced nursing during the Thirty Years' War and throughout the bubonic plague epidemic. In 1640, a cousin told her of missionary efforts in what was then called New France, and she determined to join the effort. She then traveled to Paris to seek spiritual and financial assistance and met missionaries who planned to found a town in New France. She also met Angélique Faure de Bullion, who offered her funds to build a hospital at the settlement. Mance and the other colonists left for Quebec on May 9, 1641, and arrived that August.

Ville-Marie, which would become Montreal, was founded in the spring of 1642. The first Hôtel-Dieu, a small dispensary, was established later that fall, and a permanent hospital building was built in 1645, outside the fort of Ville-Marie. As the hospital's nurse, Mance cared for ill settlers and those wounded in battle with the native Iroquois. She made several trips back to France to secure financing and support for the hospital and for Ville-Marie. In 1659, she oversaw the expansion of the building and brought from France three nuns from the order of Hospitallers of St. Joseph to assist in nursing duties at the hospital.

Mance died in Montreal in June 1673. The Hôtel-Dieu continues today as part of the Centre Hospitalier de l'Université de Montréal.

References

Daveluy, Marie-Claire. 1939. "Life of Jeanne Mance." *British Journal of Nursing* 87 (August):219–220, (September): 247–248, (November):282–283.

Daveluy, Marie-Claire. 1966. "Mance, Jeanne." In *Dictionary of Canadian Biography: Volume 1, 1000–1700*, edited by G.W. Brown. Toronto: University of Toronto Press.

Parks Canada Backgrounder. *Jeanne Mance, a Prominent Figure in the History of Montréal.* Online. http://parkscanada.pch.gc.ca/library/background/72 .htm. 17 February 2001.

LS

Marshall, Clara (1847–1931)
Physician

Clara Marshall was dean of the Woman's Medical College of Pennsylvania in Philadelphia for nearly 30 years. She was born on May 8, 1847, in London Grove Township, Chester County, Pennsylvania, one of three daughters of Pennock and Mary (Phillips) Marshall. Like many other early women physicians, she taught school before deciding to become a medical doctor. In 1871, she enrolled at the Woman's Medical College. While still a student, she taught pharmacy at the college (1874).

Upon graduation in 1875, Marshall was appointed demonstrator of materia medica and practical pharmacy at Woman's Medical. To further her knowledge of pharmaceuticals, she enrolled at the Philadelphia College of Pharmacy, the first woman admitted to the college. She was appointed chair of materia medica and therapeutics at Woman's Medical College in 1876, a position she held until 1905. In addition to her work at her alma mater, Marshall was demonstrator of obstetrics at Philadelphia Hospital (1882–1895). As such, she was the first woman appointed to the hospital's staff. In 1886, she became attending physician at the girls' department of the Philadelphia House of Refuge, making her one of the first woman doctors appointed to the staff of a state charitable institution.

She also maintained a private practice, which had grown so large by 1906 that she ceased teaching classes at Woman's Medical.

In 1888, after the unexpected death of the dean of the Woman's Medical College, Marshall was appointed dean. She inherited the job at a time when medical education in the United States was undergoing reform. The American Medical Association set new and higher standards for medical schools, including increased scientific and clinical training. In this era of reform, Marshall recognized that Woman's Medical College must modernize in order to survive, and she ably met the challenge. In 1893, she lengthened the course of study from three to four years and required additional laboratory work in chemistry and physiology. She also established a professorship in science and built a well-equipped bacteriologic laboratory (1896).

The greatest challenge for Marshall was providing clinical instruction for the college's students. The American Medical Association strongly emphasized that a medical school faculty should have a hospital in which to teach. Since 1862, Woman's Medical College had utilized Woman's Hospital, founded by Dean Ann Preston, for clinical training. The two institutions were governed by separate boards, however, and disagreement between

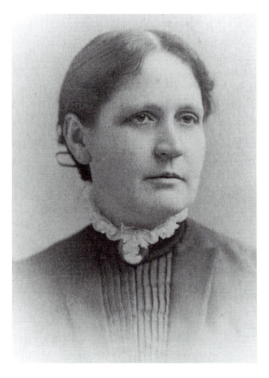

Clara Marshall. Archives & Special Collections on Women in Medicine, MCP Hahnemann University.

them led to decreased opportunity for the college's students to gain clinical experience at the hospital. Responding to the situation, in 1904 Marshall opened a small hospital in a private house staffed by the faculty. In 1907, construction of a new hospital began, and she fervently campaigned for its funding. Despite her efforts, funds came in slowly, and College Hospital was not completed until 1913.

Nevertheless, Marshall's efforts to modernize Woman's Medical College paid off when, in 1906, the American Medical Association Council on Medical Education rated the school "Class A." Additionally, the Flexner Report of 1910, which evaluated all North American medical schools and resulted in the closing of many schools, reported favorably on Woman's Medical. The college was the only all-female medical school to remain open. After more than 40 years of service to Woman's Medical College, Marshall retired in 1917.

Marshall died on March 13, 1931, in Bryn Mawr, Pennsylvania of myocarditis and artiosclerosis.

See also Preston, Ann

References

Alsop, Gulielma Fell. 1950. *History of the Woman's Medical College Philadelphia, Pennsylvania 1850–1950*. Philadelphia: J.B. Lippincott Company.

Alsop, Gulielma Fell. 1971. "Marshall, Clara." In *Notable American Women, 1607–1950: A Biographical Dictionary*, edited by E.T. James, J.W. James, and P.S. Boyer. Cambridge: Belknap Press of Harvard University Press.

Marshall, Clara. 1897. *The Woman's Medical College of Pennsylvania: An Historical Outline*. Philadelphia: P. Blakiston, Son.

Peitzman, Steven J. 1984. "Marshall, Clara." In *Dictionary of American Medical Biography*, edited by M. Kaufman, S. Galishoff, and T.L. Savitt. Westport, Conn.: Greenwood Press.

LS

Mason, Biddy [Bridget] (1818–1891)
Midwife

Biddy Mason was an African American midwife in the nineteenth century, one of the few born into slavery about whose life much is known. She was born on August 15, 1818, probably in Georgia. She was the slave of Robert Marion Smith, who owned a plantation in Mississippi, and his wife, Rebecca.

The Smiths had six children, and it is likely that Mason was midwife at their births. Rebecca Smith was frequently ill, and Mason often cared for her. Mason probably learned the art of nursing and midwifery from other slaves on the plantation.

In 1847, Smith converted to Mormonism,

and the next year he migrated to the Utah Territory with other converted Mississippians. Ninety people, 34 slaves and 56 whites set out March 10, 1848, on the 2,000-mile journey; they arrived in Salt Lake City in November. Mason, with her 10-year-old daughter, Ellen, her 4-year-old daughter, Ann, and her baby Harriet, walked the entire way. She was in charge of herding livestock and may have also been present at births that occurred on the journey. The Smith party was not in Utah long before Robert Smith decided to move to San Bernardino, California, to another Mormon colony (1851).

California had been admitted to the union as a free state in 1850. By 1855, Smith began making preparations to move his family and his slaves to the slave state of Texas. Alarmed, Mason sought help from free blacks in Los Angeles. She took Smith to court and in 1856 successfully sued for her family's freedom and the freedom of 13 other slaves. Afterward, Dr. John Strother Griffin asked her to work for him as a nurse and midwife. She agreed and earned a reputation for her skill and courage.

Mason was very successful and was able to buy a homestead 10 years after being freed. By 1884, she had built a commercial building with rental spaces on her land. She used her home as a base for charitable and philanthropic work, and with her son-in-law she founded the Los Angeles branch of the First African Methodist Episcopal (FAME) Church in 1872.

Mason died on January 15, 1891. A public art project and park are now on the site of her old homestead on South Spring Street in Los Angeles.

References

Hayden, Dolores. 1989. "Biddy Mason's Los Angeles, 1856–1891." *California History* 68 (Fall):86–99, 147–149.

Sims, Oscar L. 1992. "Biddy Mason." In *Notable Black American Women*, edited by J.C. Smith. Detroit: Gale Research.

LS

Matheson, Elizabeth Beckett Scott (1866–1958)
Physician

Elizabeth Matheson was a pioneer physician in Canada's Northwest Territories. She was born in 1866 on a farm near Campbellford, Ontario, to Scottish emigrants, James and Elizabeth Scott. Her early education was in local schools, and she received a teaching certificate in 1883 from a school in Winnipeg, Manitoba. She then taught in Manitoba until 1887, when she returned to Ontario to work in an orphanage. In 1888 the founder of the orphanage sent her to the Women's Medical College in Kingston, Ontario, for one year. Despite excellent grades, she lacked funding to continue her medical education.

In 1889 Matheson returned to teaching in Manitoba to finance the remainder of her studies. After a few weeks, however, she embarked for central India to serve as a teacher for the Presbyterian Board of Missions of Toronto, Canada. In 1891 she contracted malaria and was forced to return to Canada. Following her recovery, in December 1891, she married missionary John Grace Matheson. Together they established a mission in remote Onion Lake, Saskatchewan, with Matheson serving as teacher.

In Onion Lake, while pregnant with her second child, Matheson suffered an attack of mastitis. Seeking treatment, she made a three-day journey to find the only physician within 100 miles drunk and unable to attend her. He arrived the following day, crudely lanced her afflicted breast, and left her to be tended by a friend. This incident, plus two senseless deaths on the Indian Reserve near Onion Lake, combined with being accused of cowardice by a man whose gangrenous foot she refused to amputate, inspired her to continue her medical education.

In 1895 Matheson entered Manitoba

Medical College in Winnipeg as the only female student in her class. In the fall of 1896 she transferred to the Ontario Medical College for Women in Toronto, graduating in 1898. She refused to take the medical licensing examination of the College of Physicians and Surgeons of the North-West Territories because two licensed men in the area had not been required to do so. Although it was not unusual for an unregistered physician to practice in the late 1890s in northern Canada, Matheson found it difficult to be accepted in Onion Lake. Besides caring for her family and the children of the mission, her skills went unused until 1899, when she was called to set a broken leg. She traveled 75 miles across frozen terrain to the case, bringing her nursing infant with her. Afterward, the news of her ability spread, and her practice began to grow. In 1901, her successful management of a smallpox epidemic led the Department of Indian Affairs to appoint her as a government doctor.

In 1903, 2,000 immigrants, including registered physicians, from Liverpool, England, settled in the Onion Lake region. To compete with the incoming physicians, Matheson believed it necessary to take the licensing examination and become registered by the College of Physicians and Surgeons. To prepare, in 1904 she repeated a year of medicine at the closest school, Manitoba Medical College in Winnipeg, the only woman in the class.

Despite passing the necessary oral examinations and becoming registered in Manitoba, she was refused registration by the North-West Territories College, unless she took another examination in Calgary, Alberta. Exasperated, her husband sent a $50 check for the registration fee, and in the next mail, her registration arrived without explanation. Matheson concluded that her husband's status as a famous missionary led to the acceptance of her application. She spent the next 16 years providing medical care for the people living within a 100-mile radius of Onion Lake. She left the Onion Lake mission in 1918 to become one of two female school medical inspectors for the public schools in Winnipeg.

Matheson retired in 1941 and divided her time between her nine children's homes in Texas and Canada. She died in January 1958.

References

Buck, Ruth Matheson. 1974a. *The Doctor Rode Side-Saddle.* Toronto: McClelland and Stewart.

Buck, Ruth Matheson. 1974b. "The Mathesons of Saskatchewan Diocese." *Saskatchewan History* 28 (2):41–62.

Hacker, Carlotta. 1974. *The Indomitable Lady Doctors.* Toronto: Clarke, Irwin.

McGinnis, Janice P. Dickin, and Mary Percy Jackson. 1995. *Suitable for the Wilds: Letters from Northern Alberta, 1929–1931.* Toronto: University of Toronto Press.

CMB

Maxwell, Anna Caroline (1851–1929)
Nurse

Anna Maxwell, one of America's nursing pioneers, established two schools of nursing in New York City. She was born in Bristol, New York, on March 14, 1851, the oldest daughter of John Eglinton Maxwell and Diantha Caroline (Brown) Maxwell. After receiving her early education at home, Maxwell took three months of training (1874) in obstetrics at Boston's New England Hospital for Women and Children. She remained at New England Hospital as assistant matron until

1878, when she began her nurse education under Linda Richards at the Boston City Hospital Training School for Nurses.

After graduating in October 1880, Maxwell accepted an offer to establish a nursing education program at Montreal General Hospital in Canada. However, the hospital's physicians and administrators resisted the necessary changes that she proposed, and she resigned in June 1881. After spending three months touring hospitals in England, she served as superintendent of the Boston Training School for Nurses at Massachusetts General Hospital. In 1889 she went to New York City to become superintendent of nurses at St. Luke's Training Hospital, where she also completed the organization of the hospital's Training School for Nurses.

In 1892, Maxwell was asked to establish the School of Nursing at New York's Presbyterian Hospital. The school opened in May 1892, and for the next 30 years she ably served as its director. In 1898, the nursing course was expanded from two to three years. By abolishing traditional student allowances (1904) and by implementing tuition (1918), Maxwell could afford to increase the quality of paid instructors and also establish the school as a place of learning, rather than as a service of the hospital. She improved the quality of life for her students by adding a residence, reducing hours of duty, and hiring a student physician. Her demands for the highest quality among students and staff earned the school prestige and led to cooperative educational affiliations with the Henry Street Visiting Nurse Service (1918), the American Red Cross Training Camp at Vassar College (1918), and the nursing program at Teachers College, Columbia University (1918).

For most of Maxwell's career, she was also involved in increasing military opportunities for trained nurses. In 1898, the surgeon general of the United States Army accepted her request to allow trained nurses to care for the wounded of the Spanish-American War. Up to this time, nurses had never officially served in American military hospitals during wartime. She took leave from Presbyterian to organize 160 graduate nurses, chosen from the New York City auxiliary of the Red Cross, to care for the wounded and sick at Camp Thomas in Chickamauga Park, Georgia. After the war, she was actively involved in campaigns to establish an Army Nurse Corps and to secure military rank for nurses. Her efforts saw the creation of the Army Nurse Corps (1901) and the granting of relative rank for nurses in the armed forces (1920). To increase the number of qualified nurses availa-

ble for emergency duty through the Red Cross, she served on the National Committee on Red Cross Nursing Service to establish standards and evaluate credentials of nurses accepted by the Red Cross for service in the army and navy reserves. At the outbreak of World War I, she became chief nurse of the Presbyterian Hospital unit (U.S. Base Hospital Number 2). In 1916, she visited war zones on three fronts, but when the United States entered the war in 1917, she was too old to serve in active duty. She did, however, continue the organization of nurses for the Presbyterian Hospital unit in France.

Maxwell was active in the national nursing organizations from their beginnings. She was a charter member (1893) of the American Society of Superintendents of Training Schools for Nurses (renamed the National League of Nursing Education in 1912) and a charter member (1897) of the Nurses' Associated Alumnae of the United States (renamed the American Nurses Association in 1911). In 1899, she was a charter member of the American Red Cross Nursing Service and of the International Council of Nurses and was also active in the creation of the *American Journal of Nursing.*

Maxwell retired from Presbyterian in 1921. She remained active in nursing associations and attended the International Council of Nurses meeting in Finland in 1925. As honorary member of the Nurses' Campaign Committee, she helped raise over $1 million for a school of nursing residence for the new Columbia-Presbyterian Medical Center. In 1928, the residence was dedicated as Anna C. Maxwell Hall.

Maxwell died at Presbyterian Hospital on January 2, 1929.

See also Richards, Linda Ann Judson

Selected Additional Achievements

Her book *Practical Nursing* (with Amy E. Pope, 1907) went through four editions. Médaille d'Honneur d'Hygiène Publique, France; honorary M.A. degree from Columbia University.

References

"Anna Caroline Maxwell, R.N., M.A." 1921. *American Journal of Nursing* 21 (10):688–697.

"Anna Caroline Maxwell, R.N., M.A. 1851–
   1929." 1929. *American Journal of Nursing* 29
   (2):187–194.
Conrad, Margaret E. 1971. "Maxwell, Anna
   Caroline." In *Notable American Women, 1607–
   1950: A Biographical Dictionary*, edited by
   E.T. James, J.W. James, and P.S. Boyer. Cam-
bridge: Belknap Press of Harvard University
   Press.
Downer, Joan LeB. 1988. "Anna Caroline Max-
   well." In *American Nursing: A Biographical
   Dictionary*, edited by V.L. Bullough, O.M.
   Church, and A.P. Stein. New York: Garland.

                                          JSB

Mayo, Sara Tew (1869–1930)
Physician

Sara Mayo was one of the first female physicians to practice in the American South. She
was born on May 26, 1869, near Vidalia,
Louisiana, the second of four daughters of
George Spencer and Emma (Tew) Mayo. She
received her early education in New Orleans
and later graduated from Millwood High
School in Jackson, Louisiana. She applied to
Tulane University Medical School in New
Orleans but was rejected because the school
would not accept women students. Instead,
she earned her medical degree from the
Woman's Medical College of Pennsylvania in
Philadelphia (1898).

Mayo returned to New Orleans to begin a
medical career but was denied work in hospitals and clinics and was not allowed into
medical societies because of her sex. In response, Mayo, Dr. Elizabeth Bass, and a
small group of other women physicians
opened the New Orleans Dispensary for
Women and Children in 1905. Mayo served
as board president for the first two years and
thereafter as treasurer. The dispensary, the
only hospital in the South to be managed entirely by women, was established in a loaned
house in a heavily populated area of New Orleans and provided low-cost medical care for
poor women and children. These women
doctors worked "under great handicaps but
with such enthusiasm and fortitude" that after only three years, they could afford to
build their own hospital (Bass, p. 561). A
nursing school was added, as well as a District Nursing Service. By 1908, the dispensary had been renamed New Orleans
Hospital and Dispensary for Women and
Children. During the hospital's early years,
Mayo repeatedly sought admission to the
Orleans Parish Medical Society but was denied admittance because of her gender until
1913.

In addition to her duties at the dispensary,
Mayo was physician at St. Anna's Asylum for
destitute women and children and was on
staff at Touro Infirmary and at Baptist Hospital. She was also appointed to the board of
the Sickles Commission after persuading its
founder to provide free drugs and a clinic at
New Orleans Hospital and Dispensary. In
1910, she became the first medical woman
to earn the New Orleans *Times-Picayune*
"Loving Cup," awarded for outstanding civic
service.

Mayo died from angina pectoris in 1930.
Shortly after her death, the dispensary
changed its name to Sara Mayo Hospital.

See also Bass, [Mary] Elizabeth

References

Bass, Elizabeth. 1947. "Dispensaries Founded by
   Women Physicians in the Southland." *Journal
   of the American Medical Women's Association* 2
   (12): 560–561.
Duffy, John. 1971. "Mayo, Sara Tew." In *Notable
   American Women, 1607–1950: A Biographical
   Dictionary*, edited by E.T. James, J.W. James,
   and P.S. Boyer. Cambridge: Belknap Press of
   Harvard University Press.
Duffy, John. 1999. "Mayo, Sara." In *American
   National Biography*, edited by J.A. Garraty and
   M.C. Carnes. New York: Oxford University
   Press.

                                          JSB

McDougall, Adelaide (1909–2000)
Midwife

Adelaide McDougall received high honors for her long successful career as a midwife in Canada. Her family were members of the aboriginal Oji-Cree community, of which she eventually became an elder. She was born Adelaide Flett on April 4, 1909, in St. Theresa Point, Manitoba, the 3rd of 10 children. She grew up in and around Island Lake and spent her summers in St. Theresa Point, where she would later establish her career. Her first husband, whom she wed at an early age, died soon after the marriage. On April 3, 1931, she married Charlie McDougall and eventually had 11 children.

McDougall began her career as an assistant to local midwives, but by the age of 20 she had begun her own successful practice. She was held in high esteem for her work, and in 1967 she received an award in recognition for her services as the first aboriginal midwife to have delivered a large number of babies with a high survival rate. She battled extreme weather conditions to get to her patients, and while traveling at night, she often used lit birch bark to light her path. Around 1987, she delivered her last baby, who was also her great-grandson.

In 1999, McDougall became the first Canadian to receive the Sage Femme Award from the Midwives' Alliance of North America. The Sage Femme Award is presented to someone who has been practicing since at least 1965, who has devoted most her life to the practice, and who has made an extraordinary contribution to midwifery. Despite her impressive achievements, McDougall once said, "I am not trying to make a name for myself when I deliver a baby. The one who gave us life on this earth is the one I think of when I deliver a baby. I have guided all of the children that I have delivered. I encourage them to be good and to be understanding when dealing with their children" (quoted in "Honour Songs," p. 13).

McDougall died on November 28, 2000, in St. Theresa Point.

References

"Adelaide McDougall." 1999. Unpublished biographical sketch from Midwives Alliance of North America.

"Honour Songs." 1999. *First Nations Messenger* 2 (1):13.

JSB

McGee, Anita Newcomb (1864–1940)
Physician

Anita Newcomb McGee was the physician who established the United States Army Nurse Corps. She was born on November 4, 1864, in Washington, D.C., the oldest of three daughters of Mary Caroline (Hassler) and Simon Newcomb, a Harvard graduate and astronomer at the U.S. Naval Observatory. She obtained her primary education at home and in private schools. In 1882, she left for Europe to study at Newnham College in Cambridge, England, and at the University of Geneva. She returned to Washington in 1885 and pursued an interest in history, which included writing several articles for

Appleton's Cyclopaedia of American Biography. In 1888, she married William John McGee, a geologist for the U.S. Geological Survey. The couple had two surviving children, Klotho and Eric.

McGee earned a medical degree from Columbian (later, George Washington) University in 1892, where, during her senior year, the medical faculty barred the entrance of future women students. She completed an internship at the Women's Clinic in Washington, D.C., and studied gynecology at Johns Hopkins University in Baltimore. She then maintained a private practice until

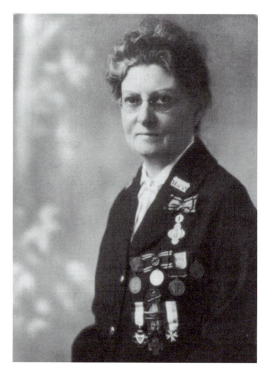

Anita Newcomb McGee. National Library of Medicine.

1895. The following year, she joined the staff of Washington's Women's Dispensary, where she remained for many years. During this time, she also served in executive positions for the American Association for the Advancement of Science and for the Women's Anthropological Society of America. For the Daughters of the American Revolution, she was surgeon general (1894–1896), the first librarian general (1896), vice president general (1898), and historian general for one year.

At the outbreak of the Spanish-American War in 1898, McGee assisted the United States Army surgeon general, George Sternberg, in assembling a group of about 1,600 highly qualified nurses for war duty. In August of the same year, Sternberg appointed her acting assistant surgeon general, making her the only woman authorized to wear an officer's uniform. At the close of the war, McGee drafted Section 19 of the Army Reorganization Act of 1901, which established a permanent Army Nurse Corps and ap-

pointed nurse Dita H. Kinney as the Corps' first superintendent. Two years later, she assisted the navy in writing legislation for its nursing corps. In 1899, she wrote a nursing manual used by both the army and the navy until 1947.

After leaving the corps in 1900, McGee organized the Society of the Spanish-American War Nurses, serving as its president for six years. She and nine members of the society traveled to Japan for six months to assist Japanese nurses during the Russo-Japanese War of 1904–1905. There, she served as superior of nurses, with the rank of a Japanese officer. She also went on an inspection tour of hospitals in Japan, Korea, and Manchuria.

In her later years, McGee lived in Washington, D.C., Woods Hole, Massachusetts, and Southern Pines, North Carolina. She lectured for a short time on hygiene at the University of California at Berkeley in 1911. She died at age 70 of arteriosclerosis in a Washington, D.C., nursing home on October 5, 1940. She was buried beside her father in Arlington Cemetery with full military honors.

See also Kinney, Dita Hopkins

Selected Additional Achievements

For her services in the Spanish-American War, McGee received the Spanish War Medal. The Japanese government awarded her the Imperial Order of the Sacred Crown, the Japanese Red Cross Decoration, and two Russo-Japanese War medals. The Dr. Anita Newcomb Award was established by the army in 1967.

References

Chaff, S.L. 1984. "McGee, Anita Newcomb." In *Dictionary of American Medical Biography*, edited by M. Kaufman, S. Galishoff, and T.L. Savitt. Westport, Conn.: Greenwood Press.

Dearing, Mary R. 1971. "McGee, Anita Newcomb." In *Notable American Women, 1607–1950: A Biographical Dictionary*, edited by E.T. James, J.W. James, and P.S. Boyer. Cambridge: Belknap Press of Harvard University Press.

Gurney, Cindy, and Dolores J. Haritos. 1988. "Anita Newcomb McGee." In *American Nursing: A Biographical Dictionary*, edited by V.L. Bullough, O.M. Church, and A.P. Stein. New York: Garland.

Oblenskey, Florence E. 1968. "Anita Newcomb McGee, M.D." *Military Medicine* 133 (5):397–400.

Reeves, Connie L. 1999. "McGee, Anita New- comb." In *American National Biography*, edited by J.A. Garraty and M.C. Carnes. New York: Oxford University Press.

JSB

McKane, Alice Woodby (1865–1948)
Physician

Alice Woodby McKane was an early African American woman physician and educator notable for her work with the poor. She was born in Bridgewater, Pennsylvania, in 1865 to Charles and Elizabeth B. (Frazier) Woodby. She attended local schools in Bridgewater, the Hampton Institute in Virginia (1884–1886), and the Institute for Colored Youth in Philadelphia, (1886–1889).

McKane must have desired to become a physician from an early age; in an 1897 letter to the *Southern Workman* she wrote that she did not graduate from Hampton because "about that time the students were sent out to teach one year before graduating. Not wishing to become a teacher, I thought it best not to begin, for fear the temptation to continue might thwart my plans for obtaining my profession" (Black Women Physicians Collection, MCP Hahnemann University). Her plans materialized when she matriculated at the Woman's Medical College of Pennsylvania in Philadelphia (now MCP Hahnemann University) in October 1889 and graduated soon thereafter (May 1892).

After graduation, McKane moved to Augusta, Georgia, and set up a medical practice. She also taught nursing classes and chemistry and physiology at the Haines Institute. On February 2, 1893, she married Cornelius McKane, a physician from Savannah. The couple founded McKane Hospital for Women and Children and Training School for Nurses in 1893, and the first students graduated two years later. The McKanes also provided health care to the destitute through their teaching hospital.

At some point during their time in Savannah, the couple traveled to Monrovia, Liberia, where they helped to organize health care facilities. While there, McKane was assistant U.S. pension medical examiner for Civil War veterans living in the country and co-organizer and head of the Department of Diseases of Women at the Monrovia hospital. She became ill while in Africa, and the couple returned to Savannah. Soon they moved to Boston to provide a better education for their children, Cornelius Jr., William Francis, and Alice Fanny. There the McKanes established a private practice, with Alice McKane primarily treating women. She also lectured to nurses in training at Plymouth Hospital.

McKane died on March 6, 1948, of arteriosclerosis.

Selected Additional Achievements

The Fraternal Society Sick Book (1913); *Clover Leaves* (a book of poems, 1914). Boston Okolona Hospital Club; St. Martin's Day Nursery Association (Boston). Business and Professional Women's Republican Club (Boston); League of Colored Poets of the World; National Association for the Advancement of Colored People (NAACP); National Equal Rights League; Republican Women's Council of Massachusetts.

References

Black Women Physicians Collection, Special Collections on Women in Medicine, Archives and Special Collections, MCP Hahnemann University, Philadelphia.

LeRoy, Casper. 1992. "Alice Woodby McKane." In *Notable Black American Women*, edited by J.C. Smith. Detroit: Gale Research.

[McKane, Alice]. 1897. "Training School for Nurses in Savannah." *Southern Workman* (August). Black Women Physicians Collection, Special Collections on Women in Medicine, Archives and Special Collections, MCP Hahnemann University, Philadelphia.

LS

McKinney Steward, Susan Maria Smith (1847–1918)
Physician

Susan McKinney Steward was the first African American woman physician in New York state and the third in the United States (after Rebecca Crumpler and Rebecca Cole.) She was born in 1847 in Brooklyn, New York, the 7th of 10 children of Sylvanus and Anne (Springsteel) Smith. Her father was a prosperous pig farmer, and the family was part of the Brooklyn black elite. Although it is not known why she chose to become a physician, it has been speculated that the death of two of her brothers during the Civil War, the high death rate in Brooklyn from the 1866 cholera epidemic, and her experience tending to a sick niece pointed her toward medicine.

In 1867 McKinney Steward entered the New York Medical College and Hospital for Women (Homeopathic), founded by Dr. Clemence Lozier in 1863. Although her father could have paid her tuition, she taught school in Manhattan to pay her way through medical school; she graduated in 1870 as the class valedictorian. She then opened a practice in Brooklyn and an office in Manhattan, making her the first African American woman to practice in New York. After a slow start, her practice grew and made her wealthy. She treated black and white patients and was known for her success in treating malnutrition in children. She practiced in Brooklyn until 1895, first as Dr. Susan Smith and then as Dr. Susan McKinney, after marrying Rev. William G. McKinney in 1871.

In addition to her private practice, McKinney Steward helped found and was on staff at Brooklyn Woman's Homeopathic Hospital and Dispensary (1881–1895). She was also on staff at her alma mater during the 1882–1883 school year and was physician and board member at the Brooklyn Home for Aged Colored People (1892–1895). During the 1887–1888 term, she did postgraduate work at Long Island Medical College Hospital, the only woman in the class.

In 1890, McKinney Steward's husband was stricken with a cerebral hemorrhage, and he died four years later. On November 26, 1896, she married army chaplain Theophilus Gould Steward. After her second marriage, she Steward traveled extensively with Rev. Steward in the western United States, but little is known about her experiences during that time. From 1898 to 1902, her husband was in Cuba and the Philippines, and she took a job as resident physician and faculty member at Wilberforce University in Ohio. She spent the majority of the rest of her life at the university.

In addition to practicing medicine, McKinney Steward was active in the suffrage and temperance movements and occasionally gave public lectures. In 1914, she gave a lecture to the National Association of Colored Women's Clubs in Wilberforce. The speech was scheduled to be on tuberculosis, but she chose instead to speak on the history of women in medicine. In discussing the early women physicians she said that "this noble band of heroic and energetic women . . . with great personal sacrifice and often humiliation, by hard work overcame the obstacles that embarrassed them . . . and opened up the road of opportunity" for women to follow (Steward, p. 16). She further noted that women of color had also become physicians, saying that "these women have measured up with their sisters in white, and in some instances have, as students, carried off the highest honors of their classes" (pp. 17–18).

McKinney Steward died suddenly on March 7, 1918, at Wilberforce.

See also Cole, Rebecca J.; Crumpler, Rebecca Davis Lee; Lozier, Clemence Sophia Harned

Selected Additional Achievements

Presented two papers (1883 and 1886) before, and was a member of, the New York State Homeopathic Medical Society; member of the Kings County (New York) Homeopathic Medical Society. Presented a paper, "Colored American Women," at First Universal Race Congress, London (1911). In 1975, the Susan Smith McKinney

Steward Medical Society was founded in her honor.

References

Alexander, Leslie L. 1975. "Susan Smith McKinney, M.D., 1847–1918." *Journal of the National Medical Association* 67 (2):173–175.
Seraile, William. 1985. "Susan McKinney Steward: New York State's First African-American Woman Physician." *Afro-Americans in New York Life and History* 9 (2):27–44.
Steward, S. Maria. 1914. *Woman in Medicine: A Paper Read before the National Association of Colored Women's Clubs at Wilberforce, Ohio, August 6, 1914.* Wilberforce, Ohio: Steward.

LS

McLean, Mary Hancock (1861–1930)
Physician

Mary McLean was one of the first women physicians to practice in St. Louis, Missouri. She was born on February 28, 1861, in Washington, Missouri, the daughter of Mary C. (Stafford) and Dr. Elijah McLean, a physician. Dr. McLean gave his daughter the best education available to young women at the time. She was tutored until the age of 13, then graduated from Lindenwood College in St. Charles, Missouri, in 1878. She studied at Vassar College until 1880, before enrolling in the University of Michigan Medical School.

McLean earned her medical degree from Michigan in 1883, in the same class as Canadian physician Amelia Yeomans. McLean then moved to St. Louis, hoping to establish an obstetrical and gynecological practice. Bertha Van Hoosen, one of the young women whom McLean mentored during her career, lived with McLean during her first year in St. Louis. In her autobiography, *Petticoat Surgeon* (1947), Van Hoosen described this trying time: "No real estate firm would rent Dr. McLean a house unless she signed a contract never to put a sign on it, or even a doorplate with Dr. or M.D. attached to her name. The reason they gave was the fear that it would place such a stigma on the house that they could never rent it again" (p. 59).

After a year of waiting, no patients came, so in 1884, McLean took a position as assistant physician at St. Louis Female Hospital and thus became the first woman to hold an official position in a St. Louis hospital. She worked in this capacity for one year, specializing in women's diseases. After leaving her post in 1885, she was able to establish a successful private practice thanks to the reputation that she earned from her hospital service. The same year, she was the first woman admitted to the St. Louis Medical Society and remained the only female member of the society for 15 years.

After the turn of the century, McLean focused her energies on the health and well-being of young girls in St. Louis. She donated her inheritance to Bethesda Hospital, an institution devoted to providing health care to the disadvantaged. She served on Bethesda's staff and also performed surgery at St. Luke's Hospital. In 1904, when the St. Louis World's Fair brought many vulnerable young women into the city, she sponsored the Emmaus Home for Girls to provide safe living quarters for the women. The home became the St. Louis Young Women's Christian Association (YWCA) the following year. McLean served on the YWCA board and worked with the association to provide health services to young women. She introduced sex education and routine medical examinations to many women who would have otherwise gone without such care. Her interest in women also included a desire to help other women enter medicine. In 1908, she formed a free clinic for working-class women staffed entirely by women.

Later in life, McLean studied medicine in China and Japan. She hoped to move to Japan to establish a surgical practice, but ill health thwarted her plans. Rather, she taught Japanese students in St. Louis so they could practice in their own country. She made several trips to China to assist medical missionaries and financed the medical education of about 20 young Chinese men and women.

McLean was a member of the American Medical Society and a fellow of the American College of Surgeons. She continued to perform surgery until a broken wrist forced her to quit in 1928. She practiced medicine until just before her death on May 17, 1930.

See also Van Hoosen, Bertha; Yeomans, Amelia Le Sueur

References

Fisher, Linda. 1986. "Mary Hancock McLean: 19th Century Trailblazer." *St. Louis Metropolitan Medicine* 8:467.

Hunt, Marion. 1980. "Woman's Place in Medicine: The Career of Dr. Mary Hancock McLean." *Missouri Historical Society Bulletin* 36 (4):255–263.

Hunt, M. 1984. "McLean, Mary Hancock." In *Dictionary of American Medical Biography*, edited by M. Kaufman, S. Galishoff, and T.L. Savitt. Westport, Conn.: Greenwood Press.

Johnson, Anne André. 1914. *Notable Women of St. Louis.* St. Louis: Woodward.

"McLean, Mary." Vertical file. Special Collections on Women in Medicine, Archives and Special Collections, MCP Hahnemann University, Philadelphia.

Van Hoosen, Bertha. 1947. *Petticoat Surgeon.* Chicago: Pellegrini and Cudahy.

JSB

McMaster, Elizabeth Jennet (1847–1903)
Nurse

Elizabeth McMaster founded Canada's first children's hospital, Toronto Hospital for Sick Children. She was born in Toronto on December 27, 1847, the second child of George and Mary Ann (Reid) Wyllie. She married Samuel Fenton McMaster in 1865 and later gave birth to two daughters and two sons.

During the early years of her marriage McMaster was involved in religious and social reform causes. Her volunteer work with society's less fortunate convinced her that Canada needed a hospital devoted to sick children. In 1875 she formed a committee of upper-middle-class women to establish such an institution. In March of the same year, the Hospital for Sick Children opened in Toronto in a rented house equipped with six cots. In the first year, 44 children were admitted to the hospital, and 67 others were treated in outpatient clinics.

McMaster believed that she had been called by God to found the Hospital for Sick Children. Under her leadership, young patients received health care as well as religious instruction. Children from poor families were not charged. While financial difficulties continually plagued the hospital, McMaster twice moved the operation to larger quarters before 1878. She also established the hospital's Training School for Nurses in 1886. The school was directed by Hannah Cody, a formally trained nurse, and graduated its first student, Josephine Hamilton, in 1888.

In 1883, newspaper owner John Ross Robertson donated money for construction of the Lakeside Home, a summer convalescent facility associated with the hospital. In 1886 Robertson joined the hospital's male Board of Trustees and led the fund-raising for a new building, large enough to accommodate 100 children. While construction was in progress, McMaster studied for two years at the Illinois Training School for Nurses in Chicago to better prepare herself for administering the larger facilities. After graduating in 1891, she returned to Toronto and became the new hospital's first superintendent. She also served as instructor in the nursing school and is credited with teaching Toronto's original first-aid courses. She resigned early the next year, following a bout with diphtheria and ongoing disagreements with the Board of Trustees over financial and medical matters.

McMaster settled in the United States, where she may have been involved in the establishment of Hospital of the Good Samaritan in Los Angeles and in the reorganization of Children's Hospital in Schenectady, New York. She died in Chicago on March 3, 1903. The Hospital for Sick Children continues to exist in Toronto.

References

Feldberg, Gina. 1994. "Wyllie, Elizabeth Jennet (McMaster)." In *Dictionary of Canadian Biography: Volume 13, 1901–1910*, edited by R. Cook. Toronto: University of Toronto Press.

Young, Judith. 1990. "Women Founders, Nurses and the Care of Children at the Hospital for Sick Children in Toronto, 1875–1899." In *Florence Nightingale and Her Era: A Collection of New Scholarship*, edited by V. Bullough, B. Bullough, and M.P. Stanton. New York: Garland.

Young, Judith. 1994. "A Divine Mission: Elizabeth McMaster and the Hospital for Sick Children, Toronto, 1875–1892." *Canadian Bulletin of Medical History* 11 (1):71–90.

JSB

McNaught, Rose Madeline (1893–1978)
Nurse-midwife

Rose McNaught helped to develop the first school of nurse-midwifery in the United States and was the first American nurse-midwife to practice in New York City. She was born on March 6, 1893, in Holyoke, Massachusetts, one of five children of William and Mary (Hurley) McNaught. She graduated from Holyoke High School and then attended Westfield (Massachusetts) Normal School. After receiving a teaching certificate in 1913, she taught in the public schools of Holyoke and Whately, Massachusetts, for about four years. She would have preferred not to teach, however, as she wanted to see the world.

When the United States entered World War I and Army School of Nursing recruiters visited Holyoke, McNaught saw her chance to go overseas. Despite disapproval from friends and family, she chose to attend the school, directed by nurse Annie Goodrich. She graduated after the war ended, around 1920, and took a position as head nurse in obstetrics at Holyoke Hospital. She soon wrote Goodrich, asking for help in finding a public health nursing position. With Goodrich's assistance, she began work as a staff nurse at Lillian Wald's Henry Street Visiting Nurse Service in New York City in 1922.

Part of McNaught's job involved assisting physicians in home births. She complained that the physicians would frequently leave nurses to conduct the births while they continued to collect medical fees. The situation made her realize the importance of advanced training in midwifery. While at Henry Street, she attended a program about midwifery by nurse Hazel Corbin, director of New York's Maternity Center Association (MCA), and she met two nurse-midwives from the Frontier Nursing Service in Kentucky who were in New York for training. She became intrigued with the idea of nurse-midwifery and decided to go into the Frontier Nursing Service.

McNaught left New York in the fall of 1926 for Leslie County, Kentucky, the home of nurse-midwife Mary Breckinridge's Frontier Nursing Service. There McNaught served as a nurse and had a firsthand introduction to the work of nurse-midwives, as well as their rugged life in the mountains. Because there was no midwifery training available in the United States, in late 1927 she traveled to London, England, to attend the York Road Lying-In Hospital's midwifery program. She received her certificate in 1928 and returned to practice in Kentucky for several years. In 1931, Mary Breckinridge encouraged her to go to New York City to help establish the Lobenstine Midwifery Clinic and School. McNaught agreed and moved back to New York that year.

McNaught's first task was to find a suitable

location on New York's West Side for the facility, as the East Side had been reserved for the training of medical students. When the clinic opened in the spring of 1932, she became the first American-born nurse-midwife to practice in New York City. In her job, she had the difficult task of introducing nurse-midwifery to skeptical New York physicians, as well as winning the respect of the city's lay midwives. When questioned by physicians about why she became a midwife, she replied that she liked the job and that women had always assisted other women in childbirth. The Lobenstine School opened in the fall of 1932 and was the first American school of nurse-midwifery. McNaught was the first supervisor of the school and clinic and was known as a firm, but fair, instructor. She strongly believed that a midwife must enjoy her work and must be in the profession out of a desire to help women in childbirth.

When the facility moved to the John E. Berwin Clinic in 1945, McNaught continued practicing and teaching there. The clinic moved again in 1952 to the MCA headquarters building, but by 1958, a lack of demand resulted in the end of home delivery service. McNaught continued to work as a consultant to the MCA until 1962 and, upon her retirement, was given life membership in the American College of Nurse-Midwives. She received the organization's Hattie Hemschemeyer Award in 1977.

McNaught died in August 1978.

See also Breckinridge, Mary; Corbin, Hazel; Goodrich, Annie Warburton; Wald, Lillian D.

References

Friedman, Alice Howell. 1988. "McNaught, Rose Madeline." In *Dictionary of American Nursing Biography*, edited by M. Kaufman. New York: Greenwood Press.

Tom, Sally Austen. 1978. "With Loving Hands: The Life Stories of Four Nurse-Midwives." Master's thesis, University of Utah.

LS

Mendenhall, Dorothy Reed (1874–1964)
Physician

Dorothy Reed Mendenhall's career was distinguished by her research on Hodgkin's disease and for her work in maternal and child health. She was born on September 22, 1874, in Columbus, Ohio, the youngest of three children of William Pratt and Grace (Kimball) Reed. She received her early education at home and then graduated from Smith College with a B.L. degree in 1895.

After taking chemistry and physics at the Massachusetts Institute of Technology, Mendenhall graduated from Johns Hopkins Medical School in Baltimore, in 1900. She continued at Johns Hopkins, completing a pathology internship and then a fellowship in pathology. As fellow, Mendenhall taught bacteriology, assisted with autopsies, and studied Hodgkin's disease, then thought to be a form of tuberculosis. Mendenhall discovered a cell that disproved this theory, and her research received international acclaim.

The cell was named the Reed cell (also called the Reed-Sternberg or Sternberg-Reed cell).

Mendenhall began an internship in 1902 at the New York Infirmary for Women and Children, and the following year began a pediatrics residency at Babies Hospital in New York. In 1906 she married Charles Elwood Mendenhall, a professor of physics at the University of Wisconsin in Madison. The couple settled in Madison, and Mendenhall gave up her career for the next eight years to raise a family. The couple had four children: Margaret (1907), Richard (1908), Thomas (1910), and John (1912). Only Thomas and John survived to adulthood.

In 1913 Mendenhall began giving medical lectures for the University of Wisconsin's Department of Home Economics. She instructed rural women on maternal and prenatal health, postpartum care, and infant nutrition. She also researched infant deaths for the Wisconsin State Board of Health and was instrumental in organizing Madison's first infant welfare clinic (1915). Four similar clinics were opened, and by 1937 Madison boasted the lowest infant mortality rate in the country. In addition to her work with the university, she developed nutrition courses and wrote many bulletins on child nutrition for the Department of Agriculture, as well as a Red Cross guide on the nutritional value of powdered milk (1918). During the 1920s she established the university's first sex education courses.

In 1917, Mendenhall began dividing her work between the U.S. Children's Bureau in Washington, D.C., and the University of Wisconsin. She completed a bureau study (1919) of war orphanages in Belgium and France and also participated in a campaign to weigh and measure all children under the age of six (1918–1919). The latter project highlighted the importance of child nutrition and led to the establishment of height and weight norms for children.

Mendenhall wrote many widely read bureau publications, including *Milk: The Indispensable Food for Children* (1918) and six chapters for *Child Care and Child Welfare: Outlines for Study* (1921). Her most famous publication was the result of her 1926 study comparing infant and maternal mortality rates in Denmark and the United States. In *Midwifery in Denmark* (1929), she concluded that many childbirth deaths in the United States were the result of the unnecessary medicalization of childbirth. In Denmark, where the midwife was in charge of

childbirth, the neonatal death rate was one-third that of the United States.

Mendenhall moved to Tryon, North Carolina, after her husband's death in 1935. She eventually settled in Chester, Connecticut, where she died of arteriosclerotic heart disease on July 31, 1964.

Selected Additional Achievements

Mendenhall's publications include "On the Pathological Changes in Hodgkin's Disease with Especial Reference to Its Relation to Tuberculosis," *John Hopkins Hospital, Reports* 10(3) (1902): 133–196; "A Case of Acute Lymphatic Leukaemia without Enlargement of the Lymph Glands," *American Journal of Medical Sciences* 124 (1902): 653–669; and "Prenatal and Natal Conditions in Wisconsin," *Wisconsin Medical Journal* 25 (1917): 353–369. The Dorothy Reed Mendenhall Scholarship Fund was established at Johns Hopkins University in 1957.

References

Conway, Jill Kerr, ed. 1992. *Written by Herself: Autobiographies of American Women: An Anthology.* New York: Vintage Books.
Corea, Gena. 1974. "Dorothy Reed Mendenhall: 'Childbirth Is Not a Disease.'" *Ms. Magazine* 11 (April):98–104.
Morantz-Sanchez, Regina. 1999. "Mendenhall, Dorothy Reed." In *American National Biography*, edited by J.A. Garraty and M.C. Carnes. New York: Oxford University Press.
Robinton, Elizabeth D. 1980. "Mendenhall, Dorothy Reed." In *Notable American Women: The Modern Period: A Biographical Dictionary*, edited by B. Sicherman and C.H. Green. Cambridge: Belknap Press of Harvard University Press.

JSB

Mergler, Marie Josepha (1851–1901)
Physician

Marie Mergler was one of the most successful and influential women in American medicine at the end of the nineteenth century. She was born on May 18, 1851, in Mainstockheim, Bavaria, the youngest of three children of Francis R. and Henriette (von Ritterhausen)

Mergler. In 1853, the family emigrated to the United States and settled in Palatine, Illinois. Mergler's physician father provided most of her early education and allowed his daughter to assist him in his medical work. She also graduated from normal schools in

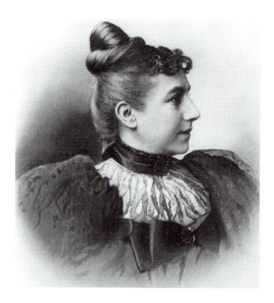

Marie Josepha Mergler. National Library of Medicine.

Illinois and New York. Afterward, she taught school and was assistant principal at a high school in Englewood, Illinois. Finding limited opportunities for advancement in the teaching profession, she turned to medicine.

In 1877, Mergler entered the Woman's Medical College of Chicago, founded, in part, by physician Mary Harris Thompson seven years earlier. She graduated as valedictorian in 1879. During her final year of study, five seniors were invited to take the Cook County Hospital internship examination. Although the women knew that they were not likely to be accepted as interns, they believed that they must attempt the examination. Mergler later wrote of the dilemma, "Not to go meant that we should perhaps never be asked again. To go meant to fail" (p. 87). While taking the exam, the students endured harassment, including "the gynecologist and obstetrician trying to get [them] off the balance by making vulgar jokes" (Mergler, p. 87). None of the women earned an internship, and it would be two years before Mary Elizabeth Bates became the first woman intern at Cook County. Mergler also competed for a Cook County Insane Asylum internship, and though her scores entitled

her to the position, the hospital board refused to accept her because of her gender.

After her unsuccessful attempts to secure an internship, Mergler went to Zurich, Switzerland, for a year of postgraduate study in pathology and clinical medicine. She returned to Chicago in 1881 and opened a practice, eventually specializing in obstetrics and gynecology. She was also surgical assistant to noted gynecologist William H. Byford. In 1882, she was named professor of materia medica and adjunct professor of gynecology at her alma mater. The same year, she became the second woman physician to join the staff of Cook County Hospital, after Sarah Stevenson. In 1886, Mergler became attending surgeon at Chicago Hospital for Women and Children, founded by Mary Harris Thompson in 1865.

In 1890, Mergler became chair and professor of gynecology at the Woman's Medical College, and in 1895 she was made head physician and surgeon at Mary Thompson Hospital (formerly Chicago Hospital for Women and Children). From 1895 to 1901 she was also professor of gynecology at the Post-Graduate Medical School of Chicago. In 1899, she was made dean of Northwestern University Woman's Medical College (the name having been changed in 1892) but was unable to hold the position long due to ill health.

Mergler died in Los Angeles, on May 17, 1901, of pernicious anemia.

See also Bates, Mary Elizabeth; Stevenson, Sarah Ann Hackett; Thompson, Mary Harris

Selected Additional Achievements

Numerous articles for medical journals; *A Guide to the Study of Gynecology* (1893); "Diseases of the New Born," in *An American Textbook of Obstetrics* (coauthor, 1895); two essays in *Woman's Medical School, Northwestern University (Woman's Medical College of Chicago): The Institution and Its Founders: Class Histories, 1870–1896.* Secretary of the college faculty, Woman's Medical College of Chicago/Northwestern University Woman's Medical College (1885–1899). Editorial staff, *Medical Woman's Journal.* Member, Illinois State Medical

Society, Chicago Medical Society, Chicago Pathological Society, American Medical Association.

References

Bonner, Thomas Neville. 1971. "Mergler, Marie Josepha." In *Notable American Women, 1607–1950: A Biographical Dictionary*, edited by E.T. James, J.W. James, and P.S. Boyer. Cambridge: Belknap Press of Harvard University Press.

Fine, Eve. 1999. "Mergler, Marie Josepha." In *American National Biography*, edited by J.A. Garraty and M.C. Carnes. New York: Oxford University Press.

Mergler, Marie J. 1896. "History of Competitive Examinations." In *Woman's Medical School, Northwestern University (Woman's Medical College of Chicago): The Institution and Its Founders: Class Histories, 1870–1896*. Chicago: H.G. Cutler.

LS

Merrick, Myra King (1825–1899)
Physician

Myra Merrick practiced medicine in Cleveland, Ohio, and was instrumental in the formation of a women's medical school and a hospital for women and children in that city. She was born in Hinckley, Leicestershire, England, on August 15, 1825, to Richard and Elizabeth King. The family left England and moved to Taunton, Massachusetts, when Merrick was one year old. At the age of eight, she worked in textile mills to help support her family. After her family moved to Cleveland in 1841, she worked as a nurse for area physicians and became interested in studying medicine.

In June 1848, she married builder Charles H. Merrick, and the couple moved to Connecticut. There she studied medicine privately with physicians Eli and Levi Ives. She then attended medical lectures at Hyatt's Academy Rooms in New York City and studied with hydropathic physician Mary Gove Nichols. In 1851, she was admitted to the sectarian Central Medical College in Rochester, New York, which was the first medical school in the United States to adopt a policy of coeducation. On May 27, 1852, Merrick graduated from the school, and the New York State Eclectic Medical Society awarded her a prize for her proficiency during the spring term.

In August 1852, Merrick became the first woman to establish a medical practice in Cleveland. Not long after, she gave birth to two sons (1854 and 1858). When her husband joined the Union army during the Civil War, she moved to rural North Eaton, Ohio, to manage his sawmill and lumber business. She also practiced medicine there. Due to financial difficulties, she returned to her practice in Cleveland in 1863.

Merrick was interested in homeopathic medicine, which is based on the use of minute doses of drugs administered according to the principle of "like cures like." When the Cleveland Homeopathic Medical College denied entrance to women in 1867, she helped found the Cleveland Homeopathic Hospital College for Women. She served as professor of obstetrics and diseases of women (1867–1871) and president of the college (1869–1871). In addition to offering medical education to women, the school presented lecture programs for women who wanted to give better care to family members. When Cleveland Homeopathic College began admitting women in 1871, the two schools merged to form the Cleveland Homeopathic Hospital College, and Merrick was appointed special lecturer in obstetrics. She resigned, however, upon learning that she would not be permitted to teach male students.

Merrick and several other women physicians founded the Cleveland Medical and Surgical Dispensary Society to provide health care to Cleveland's poor women and children. In 1878, the society opened a free dispensary, referred to as the "Open Door," which eventually became the Women's and

Children's Free Medical and Surgical Dispensary. Like many other medical institutions founded by women, the dispensary not only provided women a place to receive health care, but also gave women medical students the opportunity to gain clinical experience. Merrick worked at the dispensary one morning each week and served as its president until her death on November 10, 1899, in Cleveland.

See also Nichols, Mary Sargeant Neal Gove

Selected Additional Achievements

One of the first women members, American Institute of Homeopathy. Contributed $10,000 to building of Huron Road Hospital, where she was a staff member.

References

Gibbons, Marion Noville. 1932. "A Woman Carries the Caduceus—Myra K. Merrick." In *Pioneer Medicine in the Western Reserve*, edited by H. Dittrick. Cleveland, Ohio: Academy of Medicine of Cleveland.

Jenkins, Glen. 1977. "Women Physicians and Women's General Hospital." In *Medicine in Cleveland and Cuyahoga County: 1810–1976*, edited by K.L. Brown. Cleveland, Ohio: Academy of Medicine of Cleveland.

Kirschmann, Anne Taylor. 1999. "Merrick, Myra King." In *American National Biography*, edited by J.A. Garraty and M.C. Carnes. New York: Oxford University Press.

"Pioneer Medical Women of Cleveland and the Story of the Women's and Children's Free Medical and Surgical Dispensary." 1951. *Journal of the American Medical Women's Association* 6 (5):186–189.

Selmon, Bertha L. 1946. "The Homeopathic Medical College for Women, Cleveland—1868–1870." *Medical Woman's Journal* 53 (5):29–32.

LS

Milton, Gladys (1924–1999)
Midwife

Gladys Milton was an African American midwife in the Florida Panhandle for 40 years. In the late 1980s and early 1990s, she was at the center of a debate in Florida over who could practice midwifery. She was born to Lonnie and Lillie Mae (Anderson) Nichols on May 26, 1924, in Caney Creek, Florida. For several years during her childhood she lived with her aunt, whose collection of midwifery books Milton secretly read. In 1941, while attending Tivoli High School, she became pregnant with her first child, and while breast-feeding him, became pregnant again. She completed her high school education a few years later and soon became reacquainted with Huey Milton, a former classmate. The couple married and settled in Flowersview, Florida, eventually having five more children.

In 1958, Milton attended a mothers' meeting at her children's school, where a nurse from the health department spoke about the need for trained midwives in the rural area. She initially rejected the idea of midwifery but came to believe that it was her calling. She studied and trained at the Florala Medical and Surgical Clinic on the Florida–Alabama border. In October 1959, she received a license from the state of Florida and began 17 years of traveling and attending home births in Walton and Okaloosa Counties in Florida and Covington County in Alabama. During this time, she also worked at Florala Memorial Hospital and Mizell Hospital in Opp, Alabama.

Milton believed that pregnancy was normal, not a state of illness. She said that "the good Lord equipped us females to have our young" and believed that if pregnant women took care of themselves, it was unnecessary to treat them as if they were "about to die" by hooking them up to monitors and IVs during delivery ("Defending"). In 1968, she passed the licensed practical nurse exam, based solely on her experience. In 1973, she was half-finished with course work to be a registered nurse when two of her children were killed in a car accident, and another was seriously injured. To honor them and to allow herself to spend less time traveling to births, she built a birthing center onto her home, which opened in April 1976. Four months later, the house was struck by lightning, and the entire building was destroyed. With community help, it was rebuilt but burned a second time in May 1979. Milton persevered and opened the clinic a third time in August 1980.

As her midwifery career progressed, Milton's clientele shifted from the poverty-stricken women who could afford no other alternative, to well-educated women who chose to give birth with a midwife. She believed that physicians felt this shift, too, which resulted in their cracking down on the practice of midwifery. In 1984, the Florida legislature passed a Midwifery Practice Act, which made it difficult for lay midwives to continue their work. In August 1985, the health department began a crackdown on her clinic. The department forced her to pay high fees for licensing and inspection and shut down her clinic, citing poor paperwork, a lack of a room divider between beds, and an inadequate heating and cooling system. The clinic was closed for about a year before the community was able to raise money for the repairs.

In 1988, Milton's license to practice midwifery was suspended after a baby died during childbirth. The birth had proceeded normally until the baby's shoulders became lodged in the birth canal, an uncommon, but dangerous, complication of childbirth. Milton followed procedure by turning the woman onto her hands and knees to help dislodge the baby, but she was ultimately forced to perform an episiotomy to deliver the 10-pound stillborn child. After a legal hearing, which pitted the health department and medical establishment against Milton and lay midwives, Milton's license was reinstated, and she was found not responsible for the death. Only after two years of appeals, however, was she finally able to resume her practice. In 1993, she wrote *Why Not Me?*, an autobiographical account of her life and the ordeal of her legal battle.

Milton died on June 17, 1999, in Flowersview, having delivered 3,000 babies. Her daughter, Maria, is a midwife and continues to run the clinic.

Selected Additional Achievements

Sage Femme Award, Midwives' Alliance of North America (1976); Florida Women's Hall of Fame (1994).

References

"Deaths Elsewhere." 1999. *Tampa Tribune* (June 21, Nation/World Section): 2.
"Defending Her Birthright." 1988. *St. Petersburg Times* (October 16):1F.
Griffin, Katherine. 1992. "Gladys Delivers." *Health* 6 (May/June):54–60.
Milton, Gladys, and Christine Fulwylie. 1997. *Beyond the Storm: An Extraordinary Journey*. Pensacola, Fla.: Boaz Fulwylie Press.
Milton, Gladys, and Wendy Bovard. 1993. *Why Not Me? The Story of Gladys Milton, Midwife*. Summertown, Tenn.: Book Publishing.

LS

Minnigerode, Lucy (1871–1935)
Nurse

Lucy Minnigerode was the first superintendent of nurses for the U.S. Public Health Service. She was born near Leesburg, Virginia, on February 8, 1871, the 2nd of 11 children of Charles and Virginia Cuthbert (Powell) Minnigerode. After receiving her early education at local private schools, she earned a nursing diploma from the Bellevue Hospital Training School for Nurses in New York City in 1899.

After 10 years as a private-duty nurse, Minnigerode was superintendent of nurses at Episcopal Eye, Ear and Throat Hospital and at Columbia Hospital for Women and Chil-

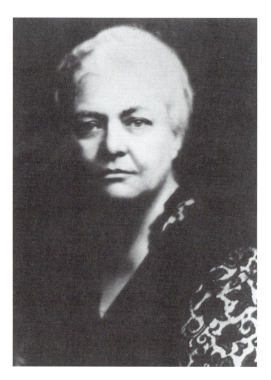

Lucy Minnigerode. National Library of Medicine.

dren (1910–1912), both in Washington, D.C. She also served as superintendent of nurses at Savannah (Georgia) Hospital.

Minnigerode's career as a public health nurse began during the outbreak of World War I, when she was appointed supervisor of the American Red Cross Unit C (1914–1915). In this capacity, she led a group of nurses to Kiev, Russia, in order to care for those suffering from the ravages of the world war and the Russian Revolution. For her work on behalf of the Russian people, Czar Nicholas II awarded Minnigerode the Cross of St. Anne (1915).

After a period as director of nurses at Columbia Hospital for Women (1915–1917), Minnigerode joined the American Red Cross Nursing Service (1917–1919). During the 1918 influenza epidemic, with the assistance of the Red Cross and the U.S. Public Health Service (USPHS), she organized nursing staff for the emergency F Street Hospital in Washington, D.C. The USPHS asked the Red Cross to appoint her as delegate of a super-

visory tour of USPHS hospitals. Her report on this tour led to the creation of a USPHS department of nurses and her appointment to its directorship in 1919. The same year, an act of Congress (Public Act 326) placed the care of veterans under the USPHS. In order to handle this huge task, Minnigerode assembled a staff of about 1,800 nurses in 76 hospitals to supply veterans with necessary care. She also instituted a graduate course for these nurses so they might better provide this service.

When the Veteran's Bureau took over the responsibility of veterans in 1922, many of Minnigerode's nurses transferred to the bureau, continuing the work that she had begun. The nurses who left to pursue other public health work were more ably prepared as a result of the education and experience that they had received under her tutelage. She continued to hold the position of superintendent, overseeing 650 nurses in 26 hospitals, caring for the beneficiaries remaining under her responsibility. She also served as a member of the advisory committee of the medical council of the Veterans Administration.

Minnigerode established and chaired the first American Nurses Association (ANA) section for government nurses and was responsible for seeing that nursing superintendents in that section became members of the association's advisory committee. In this way, she brought the needs and special talents of government services to the attention of other members of the profession. From 1923 to 1928, she served as chairperson of the ANA's committee on federal legislation.

Minnigerode died of a stroke on March 24, 1935. The pallbearers at her funeral included officers of the Red Cross and the USPHS and the U.S. surgeon general.

Selected Additional Achievements

Member, Women's Joint Congressional Committee; chair, Delano Memorial Committee; member, National Committee on Red Cross Nursing Service (1919); Florence Nightingale Medal, International Red Cross Committee (1925); chair, local committee of Red Cross nursing service

(1931); member, executive committee, District of Columbia Chapter, American Red Cross.

References

Higgins, Loretta P. 1988. "Minnigerode, Lucy." In *Dictionary of American Nursing Biography*, edited by M. Kaufman. New York: Greenwood Press.

"Obituary." 1935. *New York Times* (March 25): 15.

Paullin, Charles O. 1944. "Minnigerode, Lucy." In *The Dictionary of American Biography*, ed-

ited by H.E. Starr. New York: Charles Scribner's Sons.

Pennock, Meta Rutter, ed. 1940. *Makers of Nursing History; Portraits and Pen Sketches of One Hundred and Nine Prominent Women*. New York: Lakeside.

Stein, Alice P. 1988. "Lucy Minnigerode." In *American Nursing: A Biographical Dictionary*, edited by V.L. Bullough, O.M. Church, and A.P. Stein. New York: Garland.

JSB

Minoka-Hill, Lillie Rosa (1876–1952)
Physician

Lillie Rosa Minoka-Hill was the second Native American female physician, after Susan La Flesche Picotte. Born a Mohawk Indian, she was later adopted by the Oneida tribe in appreciation for the years of medical care that she provided them. She was born on August 30, 1876, on the St. Regis reservation in New York, the daughter of Joshua G. Allen, a Quaker physician. Her mother, a Mohawk Indian, died following childbirth. Maternal relatives raised her until she enrolled in the Grahame Institute, a Quaker boarding school for girls in Philadelphia, at age five. After graduating in 1895, she spent one year studying French at a convent in Quebec, Canada, where she converted to Catholicism.

Minoka-Hill planned on a nursing career, but her family urged her to enter medicine. In 1896, she enrolled in the Woman's Medical College of Pennsylvania in Philadelphia (now MCP Hahnemann University) and earned her medical degree in 1899. She was the second Native American woman to graduate from Woman's Medical, 10 years after Susan La Flesche Picotte. Minoka-Hill interned at the Woman's Hospital in Philadelphia and at the Woman's Clinic of the Woman's Medical College. Afterward, she and Frances Tyson, a medical school classmate, opened a joint private practice.

Minoka-Hill also worked at the Lincoln Institute, a Native American government

boarding school. There, she met Charles Abram Hill, an Oneida Indian, whom she married in 1905. Charles wanted a farmer's wife, and Minoka-Hill agreed to give up her practice. The couple moved to his farm on a reservation in Oneida, Wisconsin. However,

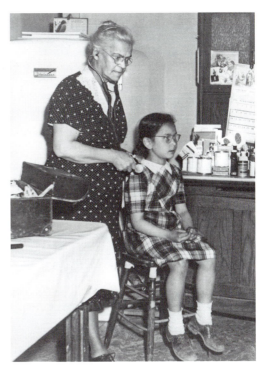

Lillie Rosa Minoka-Hill. Archives & Special Collections on Women in Medicine, MCP Hahnemann University.

Minoka-Hill could not ignore the appalling conditions of the reservation's government hospital, where a single doctor served the entire community. She began providing medical care to the Oneida and eventually became invaluable to the Oneida and local white residents.

Between 1906 and 1915, the Hills had six children. Charles Hill died suddenly of appendicitis in 1916, leaving the family with only a mortgaged farm. Rather than return to Philadelphia, where she could practice medicine profitably, Minoka-Hill remained dedicated to the Oneida. She worked out of her home, known as the "kitchen-clinic," where native herbal remedies were stocked alongside modern medicines. She often traveled long distances to administer medical care and to teach preventive medicine to her patients. Some patients paid her a small sum of money, while others could offer only goods or services. During most of her career in Wisconsin, Minoka-Hill was not licensed to practice medicine because financial constraints made it impossible for her to afford the application fee. It was not until 1934, after a group of local physicians donated the necessary $100, that she earned her medical license.

Minoka-Hill practiced medicine through a Spanish influenza epidemic and the hardships of the depression. Although a heart attack in 1946 curtailed many of her activities, she continued to practice until her death in Fond du Lac, Wisconsin, in 1952. For her work, the Oneida gave her the name You-da-gent, meaning "she who serves." A memorial to her stands outside Oneida, Wisconsin, which reads: "Physician, good samaritan, and friend to all religions in this community, erected to her memory by the Indians and white people. 'I was sick and you visited me' " (Apple, p. 483).

See also Picotte, Susan La Flesche

Selected Additional Achievements

First female member, Wisconsin Medical Society; American Indian of the Year, Indian Council Fire (1947); honorary medal, Woman's Medical College (1949); honorary membership, Outagamie Medical Society. The Dr. Rosa Minoka Hill Fund, established by her family, exists to provide opportunity and inspiration to young Native Americans.

References

American Indian Science and Engineering Society. *Rosa Minoka Hill Fund.* Online. http://www.colorado.edu/AISES/minoka.htm. 5 July 1998.

Apple, Rima D. 1980. "Minoka-Hill, Lillie Rosa." In *Notable American Women: The Modern Period: A Biographical Dictionary,* edited by B. Sicherman and C.H. Green. Cambridge: Belknap Press of Harvard University Press.

McReynolds, Jo. 1987. "Lillie Rosa Minoka-Hill." *Wisconsin Woman* (July): 28–29.

Minoka-Hill, Rosa. Deceased Alumnae Files, Special Collections on Women in Medicine, Archives and Special Collections, MCP Hahnemann University, Philadelphia.

Perry, Marilyn Elizabeth. 1999. "Minoka-Hill, Lillie Rosa." In *American National Biography,* edited by J.A. Garraty and M.C. Carnes. New York: Oxford University Press.

"Rose [*sic*] Minoka-Hill, M.D." 1949. *Medical Woman's Journal* 56 (9): 39–40.

JSB

Morani, Alma Dea (1907–2001)
Physician

Alma Morani was one of the first female plastic surgeons in the United States. She was born in New York City on March 21, 1907, the first of four children of Salvatore Natale Morani, a sculptor and painter, and Amalia Gracci Morani. She attended a local high school and then entered the premedical course at New York University (NYU). In 1928, she graduated from NYU and matriculated at the Woman's Medical College of

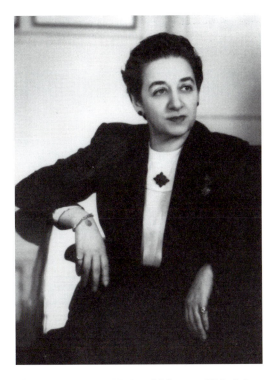

Alma Dea Morani. National Library of Medicine.

Pennsylvania in Philadelphia (now MCP Hahnemann University).

Morani earned an M.D. in 1931 and then became the first woman intern at St. James Hospital in Newark, New Jersey. Afterward, she returned to Woman's Medical to become its first female surgical resident (1932–1935). She subsequently served as assistant surgeon (1935–1938), as clinical professor of surgery (1940–1950), and as lecturer and demonstrator of operative surgery (1940–1946).

Morani eventually found the routine operative procedures of the general surgeon monotonous and decided to pursue the more creative field of plastic surgery. She completed a one-month (1939) course in plastic surgery at Polyclinic Hospital in New York City and then sought more formal training. She applied to several plastic surgery training courses but was rejected by all because of her gender. Finally, in 1946, Soroptomist International awarded her a fellowship in plastic surgery under J. Barrett Brown, a renowned St. Louis plastic surgeon. Brown "had little use for women surgeons" and allowed Mor-

ani only to observe, but not perform, plastic surgeries (quoted in Morantz-Sanchez, et al. p. 88). Despite this setback, she became the first woman admitted into the American Society of Plastic and Reconstructive Surgeons (1947).

In 1948, Morani returned to Philadelphia and established the city's first Hand Surgery Clinic as well as a plastic surgery clinic dedicated to the treatment of children's physical defects. At Woman's Medical (from 1970, the Medical College of Pennsylvania), she lectured in general surgery (1946–1950) and was assistant professor of surgery (1950–1954), lecturer in plastic and reconstructive surgery (1950–1970), and clinical professor of plastic surgery (1955–1975). She was also on staff at several Philadelphia hospitals and maintained a private surgical practice.

Morani's work was not confined to the United States. In 1964, the National Defense Medical Center of Taipei, Taiwan, appointed her to assist in establishing modern departments of plastic surgery in two Taiwanese hospitals. The center invited her again in 1968 and in 1974 to give lectures and perform plastic surgery. As president of the Medical Women's International Association (1972–1974), she traveled to Manila and the Philippines to organize the first Family Planning Congress of the Far East. The conference was attended by 467 women physicians from 14 countries and was instrumental in bringing family planning to full acceptance in that part of the world. Beginning in 1974, Morani spent two years traveling around the world giving lectures on plastic surgery and on topics of concern to medical women. In 1981, she helped establish the Pan American Medical Women's Congress, a group of 300 women physicians from Latin America.

Morani is also notable for her philanthropic efforts on behalf of her alma mater. In 1973, she donated $50,000 to the college to open a research laboratory for the study of surgical immunobiology. She also funded the Morani Gallery of Art (1985), which exhibits her own work and that of her father and others.

In 1983, Morani was appointed professor

emerita of plastic surgery at the Medical College of Pennsylvania, and today the institution's chair of plastic surgery is named after her. She died at her home in Philadelphia on January 27, 2001.

Selected Additional Achievements

Member, American College of Surgeons, International College of Surgeons, and Philadelphia College of Physicians; fourth woman fellow, American Board of Surgery (1947); founder and president, Robert H. Ivy Society (1955); regional director, American Medical Women's Association (1958–1962); president, American Women's Hospitals Service, Inc. (1967); first female treasurer (1969–1970) and director (1969–1972), Philadelphia County Medical Society. Awards include a citation for distinguished work in plastic surgery (first female recipient), Order of Sons of Italy (1955); Alumnae Achievement Award, Woman's Medical College of Pennsylvania (1964); Cavaliere of the Order of Merit, Republic of Italy (1968); Elizabeth Blackwell Award, American Medical Women's Association (1972); honorary doctor of humane letters degree, Chestnut Hill College, Philadelphia (1974); and honorary doctor of medical science, Medical College of Pennsylvania (1976).

References

"Alma Dea Morani, B.S., M.D., F.A.C.S." 1945. *Medical Woman's Journal* 52 (2): 50.

Kemeny, M. N. 1993. "Jonasson, Braunwald, and Morani. Three Firsts in American Surgery." *Archives of Surgery* 128 (6):643–646.

Morani, Alma Dea. Manuscript Collection MS-104, Special Collections on Women in Medicine, Archives and Special Collections, MCP Hahnemann University, Philadelphia.

Morantz-Sanchez, Regina Markell, Cynthia Stodola Pomerleau, and Carol Fenichel, eds. 1982. *In Her Own Words: Oral Histories of Women Physicians*. Westport, Conn.: Greenwood Press.

Solomon, Mark P., and Mark S. Granick. 1997. "Alma Dea Morani, M.D.: A Pioneer in Plastic Surgery." *Annals of Plastic Surgery* 38 (4):431–436.

JSB

Morton, Rosalie Slaughter (1876–1968)
Physician

Rosalie Slaughter Morton was the first woman faculty member at two medical schools and was involved in the efforts of women physicians to be of service during World War I. She was born on October 28, 1876, in Lynchburg, Virginia, the daughter of Mary Haines (Harker) and John Flavel Slaughter, an attorney and banker. Her early education was at private schools in Virginia and at a finishing school in Maryland. She had decided to become a doctor by the age of 16, even though her family strongly opposed her decision. She later wrote in her autobiography, *A Woman Surgeon* (1937), that her "entire upbringing and education had been designed, as it was for all Southern girls, to make me a capable wife—not to imbue me with a desire for a career" (p. 1).

Against her family's objections, Morton entered the Woman's Medical College of Pennsylvania in Philadelphia (now MCP Hahnemann University) in 1893. She served an internship at Philadelphia City Hospital and graduated from Woman's Medical in 1897. She accepted a position as resident physician at the Alumnae Hospital and Dispensary before going to Europe in 1899 for postgraduate study. Her trip abroad included six months in India studying the bubonic plague.

In 1902, Morton settled in Washington, D.C., and set up a private practice, specializing in gynecology. She married George B. Morton Jr., an attorney, on September 5, 1905, and moved to New York City. George Morton died only seven years later. In New York she set up a private practice and was the first woman faculty member at both the New York Polyclinic Hospital and Post-Graduate Medical School (gynecology department, 1912–1918) and Columbia University's College of Physicians and Surgeons (surgical department, 1916–1918). She also founded the Polyclinic's Social Service Department in 1917.

With World War I raging in Europe, in 1916 Morton was named a special commissioner of the American Red Cross for the Serbian army. She brought medical supplies with her to the Salonica front and provided medical and surgical assistance there. In 1917, Dr. Bertha Van Hoosen, of the American Medical Women's Association, appointed her chair of the War Service Committee, which became the American Women's Hospital Service, an organization that provided medical relief in war-torn countries. She was also appointed to the Committee of Women Physicians of the Medical Board of the Council of National Defense (1917–1918). For the committee, she registered American women doctors who were willing and able to offer wartime service. After the war, Morton continued to be involved in international activities; among her efforts was the organization of the Virginia Hospital Fund to provide relief to two Yugoslavian hospitals and to the Serbian Red Cross.

In 1930, after suffering several bouts of pneumonia, Morton moved to Winter Park, Florida, where she continued to practice medicine and remained active in professional societies. In addition to her medical practice and international work, Morton was the inventor of surgical instruments and medical appliances, including a treatment lamp, a surgical shoe, and adjustable bed-lifting blocks. She also lectured throughout the United States and in Europe, Australia, and Africa. She died in Winter Park on May 5, 1968.

See also Van Hoosen, Bertha

Selected Additional Achievements

A Doctor's Holiday in Iran (1940); numerous articles in the medical literature. President, Women's Medical Association, New York City (1917–1918); president, Women's Medical Society, state of New York (1927–1928); fellow, American Medical Association. Chevalier of the Order of St. Sava, Yugoslavia (1916); Medal of Mercy, Yugoslavia (1917); Kosovo Medal, Yugoslavia (1917); Serbian Red Cross, Yugoslavia (1918); Cross of Charity, Yugoslavia (1918, 1919); Commander of the Order of St. Sava, Yugoslavia (1919); Medal of Veterans of Foreign Wars (1920); Médaille d'Honneur, France (1922); Conspicuous Service Cross, New York (1923); honorary doctor of humanities, Rollins College, Winter Park (1929); honorary doctor of science, Rutgers University (1939).

References

Herbert Hoover Presidential Library and Museum. *Rosalie Slaughter Morton Papers*. Online. http://hoover.nara.gov/research/historical materials/other/morton.htm. 28 May 2001.

Morton, Rosalie Slaughter. 1937. *A Woman Surgeon: The Life and Work of Rosalie Slaughter Morton*. New York: Frederick A. Stokes.

Morton, Rosalie Slaughter. Deceased Alumnae Files, Special Collections on Women in Medicine, Archives and Special Collections, MCP Hahnemann University, Philadelphia.

The National Cyclopaedia of American Biography. 1930. Current Volume C. New York: James T. White.

LS

Mosher, Clelia Duel (1863–1940)
Physician

Clelia Mosher was an American physician who conducted pioneering research on the menstrual cycle and on women's sexuality. She was born on December 16, 1863, in Albany, New York, the oldest of two surviving daughters of physician Cornelius Duel and Sarah (Burritt) Mosher. Several of her uncles were also physicians, as was her older distant cousin and role model Eliza Mosher. In 1881, she graduated from Albany Female Academy and planned to go to college.

Her father, concerned about her delicate health, required Mosher to remain at home, however, and helped her establish a thriving florist shop. By 1889 she had saved enough money to attend Wellesley College in Massachusetts. She chose the scientific course at Wellesley, but by her sophomore year illness forced her to withdraw. In September 1891, she transferred to the University of Wisconsin at Madison and later to Stanford University in Palo Alto, California, where she earned an A.B. in zoology (1893) and an M.A. in physiology (1894).

After graduating from Stanford, Mosher became instructor of hygiene at the school (1894–1896). At the same time, she began her groundbreaking research on the menstrual cycle by requiring her students to keep records of their menstrual periods, measuring their blood pressure and other physiological factors, and interviewing them. In order to further her research, she decided to attend medical school; she applied to, and was accepted at, Johns Hopkins University School of Medicine in Baltimore. She graduated in 1900 and then spent one year as extern at the Johns Hopkins Hospital dispensary and assistant to renowned gynecologist Dr. Howard Kelly.

Although Kelly offered Mosher a lucrative salary to continue working with him, she declined his offer and returned to Palo Alto in 1901, hoping to further her own research. For the next nine years, however, she was unable to obtain funding for her research and operated a minimally successful private practice. In 1910, she was appointed professor of personal hygiene, medical adviser for women, and director of the Roble Gymnasium at Stanford University. Her new position allowed her to continue her menstrual research, which led her to conclude that menstruation was not an inherently disabling or pathological condition.

In numerous journal articles and in her popular book, *Woman's Physical Freedom* (3rd ed. 1923), Mosher stated her position that menstrual disorders were caused by poor posture and breathing habits, lack of muscle development, inactivity, and psychological factors. Of the last factor she said, "If every young girl were taught that menstruation is not normally a 'bad time,' . . . we might almost look for a revolution in the physical life of women" (p. 41). For those women who did suffer discomfort, she recommended a set of deep-breathing and isometric exercises that came to be known as "the moshers." She also advocated dress reform, physical activity for girls and women, and good posture. In 1915, she coinvented and patented the schematograph, a posture-analyzing device.

Mosher conducted, but never published, a longitudinal sexual survey that was discovered in her papers 30 years after her death. She initiated the survey in preparation for a talk to a women's club in 1892 by administering a candid questionnaire to women about their sexual habits. She continued her research for the next 30 years, and the resulting survey of 45 women, 70 percent of whom were born before the Civil War, refutes the Victorian notion of the passionless woman.

During World War I, Mosher served in France with the Red Cross (1917–1918). She returned to the United States in 1919 and was promoted to associate professor (1922) and then professor (1928) of hygiene at Stanford. She resigned in 1929, and devoted herself to her garden. She died on December 22, 1940, in Palo Alto.

See also Mosher, Eliza Maria

Selected Additional Achievements

Mosher's sex survey was published in 1980 as *The Mosher Survey: Sexual Attitudes of 45 Victorian Women* (edited by James MaHood and Kristine Wenburg; Arno Press). Member, American Medical Association; honorary doctorate, Mills College (1934).

References

Griego, Elizabeth. 1989. "The Making of a 'Misfit': Clelia Duel Mosher 1863–1940." In *Lone Voyagers: Academic Women in Coeducational Universities 1870–1937*, edited by G.J. Clifford. New York: Feminist Press at the City University of New York.

Griego, Elizabeth Brownlee. 1983. "A Part and Yet Apart: Clelia Duel Mosher and Professional Women at the Turn-of-the-Century." Doctoral diss., University of California, Berkeley.

Mosher, Clelia Duel. 1923. *Woman's Physical Freedom*. 3rd ed. New York: The Woman's Press. Original ed., *Health and the Woman Movement*, New York: National Board Young Women's Christian Associations, 1916.

Verbrugge, Martha H. 1999. "Mosher, Clelia Duel." In *American National Biography*, edited by J.A. Garraty and M.C. Carnes. New York: Oxford University Press.

LS

Mosher, Eliza Maria (1846–1928)
Physician

Eliza Mosher was one of the most eminent members of the third generation of women doctors in the United States. She was born in Cayuga County, New York, on October 2, 1846, the youngest of six children of Orthodox Quakers Augustus and Maria (Sutton) Mosher. She received her early education from private tutors and at the Friends' Academy in Union Springs, New York. During her childhood, she witnessed eight deaths from illness in her immediate family and, as a result, decided to study medicine. She hoped to enter the Female (later, Woman's) Medical College of Pennsylvania in Philadelphia. Her mother, however, "wonderfully broadminded in most things, stood aghast at the idea of a girl wanting to be a doctor" and would not allow it (quoted in Coster, p. 67).

In 1869 Mosher apprenticed at New England Hospital for Women and Children in Boston, founded by Dr. Marie Zakrzewska in 1862. She then spent six months studying privately with Lucy Sewall, the hospital's resident physician. In 1871 she entered the University of Michigan medical school, which had recently become a coeducational, yet sex-segregated, institution. She spent the third year engaged in clinical study in New York City and attending lectures at the Woman's College of the New York Infirmary.

Mosher graduated in 1875, and after two years of private practice, Governor Long of Massachusetts persuaded her to become resident physician at the Massachusetts Reformatory Prison for Women in Sherborn (1877). During the course of her duties, she equipped the prison hospital and established a training school for nurses. She also legally adopted one of the young female prisoners. From 1879 to 1881, Mosher was in London and Paris for further medical training. Upon her return she was asked to serve as superintendent of the reformatory. Although eager to reestablish a private practice, she reluctantly accepted the position lest "some other person fail in the work" (quoted in Coster, p. 69).

A serious knee injury forced her resignation in 1883. She was in constant pain for several years until a self-designed surgical operation was successfully performed on her knee. Despite her handicap, she established a private practice in Brooklyn, New York, with Lucy Hall, a medical school classmate and reformatory colleague. The two also held a joint position as resident physician at Vassar College (1883–1887). In 1888, Mosher founded a medical training course at Union Missionary Institute in Brooklyn and the following year began lecturing on anatomy and hygiene to women students at the Chautauqua Summer School in New York.

Throughout her career, Mosher was passionate about the physiological development of adolescents, especially the effect of posture on health. She made important observations on posture, most notably the relation of the position of the pelvis to the shape of the body. She designed streetcar seats and school chairs that encouraged proper posture and founded the American Posture League.

In 1896, the president of the University of Michigan convinced Mosher to serve as the university's first dean of women and professor of hygiene, despite resistance from some male faculty to appointing a woman. She instituted physical examinations for incoming students and organized the women's physical education department. She also delivered lectures on anatomy and sex education to her students at a time when Victorian modesty kept such information unavailable to most young women. She illustrated her anatomical lectures with hand-made silk organs, veins, and intestines draped over the corresponding parts of her body.

Mosher resigned in 1902 after learning that she had cancer but continued to remain active. She was instrumental in founding the Medical Women's National Association (now the American Medical Women's Association) in 1915. During World War I she participated in the establishment of the American Women's Hospitals Service, formed to provide postwar medical relief overseas. She also served as senior editor of the *Medical Woman's Journal* from 1905 until her death.

Mosher died on October 16, 1928, of pneumonia and a cerebral thrombosis.

See also Sewall, Lucy Ellen; Zakrzewska, Marie Elizabeth

Selected Additional Achievements

"The Influence of Habits of Posture upon the Symmetry and Health of the Body," *Brooklyn Medical Journal* (1892); "Habitual Postures of School Children," *Educational Review* (1892); *Health and Happiness: A Message to Girls* (1912). President, Women's Medical Society of New York; member, King's County Medical Society, Brooklyn Pathological Society, American Electro-Therapeutic Association, American Public Health Association, and American Association for the Advancement of Physical Education.

References

Bordin, Ruth B. 1971. "Mosher, Eliza Maria." In *Notable American Women, 1607–1950: A Biographical Dictionary*, edited by E.T. James, J.W. James, and P.S. Boyer. Cambridge: Belknap Press of Harvard University Press.

Coster, Esther A. 1925. "A Woman Doctor Who 'Stuck it Out.' " *Literary Digest* 85 (April 4): 66–69. [Interview with Dr. Mosher.]

Hazzard, Florence. 1946. Two biographical articles published in the *Quarterly Review*. Michigan Historical Collections, Bently Historical Library, Ann Arbor.

Morantz-Sanchez, Regina. 1999. "Mosher, Eliza Maria." In *American National Biography*, edited by J.A. Garraty and M.C. Carnes. New York: Oxford University Press.

The National Cyclopaedia of American Biography. 1914. Vol. 15. New York: James T. White.

Rosenberry, Lois K. M. 1934. "Mosher, Eliza Maria." In *The Dictionary of American Biography*, edited by D. Malone. New York: Charles Scribner's Sons.

JSB

Mundinger, Mary O'Neil (1937–   )
Nurse

Mary Mundinger is dean of the School of Nursing at Columbia University in New York. She was the driving force behind the formation of Columbia's Advanced Practice Nurse Association, a health care clinic run by nurse practitioners. She was born in Fredonia, New York, on April 27, 1937, the oldest child of Thomas and Dorothy O'Neil. She earned a B.S. in nursing from the University of Michigan (1959) and an M.A. in nursing education from Teachers College, Columbia University (1974).

During her early career, Mundinger served as director of the Nursing Education Department of United Hospital in Port Chester, New York (1971–1977), family nurse practitioner at the Greenwich (Connecticut) Hospital Primary Care Clinic (1979–1982), adjunct instructor of the baccalaureate nursing program at Pace University in New York (1975–1977), and assistant professor of the master's program (1977–1982).

Mundinger earned a doctorate from the Columbia University School of Public Health, Division of Health Policy and Administration in 1981. She stayed on at Columbia as professor of nursing and director of the graduate program (1982–1983), associate professor (1983–1986), associate dean of administrative affairs (1984–1985), and assistant dean of the Faculty of Medicine (1986). She began her current position as dean of the School of Nursing in 1986.

Since the time of her undergraduate studies, Mundinger "has always been stunned at the lack of peer respect [for nurses] from the medical profession" (Mundinger, 2000). In 1993, she took advantage of an opportunity to highlight nursing's professional contribution to health care delivery. When the Columbia-Presbyterian Medical Center needed physicians to run two of its inner-city clinics, she proposed that her advanced practice nursing (APN) faculty run the clinics. In return, she insisted the nurses be given hospital admitting privileges and supervision over patients' care. Columbia accepted her proposal, and the APN faculty members were the first in the country to have such authority.

In 1997, Mundinger formed the Columbia Advanced Practice Nurse Association (CAPNA). CAPNA is a health care clinic that provides medical care by APNs in collaboration with doctors at Columbia-Presbyterian Medical Center. CAPNA's staff, who are also faculty at the School of Nursing, have master's degrees in a primary care specialty and two more years of clinical training than registered nurses. They offer standard services such as diagnosis and treatment of illness and are legally allowed to write prescriptions. Mundinger believes that there are benefits to seeing an APN for routine health care: "Nurses are more likely to talk with patients and adapt medical regimens to a patient's preferences, family situation, and environment. They are also more likely to provide disease-prevention counseling, health education, and health-promotion activities" (Mundinger, 1994, p. 212).

Outside of her work as dean, Mundinger is a nationally recognized speaker in public health policy. She has been health care reform adviser to Senator Edward Kennedy and to President Bill Clinton. Today, she lives in Rye, New York, with her husband, Paul Mundinger, a biology professor. The couple has four children and six grandchildren.

Selected Additional Achievements

Mundinger has written numerous professional articles. Her two books, *Autonomy in Nursing* (1980) and *Home Care Controversy: Too Little, Too Late, Too Costly* (1983), earned the Book of the Year Award from the American Journal of Nursing Company. Fellow, Robert Wood Johnson Health Care Policy Program (1990), American Academy of Nursing (1983), and New York Academy of Medicine (1995). Board member, United HealthCare Corporation (1997–2000); first Centennial Professor in Health Policy, Columbia School of Nursing (1995); member, Institute of Medicine (1995). First nurse to receive the Distinguished Alumni Award, University of Michigan Medical Center (1983); honorary degree, Hamilton College (1996); Nurse Practitioner Award, *The Nurse Practitioner Journal* (1998).

References

Degree information provided by the University of Michigan, Office of Alumni Relations, Ann Arbor, Mich.; Teachers College, Columbia University, Office of the Registrar, New York, New York; and Columbia University School of Nursing, Office of the Registrar, New York.

Gregory, Sophfronia Scott, and Julia Campbell. 1998. "No Docs Allowed: Mary Mundinger's All-Nurse Clinic Gives Its Patients More Personal Medical Care." *Time* (September 21):117.

Mundinger, Mary O. 1994. "Advanced Practice Nursing-Good Medicine for Physicians?" *New England Journal of Medicine* 330(3): 211–213.

Mundinger, Mary O. 1996. Curriculum Vitae.

Mundinger, Mary O. 1996. "New Alliances: Nursing's Bright Future." *Nursing Administration Quarterly* 20(3): 50–53.

Mundinger, Mary O. May 6, 2000. Interview with author via E-mail.

JSB

Murdaugh, Sister Mary Angela (1940–   )
Nurse-midwife

Sister Angela Murdaugh is a leader in nurse-midwifery and is the director of Holy Family Services Birth Center in Weslaco, Texas. She was born on September 15, 1940, in Little Rock, Arkansas, the oldest of nine children of George Earl and Mary Angela (Graviss) Murdaugh. During World War II, the family moved to California, where her father worked at an aeronautics factory and her mother was a labor and delivery nurse. After the war, the family moved to Bryant, Arkansas.

Murdaugh has been a Franciscan Sister of Mary for more than 35 years. She believes that nurse-midwifery was "a calling from God and [she] would not have been happy doing anything clse" (Murdaugh, interview, 2000). In 1969, she earned a B.S. in nursing from the St. Louis University School of Nursing and Allied Health in Missouri. After graduating, she was a staff nurse in labor and delivery at St. Joseph's Hospital in St. Charles, Missouri, and a staff nurse in a pre-natal outpatient clinic and newborn nursery at St. Louis City Hospital. In 1971, she earned an M.S. in maternity nursing from Columbia University in New York. After completing her master's degree, she served a six-month nurse-midwifery internship at St. Vincent's Hospital in Philadelphia.

In May 1972, Murdaugh founded and became director of Nurse-Midwifery Services at Su Clinica Familiar in Raymondville, Texas. This was the first freestanding birth center in Texas and one of the first in the nation. Birth centers provide a homelike atmosphere in which women who have a minimum risk for obstetric complications may give birth. Murdaugh helped to establish an educational program at Su Clinica Familiar for Georgetown University nurse-midwifery students. In October 1980 she left Texas to become a legislative intern with NETWORK, a Catholic Social Justice Lobby in Washington, D.C.

From April 1981 to May 1983, Murdaugh was president of the American College of Nurse-Midwives (ACNM), also in Washington, D.C. She was the first to make the presidency a full-time position. During her tenure, she helped to establish a dialogue between nurse and lay midwives and established the first nurse-midwifery week. She also helped formulate a Joint Statement of Practice Relations between the ACNM and the American College of Obstetricians and Gynecologists, which continues today. In September 1983, Murdaugh returned to Texas and established the Holy Family Services Birth Center, where she provides affordable and accessible care to expectant mothers. She has also helped to establish a nurse-midwifery program at the Center for students from the Baylor College of Medicine.

Murdaugh has held numerous positions at nursing and nurse-midwifery programs across the country, including a two-year term (1988–1990) at the Frontier School of Midwifery and Family Nursing in Kentucky, founded by nurse Mary Breckinridge in 1939. Murdaugh was instrumental in getting the state of Texas to recognize certified nurse-midwives as reimbursable providers for Medicaid clients, a task that took her six years to negotiate. She has promoted nurse-midwifery on television and radio, testified and lobbied on behalf of the profession, and served on numerous nursing and nurse-midwifery committees. She also lectures and presents workshops on nurse-midwifery, maternal–infant care, the politics of nurse-midwifery, inspirational topics, birth centers, and midwifery care for poor women.

See also Breckinridge, Mary

Selected Additional Achievements

"Helping the Breastfeeding Mother," *American Journal of Nursing* 72 (8)(1972):1420–1423; "Experiences of a New Migrant Health Clinic," *Women and Health* 1 (6)(1976): 25–29; "Su Clinica Familiar—Georgetown University Pilot Project," *Journal of Nurse-Midwifery* 27 (5)(1982):25–33. Midwives' Alliance of North America (1983–present; life membership conferred 1989); member (1983–present), board member (1983–1985), secretary (1986–1987), National Association of Childbearing Centers. Hattie Hemschemeyer Award, American College of Nurse-Midwives (1990); Distinguished Fellow, American College of Nurse-Midwives (1993).

References

Gaskin, Ina May. 1995. "Interview with Sister Angela Murdaugh." *Birth Gazette* 12 (1):4–10.

Murdaugh, Angela. July 16, 2000. Interview with author via E-mail.

Murdaugh, Angela. N.d. Curriculum Vitae and Brief Biography.

National Association of Childbearing Centers. *Generations Library*. Online. http://www.birth centers.org/generationslibrary/. 20 August 2000.

LS

N

Nichols, [Margaret Carrie] Etta Grigsby (1897–1994)
Midwife

Etta Nichols attained near-legendary status through her practice of midwifery in the southern Appalachian mountains of Tennessee for nearly 60 years. She was born in Del Rio, Tennessee, on May 19, 1897, the 2nd of 10 children of John L. and Nova (Turner) Grigsby. She attended school for a short time and obtained the equivalent of an eighth grade education. Her father practiced what the local people called "country" medicine. He never attended medical school; rather, he learned by watching his father, physician John B. Grigsby. Similarly, Nichols accompanied her father on medical calls, particularly maternity cases.

On October 15, 1916, she married James Harrison Nichols and soon became pregnant with the first of their four children. From childhood, she wanted to be a nurse, but family obligations kept her from her goal. In 1930, when her father was unavailable to assist a laboring woman, she took his place and delivered her first baby. In her early years as a midwife, she frequently walked several miles to reach expectant mothers. Later, she added a birthing room to her home. Mothers were welcome to stay as long as necessary, although most found delivery with her easier than hospital birthing and left several hours after giving birth.

Nichols believed that the secret to successful midwifery was patience, and she allowed nature to take its course. She encouraged laboring women to walk around, as mothers who stayed in bed for a long time had more difficult labor. She did not believe in using painkillers, saying that mothers "get along better if they're not all doped up" (quoted in Eblen). She was also a strong believer in breast-feeding but accepted goat's milk as a substitute if the mother did not want to breast-feed. Her initial fee for delivery was $2, and by 1989 it was only $15. If a woman could not afford the fee, Nichols accepted goods or delivered babies free of charge.

In May 1989, Nichols delivered her last baby. A few months later, she developed congestive heart failure and never regained her health. In her career, she delivered more than 2,000 babies. She died on November 25, 1994.

References

Eblen, Tom. 1985. "She's a Legend as Midwife of the Mountains." *Atlanta Journal and Constitution* (September 8):2A.

Smith-Ledford, Sharon. 1998. *Etta "Granny" Nichols: Last of the Old-Timey Midwives.* Chapel Hill, N.C.: Professional Press.

LS

Nichols, Mary Sargeant Neal Gove (1810–1884)
Physician

Mary Gove Nichols was one of the first women to practice medicine in the United States and the first to publicly lecture on anatomy and physiology. She was born in Goffstown, New Hampshire, on August 10, 1810, one of three children of William and Rebecca Neal. Her early education was at local schools and under the direction of her father. Her older brother studied medicine, and she secretly read his textbooks until he hid them from her. To earn a living, she taught, helped her mother sew, and wrote stories, essays, and poems for such publications as the *Boston Traveller.*

On March 5, 1831, she married hatter Hiram Gove and the following year had a daughter, Elma Penn Gove. Four other pregnancies ended in miscarriage or stillbirth, and during this difficult time, Nichols' enthusiasm for medical study deepened. She later wrote, "The passion that has possessed me from my first reading on pathology I consider providential. I believe fully, that I have been set apart from birth for a peculiar work" (Nichols, p. 69). As medical schools were not yet open to women, Nichols was forced to study independently. She began to treat herself, her daughter, and a few women patients with water cure methods after reading a book describing them. Water cure, or hydropathy, was based on the belief that water was the natural sustainer of life and was a popular alternative to regular medical practice.

In 1837, Hiram's hat business failed, and the couple moved to Lynn, Massachusetts, where Nichols opened a boarding school. She lectured her students on anatomy and physiology and continued writing. Another early female practitioner of medicine, Harriot Hunt, boarded with Nichols for a short time. In the fall of 1838, Nichols gave a course of lectures on anatomy and physiology in Boston, the first such lectures given by a woman. She stressed the importance of studying anatomy and physiology because she believed that much of women's suffering resulted from ignorance of their bodies. The lectures proved extremely successful, and she repeated them in other towns on the East Coast.

Nichols soon became ill from overwork and an unhappy marriage. In 1840, she moved to Worcester, Massachusetts, to prepare her lectures for publication and to edit the *Health Journal and Advocate of Physiological Reform.* The journal failed, and she began lecturing again. In 1842, she left Hiram and returned to her parents' home. Three years later, she went to a water cure facility in Brattleboro, Vermont, where she observed for three months and lectured on physiology and preventive medicine. She was then a resident physician at a water cure institution in Lebanon Springs, New York. In May 1846, she established her own facility in New York City and became one of the best-known water cure physicians.

On Christmas Eve 1847, she met writer Thomas Low Nichols, and they married on July 28, 1848. Nichols continued lecturing and practicing medicine and in November 1850 gave birth to a daughter, Mary Wilhelmina. The same year, Thomas finished a degree in medicine that he had begun 15 years earlier. The couple moved to a larger water cure house, where Mary did most of the medical practice, and Thomas wrote about medical reform and other topics. In September 1851, the two opened the American Hydropathic Institute, a medical school offering education to men and women.

The Nicholses were increasingly interested in more than medicine and successively opened two Schools of Life, which focused on spiritual health and the development of the whole human being. Their first institution was in New York, and the next in Ohio; neither was very successful. Their publication of several frank works on marriage and sexuality, including Mary Nichols' autobiographical account of her life, *Mary Lyndon, or, Revelations of a Life* (1855), led to their disconnection from other health reformers. They started their own *Nichols' Journal of Health, Water-Cure, and Human Progress* in April 1853, which lasted a few years, and in the fall of 1855 moved to Cincinnati. After converting to Roman Catholicism in 1857, they traveled to Catholic institutions from the Great Lakes to the Gulf of Mexico, and Mary taught preventive medicine. In the fall of 1861, they fled to London, England, in opposition to the American Civil War. The Nicholses opened a water cure facility in Malvern for a short time and in 1875 moved back to London, where Nichols continued her medical practice. She began suffering from breast cancer, and a fall weakened her further. She died on May 30, 1884.

See also Hunt, Harriot Kezia

Selected Additional Achievements

Lectures to Ladies on Anatomy and Physiology (1842); *Lectures to Women on Anatomy and Physiology; with an Appendix on Water Cure* (1846); *Experience in Water-Cure* (1849); *Marriage: Its History, Character, and Results* (1854, with Thomas Nichols); *A Woman's Work in Water Cure and Sanitary Education* (1874). The novels *Uncle John, or, "It Is Too Much Trouble"* (1846, under the pseudonym Mary Orme); *Agnes Morris, or, The Heroine of Domestic Life* (1849); *The Two Loves, or, Eros and Anteros* (1849); *Uncle Angus* (1864); *Jerry: A Novel of Yankee American Life* (1872).

References

Blake, John B. 1962. "Mary Gove Nichols, Prophetess of Health." *Proceedings of the American Philosophical Society* 106 (3):219–234.

Nichols, Mary S. Gove. 1849. "Mrs. Gove's Experience in Water Cure." *Water-Cure Journal* 7 (February):40–41, (March):68–70, (April):103–105, (May):135–140, (June):165–168; 8 (August):35–38, (October):98–100, (November):129–132.

Noever, Janet Hubly. 1983. "Passionate Rebel: The Life of Mary Gove Nichols, 1810–1884." Doctoral diss., University of Oklahoma.

Stearns, Bertha-Monica. 1933. "Two Forgotten New England Reformers." *New England Quarterly* 6 (1):59–84.

LS

Novello, Antonia Coello (1944–   )
Physician

Antonia Novello was the first Hispanic and first female U.S. surgeon general. She currently serves as the first female minority commissioner of health for the state of New York. She was born on August 23, 1944, in Fajardo, Puerto Rico, the oldest of three children of Antonio and Ana Delia Coello. She was born with a painful congenital colon condition that required annual hospitalization. She was told that she would have surgery to correct the condition when she was 8 years old, but this did not happen until she was 18. Thus, she described herself as "one of those kids that got lost in the system of health, either because you're poor or either because . . . you cannot ask the right questions" (Academy of Achievement).

Novello's mother, a school principal, encouraged Novello to excel in her education. She graduated from high school at age 15 and later began premedical studies at the University of Puerto Rico in Rio Piedras. She earned a B.S. degree in 1965 and an M.D. degree from the university's medical school in San Juan in 1970. In 1970, she married physician Joseph Novello, and the couple relocated to Ann Arbor, Michigan. Novello completed a one-year internship and a two-year residency in the Department of Pediatrics at the University of Michigan Medical Center. In 1971, she became the first woman to earn the department's Intern of the Year award. She continued her training as a fellow in pediatric nephrology at the University of Michigan (1973–1974) and at Georgetown University Hospital in Washington, D.C. (1974–1975).

Novello then established a private practice in Springfield, Virginia, specializing in pediatric nephrology. In 1978 she took a position as project officer at the National Institute of Arthritis, Metabolism and Digestive Diseases of the National Institutes of Health (NIH) in Bethesda, Maryland. She rose through the ranks of the NIH and in 1986 was promoted to deputy director of the National Institute of Child Health and Human Development. During this time, she also earned a master of public health degree from Johns Hopkins University (1982). In her four years as deputy director, Novello coordinated research for children with acquired immune deficiency syndrome (AIDS) and brought public attention to the fact that pregnant women with AIDS can pass the disease on to their babies. Concurrently, she taught pediatrics at Georgetown University (1986 and 1989) and at the Uniformed Services University of Health Sciences (1989). She also cochaired the Advisory Committee on Women's Health Issues, was instrumental in the enactment of the National Organ Transplant Act of 1984, and played a role in drafting health warning labels for cigarette packages.

During her career with the NIH, Novello received many commendations for her public health work. President George Bush took note of her successes and nominated Novello to be the next U.S. surgeon general. On March 9, 1990, she was sworn in as the 14th surgeon general and achieved the distinction of being the first Hispanic and first female to achieve that position. In this role, she led approximately 6,000 commissioned officers of the U.S. Public Health Service in her quest to reduce the number of deaths caused by AIDS, breast cancer, and alcohol and tobacco abuse. She also worked to end the stigma against mental illness. Novello's personal experience with chronic childhood illness and as a female and a minority prepared her for her role as the nation's health adviser. She was one of the first in the medical profession to emphasize the public health concerns of domestic violence, AIDS, and underage drinking and smoking. She was, and continues to be, a supporter of improving health care access to minorities, who often suffer a disproportionate number of preventable health problems.

Novello stepped down as surgeon general in 1993. That year she served as adjunct professor of pediatrics and communicable diseases at the University of Michigan Medical School and began her work with the United Nations Children's Fund (UNICEF), educating people worldwide on health and nutrition (1993–1996). In 1996, she returned to Johns Hopkins University as director of community health policy in the School of Health and Hygiene and as visiting professor of Health Policy and Management. On June 15, 1999, New York governor George Pataki appointed her as commissioner of the New York State Department of Health. As the first female, minority commissioner, she continues her work as an advocate for public health, especially for women, children, and minorities.

Selected Additional Achievements

Author of more than 75 articles and book chapters on pediatrics, nephrology, and public health. Diplomate, American Board of Pediatrics. Numerous awards and honors, including more than 30 honorary degrees, the Surgeon General's Exemplary Service Medal (1989), the Public Health Service Outstanding Unit Citation (1989), Certification of Commendation, Department of Health and Human Services, Assistant Secretary for Health (1989), the Surgeon General Medallion (1990), the Nathan B. Davis Award, American Medical Association, and the Congressional Hispanic Caucus Medal.

References

Academy of Achievement. "Antonia Novello, M.D." *Hall of Public Service.* Online. http://www.achievement.org./frames.html. 5 August 2000.

Graham, Judith, ed. 1992. *Current Biography Yearbook 1992.* New York: H.W. Wilson.

Howes, Kelly King. 1993. "Antonia Novello." In *Notable Hispanic American Women,* edited by D. Telgen and J. Kamp. Detroit: Gale Research.

"Puerto Rico Profile: Antonia Novello." 2000. *Puerto Rico Herald* 4 (12). Online. http://www.puertorico-herald.org/issues/vol4n12/ProfileANovello-en.shtml. 15 August 2000.

Who's Who of American Women 1999–2000. 1998. 21st ed. New Providence, N.J.: Marquis Who's Who.

JSB

Noyes, Clara Dutton (1869–1936)
Nurse

Clara Noyes is most noted for her work with the American Red Cross during and after World War I. She was born on October 3, 1869, at Port Deposit, Maryland, the third of nine children of Laura Lay (Banning) and Enoch Dutton Noyes. Her early education was at private schools in Maryland and Connecticut.

In 1896, she graduated from the Johns Hopkins Training School for Nurses in Baltimore and remained on as head nurse at Johns Hopkins Hospital. She was then superintendent of the training school for nurses at New England Hospital for Women and Children in Boston (1897–1901) and superintendent of the Hospital and Training School for Nurses at St. Luke's Hospital in New Bedford, Massachusetts (1901–1910). In 1910, she became general superintendent of training schools at the Bellevue and Allied Hospitals in New York City. While she was at Bellevue, a school for midwives was founded, which she endorsed.

With the eruption of World War I in Europe in 1914, there was an increased demand for nurses to serve with the Red Cross. Thus, Jane Delano, chair of the National Committee on Red Cross Nursing Service, appealed to Noyes to accept a position as director of the Red Cross' Bureau of Nursing Service. After an initial reluctance to leave Bellevue, Noyes accepted the position and arrived in Washington, D.C., in September 1916. Among her duties were organizing nursing services at military hospitals and at relief organizations and selecting and assigning Red Cross nursing personnel. She also went on speaking tours to recruit nurses and had recruited 53,000 nurses by the end of her career. Additionally, she created standardized instructions for women volunteers who wished to make surgical dressings for the war effort and was responsible for seeing that Red Cross nurses had uniforms and the proper equipment for duty.

When Delano died unexpectedly in 1919, Noyes took over as director of the American Red Cross Department of Nursing and as chair of the National Committee on Red Cross Nursing. In 1920, she embarked on an inspection tour of Red Cross activities in Europe. During the tour, she encouraged local European communities to develop their own nursing operations so that service would continue after the Red Cross departed.

Noyes died suddenly on June 3, 1936, in Washington, D.C., after suffering a heart attack.

See also Delano, Jane Arminda

Selected Additional Achievements

Editor, Red Cross section, *American Journal of Nursing*. President, National League of Nursing Education (1913–1916); president, American Nurses Association (1918–1922); vice president, International Council of Nurses (1925, 1929, 1933); president, Board of Directors of the American Journal of Nursing Company (1911–1918). Patriotic Service Medal, National Institute of Social Sciences (1919); Florence Nightingale Medal, International Committee of the Red Cross (1923); Walter Burns Saunders Medal (1933); American Nurses Association Hall of Fame (1998).

References

Dock, Lavinia L., Sarah Elizabeth Pickett, Clara D. Noyes, Fannie F. Clement, Elizabeth G. Fox, and Ann R. Van Meter. 1922. *History of American Red Cross Nursing*. New York: Macmillan.

Higgins, Loretta P. 1988. "Noyes, Clara Dutton." In *Dictionary of American Nursing Biography*, edited by M. Kaufman. New York: Greenwood Press.

Pfefferkorn, Blanche. 1958. "Noyes, Clara Dutton." In *The Dictionary of American Biography, Supplement 2*, edited by R.L. Schuyler and E.T. James. New York: Charles Scribner's Sons.

LS

Nutting, [Mary] Adelaide (1858–1948)
Nurse

Adelaide Nutting was a leader in American nursing whose work at the nursing schools of Johns Hopkins Hospital and at Teachers College, Columbia University helped to define and reform nursing education. She was also a leader in nursing organizations and helped to put nursing on a firm professional foundation. She was born on November 1, 1858, in Frost Village, Quebec, Canada, the fourth of five children of Vespasion and Harriet Sophia (Peasley) Nutting. Most of her childhood was spent in Waterloo, Quebec, where her family struggled to make ends meet. Her early education was at a village academy, a convent school, and a private school in Montreal. She also received special instruction in music and art and taught music at a girls' school in Saint John's, Newfoundland, for one year (1882–1883).

In the summer of 1889, Nutting read about the opening of the Johns Hopkins Training School for Nurses in Baltimore. She wrote superintendent Isabel Hampton Robb and was soon admitted to the first nursing class at Hopkins. While a student, Nutting won a prize for writing a detailed article on a typhoid case that she had attended; the article was published in *Trained Nurse and Hospital Review* (March 1891). She graduated in 1891 and stayed at Johns Hopkins as head nurse of various wards. She was named assistant superintendent in 1893.

Within a year, Robb married and left Johns Hopkins, and Nutting succeeded her as superintendent of nurses and principal of the training school. Nutting accepted the appointment on the condition that she be allowed a year to visit nursing schools around the country and abroad. When she returned to the school in September 1895, she submitted innovative plans to increase the course length to three years, reduce the nurse's day to eight hours, and withdraw student allowances. At the time, nursing schools were located in hospitals, where students were responsible for nursing functions. Nutting wanted to reform this system, believing that a hospital's focus on economic interests did not foster an educational environment. She described the strange relationship between hospital and nurse training school by saying, that "the effort to do honest educational work in a place and a medium designed and conducted for other purposes has brought about complex situations and curiously baffling problems" (Nutting, p. vi).

In 1901, Nutting developed a six-month preliminary program for Johns Hopkins student nurses, which permitted them to learn some theory before they began hospital work. Among her other innovations at Johns Hopkins were adding graduate nurses to the staff, paying lecturers, introducing social subjects to the curriculum, and establishing a library and a history of nursing club. Nutting's interest in nursing history inspired her to work with Lavinia Dock in writing the multivolume work *A History of Nursing* (first two vols., 1907; second two, 1912). While at Johns Hopkins, Nutting also helped draft Maryland's first nurse-practice law in 1904.

Nutting believed that nurses, like other professionals, should have a thorough university education. To that end, she and Isabel Hampton Robb persuaded the dean of Columbia University's Teachers College to allow an experimental course in hospital economics at the college. Between 1899 and 1907, Nutting taught part-time at the school. In 1907, she left Johns Hopkins to become a full-time professor at Teachers College, making her the first nurse to hold a university professorship.

In 1910, the college set up a department of nursing and health, with Nutting as chair. There she developed programs in hospital administration and nursing education and added instruction in the new field of public health nursing. In 1912, she published *Educational Status of Nursing*, the first comprehensive study of American nursing. She remained at Teachers College until her retirement in 1925. By then, the school awarded bachelor's and master's degrees in nursing and had educated many of the profession's future leaders.

In addition to her work at Johns Hopkins and at Teachers College, Nutting was active in nursing organizations and was involved in nearly all early twentieth-century efforts to reform nursing education. She served on the Nurses' Associated Alumnae committee that created the *American Journal of Nursing* in 1900 and was chair of the National League of Nursing Education's Committee on Education (1903–1921), which published *Standard Curriculum for Schools of Nursing* in 1917. During World War I, she was chair of the committee responsible for coordinating the nation's nurses, the General Medical Board of the Council of National Defense's nursing committee. She was also a member of the Rockefeller Foundation's Committee for the Study of Nursing Education, which produced the Winslow-Goldmark report in 1923 (published as *Nursing and Nursing Education in the United States*). The report was an extensive study of nursing education and practice that advocated high standards in nursing schools and led to the establishment of an experimental university school of nursing at Yale University.

After her retirement from Teachers College, Nutting published several of her essays in *A Sound Economic Basis for Schools of Nursing* (1926). She died on October 3, 1948, in White Plains, New York.

See also Dock, Lavinia Lloyd; Robb, Isabel Adams Hampton

Selected Additional Achievements

Numerous articles in the nursing literature. President (1896, 1909), vice president (1897), secretary (1903, 1904), American Society of Superintendents of Training Schools for Nurses; president, American Federation of Nurses (1901–1913); president, Maryland State Association of Graduate Nurses (1903); honorary president, Florence Nightingale International Foundation (1934). Founder, Women's Faculty Club, Columbia University, American Home Economics Association (1908), and the *Journal of Home Economics.* Liberty Service Medal, National Institute of Social Sciences (1918); honorary master of arts, Yale University (1922); first recipient, Mary Adelaide Nutting Award, National League of Nursing Education (1944); American Nurses Association Hall of Fame (1976).

References

Donahue, M. Patricia. 1988. "Mary Adelaide Nutting." In *American Nursing: A Biographical Dictionary*, edited by V.L. Bullough, O.M. Church, and A.P. Stein. New York: Garland.

Dunbar, Virginia M. 1971. "Nutting, Mary Adelaide." In *Notable American Women, 1607–1950: A Biographical Dictionary*, edited by E.T. James, J.W. James, and P.S. Boyer. Cambridge: Belknap Press of Harvard University Press.

Marshall, Helen E. 1972. *Mary Adelaide Nutting: Pioneer of Modern Nursing.* Baltimore: Johns Hopkins University Press.

Nutting, Mary Adelaide. 1984. *A Sound Economic Basis for Schools of Nursing and Other Addresses.* Reprint ed. New York: Garland. Original ed., New York: G.P. Putnam's Sons, 1926.

Ward, Patricia Spain. 1974. "Nutting, Mary Adelaide." In *The Dictionary of American Biography: Supplement 4, 1946–1950*, edited by J.A. Garraty and E.T. James. New York: Charles Scribner's Sons.

LS

O

Ohlson, Agnes K. (1902–1991)
Nurse

Agnes Ohlson was a leader in the improvement of nursing education and licensure in the United States. She was born in New Britain, Connecticut, on February 20, 1902, the second of four children of Swedish immigrants Johannes and Karolina (Nelson) Ohlson. She graduated from New Britain High School in 1919 with the hope of entering nursing school. Her parents wanted her to fill the traditional female role of wife and homemaker, but her father promised his encouragement if, at the age of 21, she still wanted to be a nurse. Until then, Ohlson worked as a secretary but retained her original goal. She entered nursing school at Boston's Peter Bent Brigham School of Nursing and graduated in 1926.

In 1926, Ohlson became supervisor at Wesson Maternity Hospital in Springfield, Massachusetts. She left Wesson after nine months to attend Teachers College, Columbia University in New York City and earned a bachelor's degree in administration (1931). While she was a student, she served as assistant director of nursing service at Truesdale Hospital in Fall River, Massachusetts (1927–1929). After graduation, she became director of nursing and superintendent of the nurse training school at Waterbury Hospital in Wa-

terbury, Connecticut (1931–1936). While at Waterbury, she became a member of the Board of Directors of the Connecticut Nurses Association and was elected to the Board of Directors of the Connecticut State Board of Nursing Examiners (1935). She resigned from Waterbury the next year to begin her most memorable work as secretary and chief examiner of the state board, a position that she held for approximately 27 years. In this role, she worked to improve and strengthen the education, licensure, and registration of Connecticut's nurses.

Ohlson began her tenure by successfully lobbying for the addition of a legal definition of nursing in the state's nursing laws. Her most important work concerned the board's essay-style licensure examination, which she believed lacked objectivity. Ohlson made inquiries to other state boards and found that they used similar examinations. Concerned that the boards were not meeting their requirements to assure that nurses were adequately trained, she asked the American Nurses Association (ANA) to call a meeting of state board members. The group eventually became an association committee that, together with a similar committee of the National League of Nursing Education

(NLNE), developed the State Board Test Pool Examinations, the first national qualifying examination for nurse licensure. The test pool exams were different from the essay tests in that they were standardized, objective, and machine-graded.

Within her own state, Ohlson strengthened the standards used to evaluate nursing schools. She was instrumental in the formation of the school of nursing at the University of Connecticut in Storrs. The school opened in 1942 and was the state's first baccalaureate nursing program at a public university. Ohlson's devotion to nurse licensure and education is exhibited by her activities in professional organizations. By 1950, she had been president of the Connecticut League for Nursing Education (1946), chair of the ANA Committee for the Bureau of State Boards of Nurse Examiners, chair of the education section and president of the Connecticut State Nurses Association (1947–1949), and chair of the NLNE Committee on State Board Problems. She was also secretary (1950–1954) and president (1954–1958) of the ANA. In her 1954 presidential address, Ohlson reiterated the need for nursing to "set [its] own standards, publicize them wisely, then effectively implement ever-improved excellence of practice" (quoted in Daisy, 1996, p. 1).

Ohlson retired from Connecticut State Board of Nursing Examiners in 1963. She died in Florida in 1991.

Selected Additional Achievements

"Eight-hour Plan for Private Duty Nurses," *American Journal of Nursing* (1932). Master's degree in government, Trinity College, Hartford, Connecticut (1951). Consultant, Cadet Nurse Corps, U.S. Public Health Service (1943–1944); U.S. delegate, 8th World Health Assembly, Mexico City (1955); first president, American Nurses' Foundation (1955–1958); president (1957–1961) and vice president (1961–1965), International Council of Nurses; vice president, Citizens Committee for World Health (1956). Life membership, Foundation of the Women's Auxiliary of the American Swedish Historical Museum (1959). First recipient, Agnes Ohlson Award for Outstanding Contributions to Nursing through Political Action, Connecticut Nurses Association (1980); American Nurses Association Hall of Fame (1996).

References

"Candidates for ANA Election." 1950. *American Journal of Nursing* 50 (4):254.

Daisy, Carol A. 1992. "Agnes K. Ohlson." In *American Nursing: A Biographical Dictionary*, edited by V.L. Bullough, L. Sentz, and A.P. Stein. New York: Garland.

Daisy, Carol. 1996. "Keeping the Flame: The Influence of Agnes Ohlson on Licensure and Registration for Nurses, 1936–1963." Doctoral diss., University of Texas.

JSB

Osborne, Geneva Estelle Massey Riddle (1901–1981)
Nurse

Geneva Osborne was an African American nurse who worked to improve educational and professional opportunities for other black nurses. She was born on May 3, 1901, in Palestine, Texas, to Hall and Bettye Massey. She was the 8th of 10 surviving children, all of whom attended segregated schools in Palestine. She graduated from Prairie View State College in Texas and afterward taught for two years in rural schools. In 1920, she entered the segregated school of nursing at St. Louis City Hospital 2 (later, Homer G. Phillips Hospital).

After graduating in 1923, Osborne continued at City Hospital as head nurse of a large ward. She left this position after three years, frustrated that less qualified white nurses were advancing ahead of her. She was then appointed as a public health nurse for the St. Louis Municipal Visiting Nursing Service. Again, racial discrimination inhibited her advancement, and she made the decision to leave nursing altogether. However, a friend convinced her to take a teaching position in Kansas City, Missouri. She taught physiology and hygiene at Lincoln High School and Lincoln Junior College as well as nursing students from Kansas City and Wheatley-Provident Hospitals.

During the summers between 1927 and 1929, Osborne took nursing classes at Teachers College, Columbia University in New York City. Afterward, she attended Columbia full-time when she became the first African American to receive a Julius Rosenwald Fund scholarship. She earned a B.S. degree in 1930, and in 1931, when she received an M.A., she also earned the distinction of being the first black nurse to receive a master's degree. While completing her master's course work, she served as instructor at New York's Lincoln Hospital and was the first African American instructor at the Harlem Hospital School of Nursing.

After leaving Columbia, Osborne was appointed as the first director of nursing education at Freedmen's Hospital School of Nursing in Washington, D.C., a segregated and financially insecure institution. To combat educational disadvantages caused by financial difficulties at Freedmen's, she developed extracurricular programs and worked with Howard University to improve the hospital's science courses. In 1934, after three years, she left Washington for Akron, Ohio, to work on a Rosenwald study of poverty and health conditions in the American South. She was one of 14 investigators whose recommendations led to the establishment of federal health and educational programs in the South.

Already active in the National Association of Colored Graduate Nurses (NACGN), Osborne was elected to its presidency in 1934. As president, she improved professional and educational opportunities for black nurses who were educated in segregated, poor, and unaccredited schools.

In 1940, Osborne became the first African American superintendent of nurses and director of the Homer G. Phillips Hospital nursing school. Three years later, she left for New York City to increase military acceptance of black nurses on behalf of the National Nursing Council for War Service (later, the National Nursing Council). During her two-year tenure, the navy accepted black nurses for the first time, the army increased the number that it accepted, and the number of nurse training schools admitting both races increased from 14 to 38.

In 1945 Osborne accepted a position as assistant professor of nursing education at New York University. She remained in this position until 1954 and was the university's first African American instructor. During her later years, Osborne was active in a variety of nursing organizations. She served in several executive positions for the National League for Nursing (1954–1966). She was also the first black member of the Board of Directors of the American Nurses Association (1948–1952) and represented that organization at the 1949 congress of the International Council of Nurses in Stockholm, Sweden.

After retiring in 1966, Osborne moved to Oakland, California. She was married to Bedford N. Riddle (ca. 1935) and to Herman Osborne (ca. 1945); there were no children from either marriage. She died in Oakland on December 12, 1981. In 1982, the Nurses' Educational Fund established the Estelle Massey Osborne Memorial Scholarship, to be awarded to African American nurses seeking master's degrees in nursing.

Selected Additional Achievements

Honorary member, American Academy of Nursing; Mary Mahoney Award (1946); Nurse of the Year Award, New York University (1959); American Nurses Association Hall of Fame (1984). Advisory committee, U.S. surgeon general and U.S. Public Health Service; vice president, national health project of Alpha Kappa Alpha.

References

Hawkins, Joellen Watson. 1988. "Osborne, Estelle Geneva (Massey) Riddle." In *Dictionary of American Nursing Biography*, edited by M. Kaufman. New York: Greenwood Press.

Riddle, Estelle Massey, and Josephine Nelson. 1945. "The Negro Nurse Looks toward To-

Sloan, Patricia E. 1988. "Geneva Estelle Massey Riddle Osborne." In *American Nursing: A Biographical Dictionary*, edited by V.L. Bullough,

O.M. Church, and A.P. Stein. New York: Garland.

Yost, Edna. 1965. *American Women of Nursing.* Rev. ed. Philadelphia: J.B. Lippincott.

JSB

Osborne, Mary D. (1875–1946)
Nurse

Under the leadership of Mary D. Osborne, the state of Mississippi improved health care for its mostly poor, black population by increasing the number of public health nurses and by introducing formal licensing and education of lay midwives. She was born in Ohio on April 27, 1875. Little is known about her early life.

In 1902, Osborne graduated from the Akron City Hospital School of Nursing. She became the assistant director of nurses at the hospital in 1906 but later left this position to undertake postgraduate work in New York City at Woman's Hospital. She went on to become assistant director of nurses at Woman's Hospital. In 1912, Osborne was named supervisor of nurses for the Association for Improving the Condition of the Poor in New York.

In April 1921, Osborne became supervisor of the Division of Maternal and Child Health, which operated under the Mississippi State Board of Health. Later that year, she was given additional duties as supervisor of public health nurses. Federal funding, a result of the Sheppard-Towner Act, became available, allowing the Mississippi State Board of Health to place an increased emphasis on public heath nursing. In 1933, Osborne became the associate director of the Division for Maternal and Child Health.

The role of the public health nurse in Mississippi became much more important under Osborne's supervision. During the Great Depression, she took advantage of the funding provided by President Roosevelt's New Deal and placed at least one public health nurse in each of Mississippi's 82 counties. The num-

ber of public health nurses in Mississippi rose from 7 in 1921 to 165 in 1940. She increased the number of educational opportunities for nurses as well as requirements for nurses, including mandatory membership in the Mississippi State Nurses Association.

Osborne's biggest impact, however, was her work with midwives. She worked to improve the skills and training of the "granny" (lay) midwives, who delivered approximately 85 percent of the African American babies born in Mississippi. Though these women were greatly respected in their communities, they were often poorly educated and untrained in the basics of good hygiene, appropriate prenatal care, and nutrition. Ninety-nine percent of them were black, and 90 percent could not read or write. While the doctors and health administrators of the day were opposed to midwives, Osborne recognized that they were used because most expectant mothers were poor or lived in remote areas where doctors did not visit.

Osborne initiated public health nursing supervision of midwives. She created the *Manual for Midwives*, which outlined midwifery procedures, and she provided educational opportunities for midwives. Public health nurses trained midwives, gave them physical examinations, and followed up on the care that they provided. Midwifery permits were issued to those meeting requirements, and soon doctors and health officials gave their support to Osborne's work. The infant mortality rate among African American babies in Mississippi dropped almost 30 percent from 1930 to 1935.

Osborne remained in the position of supervisor of public health nurses until she retired on June 30, 1946. She immediately returned to Ohio but died only a week later on July 7, 1946.

Selected Additional Achievements

President, Mississippi State Nurses Association (1932); delegate, International Council of Nurses (1929); American Nurses Association Hall of Fame (1996).

References

American Nurses Association. *The Hall of Fame Inductees: Mary D. Osborne.* Online. http://www.nursingworld.org/hof/osbomd.htm. 23 March 2001.

Ferguson, James H. 1950. "Mississippi Midwives." *Journal of the History of Medicine and Allied Sciences* 5:85–95.

MNA Historical Committee. 1986. *Passing on the Flame: The History of the Mississippi Nurses' Association, 1911–1986.* Jackson: Mississippi Nurses' Association.

Morton, Margaret. 2000. "Mary D. Osborne." In *American Nursing: A Biographical Dictionary,* edited by V.L. Bullough and L. Sentz. New York: Springer.

DTW

Owens-Adair, Bethenia Angelina (1840–1926)
Physician

Bethenia Owens-Adair's career as a physician in the American West exemplifies, as she claims in her autobiography, the struggle of pioneer women to make their way. She was born on February 7, 1840, in Van Buren County, Missouri, the second of nine children of Thomas and Sarah (Damron) Owens. The family emigrated to the Pacific Northwest, settling in Oregon's Umpqua Valley in 1853.

In 1854, at the age of 14, Owens-Adair married Legrand Hill, but the couple divorced in 1859, after having one child, George. By the time of the divorce, her education consisted of three months' instruction from an itinerant teacher. At 18, she joined her younger siblings at a school in Roseburg, Oregon. Between 1860 and 1865, Owens-Adair completed her education at schools in Oregon and the Washington Territory and took washing, sewing, and teaching jobs to earn a living.

In 1867, she returned to Roseburg, set up a successful millinery business, and became active in the woman suffrage movement. Desiring more satisfying work, she announced to local doctors her availability for nursing duties. While her reputation as a nurse grew, she decided to begin a medical education. In preparation, she studied a *Gray's Anatomy.*

Owens-Adair studied medical texts in secret, for "to do so openly made a woman the subject of public ridicule" (Owens-Adair, p. 411). In 1871, when she announced her decision to her family, she "was not prepared for the storm of opposition that followed" (Owens-Adair, p. 80). Undaunted, she enrolled in Philadelphia's Eclectic School of Medicine and attended lectures at Blockley Hospital.

Owens-Adair earned her medical degree in 1874 and returned to Roseburg to practice. However, when she accepted a challenge by local male doctors to perform an autopsy on a male cadaver, a scandal ensued. Unable to practice peacefully in Roseburg, she set up practice in the more cosmopolitan Portland. She also specialized in medicated vapor baths combined with electricity. In 1875, she adopted Mattie Belle Palmer, who would earn a medical degree from Willamette University in Oregon in 1886.

Orthodox physicians looked down on the unconventional methods of the "bath doctor," prompting Owens-Adair to seek medical training at the mainstream, all-male Jefferson Medical College in Philadelphia. In 1878, after seeing her son earn a medical degree from Willamette University, she returned to Philadelphia. There she met Hannah

Longshore, a member of the first graduating class of the Female (later, Woman's) Medical College of Pennsylvania. Longshore told her plainly, "I have no faith that you can get into Jefferson College, but I want to see you try it." Owens-Adair visited Dr. Gross, a Jefferson professor, who advised her that the Board of Regents "would simply be shocked, scandalized, and enraged at the mere mention of admitting a woman" (Owens-Adair, pp. 89–90). He suggested that she try the University of Michigan, which already accepted women medical students. She was accepted there and graduated with her second medical degree in 1880. Following graduation, she spent the summer engaged in clinical work in Chicago, completed six months' postgraduate work in Michigan, and then toured hospitals in Europe with her son.

In 1881, Owens-Adair returned to her Portland practice and was active in the Oregon State Medical Society. In 1884, she married Colonel John Adair and three years later gave birth to a girl, who lived only a few days. Intense grief prompted a move to her husband's farm near Astoria, Oregon, where she regained her energy and was soon practicing medicine. In 1888, the couple adopted George's son, Victor Hill, after his mother's death. Three years later, they adopted the newborn son of a patient, whom they named John Adair Jr. The family moved to North Yakima, Washington, where George practiced in 1899. Owens-Adair set up a successful practice there, taking the summer of 1900 to receive postgraduate instruction at the Chicago Clinical School. She wrote many articles for various Oregon newspapers on such topics as fitness, suffrage, temperance, and women as physicians.

Around the turn of the century, Owens-Adair joined the controversial eugenics movement. Eugenics advocates argued that mental illness, criminality, and sickliness were hereditary and advocated laws for the sterilization of citizens with such characteristics. She retired from medical practice on October 10, 1905, and spent her later years on a farm in Warrenton, Oregon. On September 11, 1926, she died in Astoria, Oregon, from inflammation of the lining of the heart.

See also Longshore, Hannah E. Myers

Selected Additional Achievements

Lecture on Hygienic and Pre-Natal Influence: Delivered before the Woman's Christian Temperance Union (published, 1884); *Human Sterilization* (1910); *The Eugenic Marriage Law and Human Sterilization: The Situation in Oregon* (1922); *Human Sterilization, It's [sic] Social and Legislative Aspects* (1922).

References

Bingham, Edwin R. 1971. "Owens-Adair, Bethenia Angelina." In *Notable American Women, 1607–1950: A Biographical Dictionary*, edited by E.T. James, J.W. James, and P.S. Boyer. Cambridge: Belknap Press of Harvard University Press.

Currey, Linda Lorraine. 1978. "The Oregon Eugenic Movement: Bethenia Angelina Owens-Adair." Master's thesis, Oregon State University.

Dodds, G. B. 1984. "Owens-Adair, Bethenia Angelina." In *Dictionary of American Medical Biography*, edited by M. Kaufman, S. Galishoff, and T.L. Savitt. Westport, Conn.: Greenwood Press.

Miller, Helen Markley. 1960. *Woman Doctor of the West: Bethenia Owens-Adair*. New York: Julian Messner.

Owens-Adair, Bethenia Angelina. 1906. *Dr. Owens-Adair: Some of Her Life Experiences*. Portland, Ore.: Mann and Beach.

JSB

P

Palmer, Sophia French (1853–1920)
Nurse

Sophia Palmer was the first editor of the *American Journal of Nursing*. She was born in Milton, Massachusetts, on May 26, 1853, the 7th of 10 children of Simeon Palmer, a graduate of Harvard Medical School, and Maria Burdell (Spencer) Palmer. Little is known of her early life and education until 1876. That year she entered the Boston Training School for Nurses at Massachusetts General Hospital, where Linda Richards, one of the first trained nurses, was superintendent.

Two years later Palmer graduated from the Boston Training School and then spent several months in Philadelphia as a private nurse. She traveled to California with a private patient and remained there for two years. Around 1883, she became superintendent of St. Luke's Hospital in New Bedford, Massachusetts. She attempted to establish a nurse training school at St. Luke's, but the hospital's financial distress forced Palmer to resume her private practice instead. She also worked with pioneering nurse Anna Maxwell at Massachusetts General Hospital, where Palmer also undertook postgraduate studies.

In 1889 Palmer moved to Washington, D.C., where she founded and directed a nurse training school at Garfield Memorial Hospital. She then relocated to New York to assume the directorship (1896–1901) of the Rochester City Hospital and Training School (later, Rochester General Hospital).

Throughout her career, Palmer was an outspoken advocate for the creation of a national professional nursing organization and journal. In 1893, she became editor of the *Trained Nurse and Hospital Review* and helped found the American Society of Superintendents of Training Schools for Nurses of the United States and Canada (now the National League for Nursing). Palmer was also instrumental in the formation of the Nurses' Associated Alumnae of the United States and Canada (since 1911, the American Nurses Association). In 1900, Palmer, along with Mary E. P. Davis and Isabel Robb, served on the Alumnae Committee that formed the *American Journal of Nursing*. That year, she became the publication's first editor in chief, a position that she held for 20 years.

Palmer resigned from Rochester City Hospital in 1901 to devote her energies to the *Journal*. She described the reason for the creation of the *Journal*: "[W]ith the rapid strides that the profession is making in every direction, journalism would seem to be a necessary part of the trend of nursing progress" (Palmer, p. 64). She used the *Journal* as a tool for advocating professional and educational reform. Among her editorial campaigns was the need for legislation to regulate the training and practice of nurses. When New York became one of the first states to require registration of nurses (1903), she was appointed as chairman and board member of the New York Board of Nurses Examiners. Other editorials concerned the creation of university schools of nursing and the provision of rank for military nurses. Mary Roberts, Palmer's editorial successor, credits Palmer with being the first to advocate state inspectors for nurse training schools. She remained editor until her death from a cerebral hemorrhage on April 27, 1920.

Palmer never married, but in 1906 she adopted an eight-year-old girl, Elizabeth, who died of tuberculosis at the age of 20. The Sophia F. Palmer Library (1953) of the *American Journal of Nursing* and the Palmer-Davis Library (1939) at the Massachusetts General Hospital were named in her honor. She was elected to the American Nurses Association Nursing Hall of Fame in 1976.

See also Davis, Mary E.P.; Maxwell, Anna Caroline; Richards, Linda Ann Judson; Robb, Isabel Adams Hampton; Roberts, Mary May

References

Church, Olga Maranjian. 1999. "Palmer, Sophia French." In *American National Biography*, edited by J.A. Garraty and M.C. Carnes. New York: Oxford University Press.

Goostray, Stella. 1971. "Palmer, Sophia French." In *Notable American Women, 1607–1950: A Biographical Dictionary*, edited by E.T. James, J.W. James, and P.S. Boyer. Cambridge: Belknap Press of Harvard University Press.

Palmer, Sophia. 1900. "Editorial." *American Journal of Nursing* 1 (1):64.

JSB

Parker, Valeria Hopkins (1879–1959)
Physician

Valeria Parker was an early American woman physician and an active member of the social hygiene movement. She was born on February 11, 1879, in Chicago to Anson Jones and Martha (Leath) Hopkins. She studied at Augusta Hospital in Berlin, Germany, in 1892 and then studied in Switzerland until 1895. She graduated with an A.B. from Oxford (Ohio) College in 1895 and an M.D. from the Hering Homeopathic Medical College in Chicago in 1902. She practiced medicine until 1905, the year she married Dr. Edward O. Parker. The couple had two children, Mason and Leath.

Parker spent the rest of her career as an active member of the social hygiene movement. The social hygiene activists worked to end prostitution and supported sex education to stop the spread of venereal disease. In 1914 she was appointed to the staff of the Connecticut Social Hygiene Association. She worked with the state association until 1919, when she began working with the American Social Hygiene Association, founded by Dr. Rachelle Yarros. Around this time, Parker also ran a home for unmarried mothers and their babies.

In 1920, Parker was appointed as lecturer on venereal disease and social hygiene for the U.S. Public Health Service. In June of the following year, she took a one-year leave from the American Social Hygiene Association to serve as executive secretary of the U.S. Interdepartmental Social Hygiene Board. She also served as chair of the social hygiene committee for the National League of Women Voters (1919–1921) and the National Congress of Parents and Teachers (1921–1927) and was on the advisory committee for social hygiene of the General

Federation of Women's Clubs. She was also lecturer at the New York School of Social Work from 1924 to 1925.

In 1940, Parker wrote *For Daughters and Mothers* a manual for the adolescent girl on puberty, dating, sexual development and reproduction, marriage, and childbirth. She wrote the book to teach young women "the important facts . . . to enter marriage with strong healthy bodies and with such understanding as may enable them to share the experiences of married life happily and successfully" (p. 136). When this book was published, Parker was serving as director of the Bureau of Marriage Counsel and Education for Social and Family Relations in New York City. She was also director of the Institute of Marriage and the Home in East Orange, New Jersey (1936–1937).

Outside of her social hygiene work, Parker was appointed as the first woman probation officer in Greenwich, Connecticut (1913), and was later appointed by the Connecticut State Council of Defense as the first woman officer in that state's police force. She was also an active member of the woman's rights movement.

Parker died on October 25, 1959.

See also Yarros, Rachelle Slobodinsky

References

The National Cyclopaedia of American Biography. 1924. Current Volume A. New York: James T. White.

"Obituary." 1960. *Journal of the American Medical Association* 172 (3):136–137.

Parker, Valeria Hopkins. 1940. *For Daughters and Mothers.* Indianapolis: Bobbs-Merrill.

JSB

Pelletier, Henriette Blier (ca. 1864–1961)
Midwife

Henriette Pelletier had a long and very successful career as a midwife in far northern Maine in the late nineteenth and early twentieth centuries. Her life and career exemplify the importance of skillful midwifery in the life of frontier America. She was born to Mathias and Salomee Blier around 1864, probably in Sainte Alexandre, Quebec, Canada. The family moved to Saint Luce Parish (now Frenchville, Maine) in the Madawaska Territory when she was young. Henriette married Damase Pelletier, a folk healer, on January 9, 1882, and the couple had 13 children, all of whom were born with the aid of a midwife.

Pelletier apprenticed with her midwife and began delivering babies on her own in the 1880s. No matter the time of day or weather conditions, she left her home, usually on foot, to attend women in labor. When she arrived, she encouraged the laboring woman to walk around for as long as possible, unless there was a chance of bleeding. Most births were routine, with Pelletier providing moral support and encouragement. She had great patience and insisted that nature take its

course. Once the baby was delivered, she presented it to the mother briefly and then carefully examined it for abnormalities. She encouraged the mother to sip fluids and insisted that the baby breast-feed as soon as possible.

Although most deliveries were normal, complications sometimes occurred. If the baby presented in a breech position, Pelletier did what she could to manipulate it with her hands, rubbed in olive oil. A serious concern of midwives at that time was the position of the fetus before delivery. To correct abnormal positions, Pelletier tried folk remedies, such as requiring the mother to swallow three small balls of red silk with egg white, before she attempted to manually position the baby. If a patient was past her due date, she would use an infusion of blood root or wintergreen before resorting to rupturing the amniotic sac with her fingers.

In addition to practicing midwifery, Pelletier was a folk healer who used many herbal medicines. She also performed other functions in the community, such as shrouding the dead and making and repairing leather goods. She retired from midwifery when she was about 74 years old, after delivering more than 500 babies. She never lost a child, although two mothers died, one from a hemorrhage and the other from what was probably puerperal infection. Pelletier died on March 31, 1961, at Fort Kent, Maine.

References

Guimond, Leon (Frenchville, Maine). July 15, 2000. Interview with author via E-mail.

Paradis, Roger. 1981. "Henriette, La Capuche: The Portrait of a Frontier Midwife." *Canadian Folklore* 3 (2):110–126.

LS

Peplau, Hildegard E. (1909–1999)
Nurse

Often referred to as the "nurse of the century" or the "mother of psychiatric nursing," Hildegard Peplau is notable for her contributions to the theory of psychiatric nursing, which revolutionized the relationship between patient and nurse. Born in Reading, Pennsylvania, on September 1, 1909, she was the second of six children of Gustav and Ottylie Peplau, a Polish couple that emigrated from Germany. Though Peplau worked in several different jobs as an adolescent, she did not decide on nursing as a profession until her late teens.

Peplau graduated from high school in 1928 and later that year entered Pottstown (Pennsylvania) Hospital School of Nursing. Her first experience with psychiatric nursing was through lectures, demonstrations, and tours of Morristown State Hospital by Arthur Noyes. Noyes, unlike her other instructors, encouraged students to ask questions, leading Peplau to believe that psychiatric nursing might allow more flexibility and opportunity than other areas of nursing. While she was a student at Pottstown, a female physician joined the all-male staff of the hospital. Because the female doctor was excluded from socializing with other physicians, she requested that a student be allowed to play tennis with her. Peplau was assigned to become the physician's tennis partner. Through this acquaintance Peplau was recommended for the position of camp nurse at New York University's summer camp for physical education, following her graduation from Pottstown in 1931.

In 1936, Peplau was able to parlay this position into a recommendation to work at Bennington College in Vermont as school nurse. She was offered a full scholarship while working at Bennington, and she went on to earn her B.A. in interpersonal psychology in 1943. While at Bennington and during fieldwork at Chestnut Lodge, a private psychiatric hospital, she studied with Erich Fromm, Frieda Fromm-Reichmann, and Harry Stack Sullivan. It was Sullivan's work that Peplau expanded upon when she began writing her own theories of nursing education and practice.

Following the completion of her studies at Bennington, Peplau served as a first lieutenant in the Army Nurse Corps during World War II (1943–1945). She was in the neuropsychiatry unit of the 312th Station in England. After her return from England, Peplau entered Teachers College at Columbia University, and in 1947 she earned a master's degree in psychiatric nursing. She began work in psychiatric nursing at Highland Hospital in Asheville, North Carolina, but was asked to return to Teachers College to work on the development of a graduate program in psychiatric nursing. In 1949, she completed her seminal text, *Interpersonal Relations in Nursing*. Publication of the book was delayed until 1952 because the publisher was resistant to the idea of a nurse's publishing a work without a doctor as coauthor. The book led to a revolution in the way that nurses and patients interacted and signaled a change in how the nurse–patient relationship was perceived. Peplau advocated that the one-on-one relationship between the nurse and the patient had a therapeutic value.

From 1954 until 1974, Peplau was a member of the faculty at the College of Nursing at Rutgers University in New Brunswick, New Jersey. She frequently gave workshops and speeches and contributed to the literature on psychiatric nursing. She served as executive director of the American Nurses Association from 1969 to 1970 and was president from 1970 to 1972. During her tenure at Rutgers she held numerous visiting professor positions at universities in Africa, Latin America, Europe, and the United States.

Peplau died on March 17, 1999, in Sherman Oaks, California.

Selected Additional Achievements

Numerous articles in nursing and psychiatric journals. American Nurses Association Hall of Fame (1984); numerous honorary doctorates. Fellow, American Academy of Nursing and Sigma Theta Tau; board member and third vice president, International Council of Nurses, 1973–

1981; consultant, Surgeon Generals of the Air Forces of Turkey and Labrador; member, Expert Advisory Committee to the World Health Organization.

References

Barker, Phil. 1993. "The Peplau Legacy." *Nursing Times* 89 (11):48.

Barker, P. 1999. "Obituary, Hildegard E. Peplau: The Mother of Psychiatric Nursing." *Journal of Psychiatric and Mental Health Nursing* 6 (3): 175–176.

"Hildegard Peplau: Grande Dame of Psychiatric Nursing." 1986. *Geriatric Nursing* 7 (6):328–330.

"In Memoriam, Hildegard E. Peplau, RN; EdD; FAAN." 1999. *Nursing Science Quarterly* 12 (3):188–189.

Taylor, Cecelia Monat. 1990. *Mereness' Essentials of Psychiatric Nursing.* Edited by L.L. Duncan. 13th ed. St. Louis: C.V. Mosby.

Visone, Elizabeth M. B., and Olga Maranjian Church. 1992. "Hildegard Peplau." In *American Nursing: A Biographical Dictionary*, edited by V.L. Bullough, L. Sentz, and A.P. Stein. New York: Garland.

DTW

Peterson, Mary (1927–   )
Midwife

Mary Peterson's life and career are representative of the many generations of Native Alaskan women who have practiced midwifery. She practiced in the Alutiiq village of Akhiok on Kodiak Island, 250 miles southwest of Anchorage. The Alutiiq culture blends indigenous and Russian traditions, since the area was colonized by Russia before Alaska was purchased by the United States. Peterson was born in Akhiok on September 18, 1927, the oldest of 18 children of Teacon and Ephrezenea Peterson. She attended school in the towns of Karluk and Akhiok. At the age of 10, she started working at a local fish cannery.

As was customary, Peterson's parents chose an older man for her to marry not long after her first menstrual period. Thus, at the age of 15, she left school to wed Willy

Eluska, 11 years her senior. The couple had five children before Eluska drowned. She later married Walter Simeonoff and gave birth to 13 more children. Like most local midwives, Peterson learned the art of midwifery through her own experiences in childbirth and by assisting with, and witnessing, other births. She always wanted to be a nurse and found midwifery a satisfying outlet for her desire to help others. She delivered her first baby when her sister went into labor while she was alone with her. After that, she delivered about 25 more children before being elected Akhiok's midwife in 1947.

Native Alaskan midwives used various methods to help a woman through pregnancy, labor, and the postpartum period. For prenatal care, women were taken to the *banya*, or steam bath, to promote relaxation.

Midwives believed that it was very important to keep a pregnant woman warm and used scrubbers made of grass roots called *taaritet* to increase her blood flow and to heat her whole body. When a baby was born, the midwife used cooking oil to clean it and carefully watched the mother to ensure that the placenta was fully expelled. The midwife usually stayed in the woman's home for several days to help cook, clean, and care for the newborn baby and mother.

In addition to practicing midwifery, Peterson was a nurse for the local population, at first informally and then through the Community Health Aide Program. This program provided training in preventive, acute, and maternal and child health care to Peterson and to women like her. Peterson left Akhiok for Anchorage in 1980 to escape her abusive, alcoholic husband. She returned in 1992 and continues to reside in the village.

References

Mulcahy, Joanne B. 2001. *Birth and Rebirth on an Alaskan Island: The Life of an Alutiiq Healer.* Athens: University of Georgia Press.

Mulcahy, Joanne B., and Mary Petersen [*sic*]. 1993. "Mary Petersen [*sic*]: A Life of Healing and Renewal." In *Wings of Gauze: Women of Color and the Experience of Health and Illness*, edited by B. Bair and S. Cayleff. Detroit: Wayne State University Press.

LS

Phillips, Harriet Newton (1819–1901)
Nurse

Harriet Phillips was one of the first trained nurses in the United States. Little is known of her early life, except that she was born on December 29, 1819, in Pennsylvania. During the Civil War, she worked as a volunteer nurse for the Western Sanitary Commission at both General Hospital, Jefferson Barracks, near St. Louis, Missouri (1862–1863), and General Hospital, Benton Barracks, in St. Louis (1863–1864). She also worked for Nineteenth General Hospital of Nashville, Tennessee, in February 1864.

Phillips received a discharge on March 23, 1864, and later enrolled in a nurse training course at the Woman's Hospital of Philadelphia. The course was associated with the Female (later, Woman's) Medical College of Pennsylvania, and she was likely trained by Dr. Emeline Cleveland, who was in charge of nurses' training there. She finished her training sometime before 1870, several years earlier than nurse Linda Richards, who is often mistakenly identified as America's first trained nurse. From 1870 to 1871, Phillips was head nurse at Woman's Hospital and an instructor at the hospital's nurse training school. She did missionary work among the Ojibway and Sioux tribes of Wisconsin from 1872 to 1875 and then moved to San Francisco to work as a matron and at a Presbyterian mission. In 1878, she received advanced training at Woman's Hospital in Philadelphia, but nothing else is known of her subsequent career.

Phillips died on August 29, 1901, in Gladwyne, Pennsylvania.

See also Cleveland, Emeline Horton; Richards, Linda Ann Judson

References

Hawkins, Joellen Watson. 1988. "Phillips, Harriet Newton." In *Dictionary of American Nursing Biography*, edited by M. Kaufman. New York: Greenwood Press.

Large, Joan T. 1976. "Harriet Newton Phillips, the First Trained Nurse in America." *Image* 8 (1):49–51.

LS

Picotte, Susan La Flesche (1865–1915)
Physician

Susan La Flesche Picotte was the first Native American woman to earn a medical degree. She was born on the Omaha reservation in Nebraska on June 17, 1865, the youngest of seven children of the last recognized chief of the Omaha tribe, Joseph La Flesche (Iron Eye), and Mary Gale La Flesche, the half-British daughter of an army physician. Picotte received her early education at a Presbyterian mission boarding school and at a Quaker day school. With her sister, Marguerite, she then attended the Elizabeth Institute for Young Ladies in Elizabeth, New Jersey (1879–1882), and the Hampton Normal and Agricultural Institute in Virginia (1884–1886).

From childhood Picotte desired to study medicine. She wrote to Sara Kinney, president of the Connecticut Indian Association, after learning that the association had agreed to finance her medical education: "It has always been a desire of mine to study medicine ever since I was a small girl, for even then I saw the needs of my people for a good physician" (quoted in Mathes, 1982, p. 506).

Picotte enrolled at the Woman's Medical College of Pennsylvania in Philadelphia in 1886. In addition to her classes, she was active in local religious organizations and spoke to missionary groups on the plight of American Indians. She spent the summer of her second year at home caring for her aging parents and nursing the Omaha through a measles epidemic. She returned to Philadelphia and became the first Native American female physician in the country when she graduated in 1889. After graduation, she competed for, and won, an internship at Woman's Hospital in Philadelphia.

Picotte returned to the Omaha reservation in August 1889 as physician for the government boarding school. After only three months, the reservation adults sought her services, especially the women who were reluctant to see a white male doctor. She became so popular that local whites were added to her caseload. In 1891, she began a posi-

tion as medical missionary for the Women's National Indian Association. In these roles and throughout her career, she taught the Omaha preventive health practices, warned of the dangers of alcoholism, and was an adviser on many nonmedical matters. Eventually, traveling across the large, hilly reservation in extreme temperatures became too difficult for Picotte, who had never been of robust health.

She resigned from her position in 1893, and the following year she married Henry Picotte, a French Sioux Indian. The couple settled in Bancroft, Nebraska, where Picotte established a private practice open to both whites and Native Americans. She also raised two sons, Caryl and Pierre, and nursed her husband through the illness that led to his death in 1905. After Henry's death, Picotte and her sons moved to the small town of

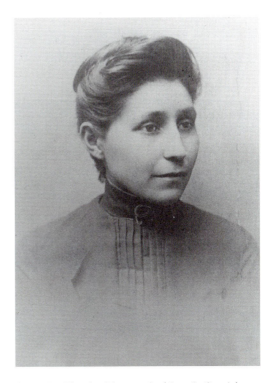

Susan La Flesche Picotte. Archives & Special Collections on Women in Medicine, MCP Hahnemann University.

Walthill, founded in 1906 on the Omaha reservation. There, she helped organize the Thurston County Medical Association and served on the Walthill health board. As chairman of the State Health Committee of the Nebraska Federation on Women's Clubs, she worked to pass health-related bills through the state legislature. She continued her temperance work and was an advocate for Native American land rights.

Picotte's greatest personal success was the founding of Walthill Hospital in 1913, only two years before her death. She had dreamed of building a hospital for the Omaha for many years and was finally successful with donations of money, land, and equipment. She served as attending physician whenever her health allowed her to do so. The hospital remained open until 1947.

Picotte died on September 18, 1915, from what was probably cancer. After her death, the Walthill Hospital was renamed Dr. Susan La Flesche Picotte Hospital. The hospital is now on the National Register of Historic Places and is named the Susan La Flesche Picotte Center.

References

Diffendal, Anne P. 1994. "The La Flesche Sisters: Victorian Reformers in the Omaha Tribe." *Journal of the West* 33 (1): 37–44.

Green, Norma Kidd. 1971. "Picotte, Susan La Flesche." In *Notable American Women, 1607–1950: A Biographical Dictionary*, edited by E.T. James, J.W. James, and P.S. Boyer. Cambridge: Belknap Press of Harvard University Press.

Mathes, Valerie Sherer. 1982. "Susan La Flesche Picotte: Nebraska's Indian Physician, 1865–1915." *Nebraska History* 63 (4): 502–530.

Mathes, Valerie Sherer. 1993. "Susan La Flesche Picotte, M.D.; Nineteenth-Century Physician and Reformer." *Great Plains Quarterly* 13 (3): 172–186.

Tong, Benson. 1999. *Susan La Flesche Picotte, M.D.: Omaha Indian Leader and Reformer.* Norman: University of Oklahoma Press.

JSB

Porn, Hanna (1860–1913)
Midwife

Hanna Porn was a trained midwife arrested in Gardner, Massachusetts, in 1907. Her arrest and trial were part of a movement to abolish midwifery and force women to have their babies delivered by physicians. While Massachusetts was the only state to actually outlaw midwifery in the early twentieth century, the rest of the United States saw a similar move to medicalize childbirth.

Little personal information is known about Hanna Porn. She was born in Mustari, Finland, on November 11, 1860, to Adam and Eva Kuniholm. While still living in Finland, she married Edward Porn. Edward died sometime before Hanna left Finland in 1895 to join her brother in Gardner, Massachusetts. She attended the Chicago Midwife Institute in Illinois and in April 1896 received a diploma that stated that "she had received theoretical and practical instruction in the art of midwifery for a period of six months, and was declared a graduated midwife" (quoted in "Commonwealth," p. 327). She returned to Gardner, presented herself as a midwife to authorities, and began attending births. Her first delivery was recorded on February 11, 1897.

Porn worked almost entirely with working-class immigrant mothers, mostly from Finland, Russia, and Sweden. She usually charged two dollars to five dollars for a delivery. Making no attempt to hide her work from authorities, Porn, unlike most midwives of the day, kept an office in Gardner. She completed birth registrations for the births that she attended, noting her title of "midwife" below her signature. In the 11 years of her practice, she registered a total of 642 births. The rate of death of newborns among children whom she delivered was less than half that of the physicians in Gardner. Presumably, she referred mothers facing difficult births to doctors for delivery.

In July 1905, criminal charges were filed against Porn for the illegal practice of medicine. The complaint was not brought by a patient but by the executive secretary of the Massachusetts Board of Registration in Medicine, Dr. Edwin B. Harvey. At Porn's trial, she was found guilty of illegally practicing medicine and of presenting herself as a medical practitioner without holding a license. She was fined $200. She appealed, but the Worcester Superior Court upheld the guilty verdict. Another appeal was not heard until 1907 in the Massachusetts Supreme Court, which resulted in a new trial in June of that year. Again Porn lost and appealed to the Massachusetts Supreme Court on the basis that midwifery was not defined by law as the practice of medicine. The court disagreed and upheld her conviction based on the 1901 Medical Practice Act. The Medical Practice Act had created legal requirements for the practice of medicine and named obstetrics as a branch of medicine. The act did not make separate allowances for midwives. The 1907 ruling by the Massachusetts Supreme Court in Porn's case upheld that midwives did not meet the requirements for practicing medicine; thus, the practice was illegal.

Porn did not cease delivering babies, however, and was arrested again in December 1907. She was found guilty the following April and fined $125. She continued to deliver babies into 1909, although it appears that she stopped signing birth records at the end of 1908. Following another arrest, Porn was found guilty in court again and fined $100 in March 1909. The appeal of this conviction was tried in the Worcester Superior Court before an all-male jury. Porn stated during the trial: "The reason I continued the business, after being told by the court to stop the work, is that I thought the law is unjust. I had to make a living" (quoted in "Mrs. Porn"). She was found guilty and sentenced to three month's imprisonment.

Porn died only four years after being released from prison, on July 8, 1913. Though she did not sign any birth records following her release from prison, it is believed that she continued to deliver babies, though in much smaller numbers. Her obituary stated that she worked as a private nurse at a residence in Gardner.

References

"Commonwealth v. Porn." 1907. In *Massachusetts Reports: Cases Argued and Determined in the Supreme Judicial Court of Massachusetts.* Vol. 196. Boston: H. O. Houghton.

Declercq, Eugene R. 1994. "The Trials of Hanna Porn: The Campaign to Abolish Midwifery in Massachusetts." *American Journal of Public Health* 84 (6):1022–1028.

Litoff, Judy Barrett. 1978. *American Midwives: 1860 to the Present.* Westport, Conn.: Greenwood Press.

"Mrs. Porn Sentenced." 1909. *Worcester Telegram* (September 1):1.

DTW

Porter, Elizabeth Kerr (1894–1989)
Nurse

Elizabeth Porter is best known for her tenure as president of the American Nurses Association, the only national nursing association composed entirely of registered professional nurses. She was born on May 21, 1894, in Pittsburgh to Richard and Catherine (Anderson) Kerr. She graduated from Fifth Avenue High School in Pittsburgh in 1911 and in 1914 married Eugene Vandergrift Porter. When her husband died in 1921, she supported herself as a music teacher. After five years, she decided to leave music and enter nursing, a field that she felt would provide "a very interesting life with real meaning and usefulness" (quoted in Rothe and Lohr, p. 475).

Porter entered the Western Pennsylvania Hospital School of Nursing in 1927. She graduated in 1930 and continued her nursing education at the Teachers College of Columbia University. She earned a B.S. degree in 1935 along with a certificate to teach in nursing schools. The following year, she went on to the University of Pennsylvania School of Nursing, where she earned two degrees in nursing education, a master's in 1936 and a doctorate in 1946.

In addition to her studies, Porter was teaching supervisor at Western Pennsylvania Hospital (1930–1935) and lecturer of nursing at Margaret Morrison Carnegie College in Pittsburgh (1933–1935). She coordinated the advanced clinical nursing program at the University of Pennsylvania School of Nursing, where she eventually achieved full professor status. She left the university in 1949 to become professor and director of Advanced Programs in Nursing Education at the Frances Payne Bolton School of Nursing at Cleveland's Case Western Reserve University. She was appointed dean of the program in 1953.

In 1950, Porter was named president of the American Nurses Association (ANA). As president, she was instrumental in "strengthening the association's economic security program; improving employment conditions for nurses; increasing nursing representation on national boards and commissions; [and]

eliminating racial restrictions to membership in the association" (ANA Hall of Fame Web Page). She also helped implement a standard 40-hour workweek. In 1952, when she was reelected president of the ANA, the association began a cooperative effort with the Federal Civil Defense Administration and the Department of National Defense to promote health care in times of emergency.

During her later years, Porter was president of the Ohio Nurses Association (1958–1960). She died in 1989.

Selected Additional Achievements

Pennsylvania Ambassadorial Award (1954); Shirley Titus Award, American Nurses Association; Florence Nightingale Award, International Red Cross; honorary doctorate degree, University of Pennsylvania. Vice president, American Nurses Foundation; board member, National Health Council.

References

American Nurses Association. *The Hall of Fame Inductees: Elizabeth Kerr Porter.* Online. http://www.nursingworld.org/hof/portek.htm. 13 November 1998.

"Nurses' Advice Is Urged." 1950. *New York Times* (July 10):23.

Rothe, Anna, and Evelyn Lohr, eds. 1953. *Current Biography Who's News and Why 1952.* New York: H.W. Wilson.

JSB

Preston, Ann (1813–1872)
Physician

Ann Preston was the first female dean of the Woman's Medical College of Pennsylvania in Philadelphia (now MCP Hahnemann University). As dean, she continually strove to give her students the same medical education available to men and thus played an invaluable role in opening the doors of medicine to women.

Preston was born on December 1, 1813, in West Grove, Pennsylvania. She was the only surviving daughter and second of seven

children of Amos Preston and Margaret (Smith) Preston. Amos was a Quaker minister, and both parents were abolitionists and supporters of women's rights. Preston received her early education at a local Quaker school. She later entered a boarding school in Chester, Pennsylvania, but was unable to complete her education, as her mother's invalidism required her to return home to care for her brothers. After her brothers were grown, she taught school and published

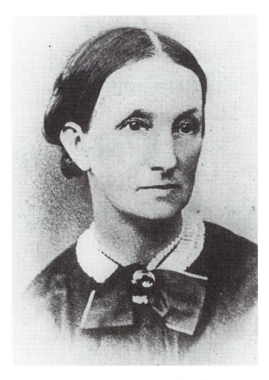

Ann Preston. National Library of Medicine.

Cousin Ann's Stories for Children (1849). She spent her leisure hours involved in temperance and women's rights societies. Also an active abolitionist, she once helped a slave through the Underground Railroad.

Preston continued her education informally by joining local literary and intellectual societies and by teaching herself Latin. She read texts on physiology and hygiene and during the 1840s taught classes on these subjects to women and girls. Soon she decided to pursue medicine because she believed that the need for qualified female physicians represented a "deep and wide-spread want of Society" (Preston). She began an apprenticeship in 1847 with Nathaniel R. Moseley of Philadelphia. She applied to four medical schools in that city but was rejected because of her sex.

In 1850, a group of Quakers founded the Female Medical College of Pennsylvania, the first women's medical school in the country. The same year, Preston enrolled in the college's first class, just before her 37th birthday. She graduated on December 31, 1851,

in a class of seven that included pioneer woman physician Hannah Longshore. Preston continued on for a year of postgraduate study and opened a private practice. She began a lifelong career at the college with her appointment as professor of physiology and hygiene in 1853.

In 1858, the Pennsylvania County Medical Society formally ostracized the college, an act that made it impossible for the students to attend clinical lectures at all-male teaching hospitals. The next year the Philadelphia State Medical Society also denounced the college. Knowing that clinical observation was imperative for a proper medical education, Preston led the establishment and funding of Woman's Hospital in connection with the college. She sent Emeline Cleveland, then instructor of anatomy, to the School of Obstetrics at the Maternité of Paris to prepare for a position as the hospital's chief resident. Although the outbreak of the Civil War forced the college to close in 1861, the hospital opened that year, staffed by college faculty and four women graduates. When the college reopened in 1862, Preston was appointed corresponding secretary and member of the Board of Managers and was on the medical staff. The same year she also established a training school for nurses.

In 1866, Preston became the first woman dean of the Female Medical College (renamed the Woman's Medical College the following year). In 1867 she wrote "Reply to Preamble and Resolutions of the Philadelphia County Medical Society," which had again denounced the school. In the reply, printed in the *Medical and Surgical Reporter* on May 4, Preston decried "the injustice which places difficulties in our way, not because we are ignorant or pretentious or incompetent or unmindful of the code of medical or Christian ethics, but because we are women" (quoted in Marshall, 1897, p. 53).

Although Woman's Medical now had its own hospital, its resources were insufficient to provide training equal to that of the large Philadelphia hospitals. Preston sought other means of hospital training, and in 1868, her students were admitted to clinics at Philadelphia Hospital, known as Blockley. Gaining entrance into Pennsylvania Hospital proved more difficult. As early as 1855, Preston applied unsuccessfully on her own behalf to the hospital clinics. As dean, she continued her efforts for the educational benefit of her students, and in 1869 Pennsylvania Hospital finally accepted her application. On November 6 the first group of students, which included future pioneering obstetrician Anna Broomall, set off for the lectures. Upon their arrival they found an angry mob of male students who protested the women's presence. As the disturbance escalated, hospital managers locked the women in a safe room, releasing them a few at a time so they might escape less noticeably. This event was soon followed by a petition signed by local physicians declaring the immorality of coeducational medical education. A reply, written by Preston and Cleveland, appeared in local papers: "We maintain . . . that science is impersonal, and that the aim of relief to suffering humanity sanctifies all duties; and we repel as derogatory to the profession of medicine, the assertion that the physician . . . need be embarrassed, in treating general diseases, by the presence of earnest women students" (quoted in Marshall, 1897, p. 26). Their response drew public sympathies to the side of the women, and the hospital managers continued to allow the women into lectures.

Preston continued her duties at the Woman's Medical College and at Woman's Hospital until her death. She also maintained a private practice, but poor health forced her to limit it to office consultation. She died from articular rheumatism at her home on April 18, 1872. She willed her medical instruments and books to the Woman's Medical College, as well as a $4,000 annual endowment for female medical students.

See also Broomall, Anna Elizabeth; Cleveland, Emeline Horton; Longshore, Hannah E. Myers

References

Alsop, Gulielma Fell. 1971. "Preston, Ann." In *Notable American Women, 1607–1950: A Biographical Dictionary*, edited by E.T. James, J.W. James, and P.S. Boyer. Cambridge: Belknap Press of Harvard University Press.
Judson, Eliza E. 1873. *Address in Memory of Ann Preston, M.D.: Delivered by Request of the Corporation and Faculty of the Woman's Medical College of Pennsylvania, March 11th, 1873.* [Philadelphia?]: N.p.
Marshall, Clara. 1897. *The Woman's Medical College of Pennsylvania: An Historical Outline.* Philadelphia: P. Blakiston, Son.
Marshall, Clara. 1915. "Ann Preston, M.D.: A Biographical Sketch." *Bulletin of the Woman's Medical College of Pennsylvania* 65 (5): 6–9.
The National Cyclopaedia of American Biography. 1900. Vol. 10. New York: James T. White.
Preston, Ann. 1856. "Letter to the Board of Managers of the Pennsylvania Hospital (May 26, 1856)." Deceased Alumnae Files, Special Collections on Women in Medicine, Archives and Special Collections, MCP Hahnemann University, Philadelphia.

JSB

Putnam, Helen Cordelia (1857–1951)
Physician

Helen Putnam was a nationally recognized advocate of children's health. She was born in Stockton, Minnesota, on September 14, 1857, the daughter of Herbert Asa and Celintha T. (Gates) Putnam. She graduated from Vassar College in 1878 and continued her education at Harvard University's Sargent School of Physical Training. She then served as director of physical education (1883–1890) at Vassar and was vice president of the American Association for the Advancement of Physical Education (1885–1888).

Putnam earned a medical degree from the Woman's Medical College of Pennsylvania in Philadelphia in 1889 (now MCP Hahnemann University) and afterward completed an internship (1890–1891) at Boston's New England Hospital for Women and Children, founded by Dr. Marie Zakrzewska in 1862. Putnam began her life as a doctor in Providence, Rhode Island, where she specialized in gynecology.

Outside of her regular medical activities, Putnam was devoted to the issue of physical education, especially its relation to the health of schoolchildren. In her 1893 book, *Supervision of School Gymnastics by Medical Specialists*, Putnam argued that lack of exercise, bad posture, insufficient nutrition, poor lighting, restrictive clothing, and lack of fresh air led to headaches, dizziness, poor eyesight, scoliosis, anemia, anorexia, and even stupidity. She argued that every school should create a physical education department, led by a medical examiner whose prescriptions should offer "much choice and variety of exercise as will afford the general recreation and development essential to mind and body of the student" (Putnam, 1893, p. 9). Between 1909 and 1912, she wrote a series of articles on school health for *Child Welfare Magazine*. Many of these articles were published in a revised format as *School Janitors, Mothers and Health* (1913), in which Putnam asserted that mothers should demand the same standard of cleanliness in schoolhouses as they did in their homes. She also argued that school janitors should take housekeeping courses.

Putnam became interested in the problem of infant mortality after serving as the American Academy of Medicine delegate to the International Conference on School Hygiene (London, 1907). Her work in this area stressed the importance of prenatal care and a sanitary milk supply. In 1908, after having been elected president of the academy, she organized the Conference on the Prevention of Infant Mortality. As a result of the conference, the American Association for the Study and Prevention of Infant Mortality was established. Working with Dr. Abraham Jacobi (husband of pioneering woman physician Mary Putnam Jacobi), Putnam organized the American Child Health Organi-

zation. The two associations merged in 1923 to form the American Academy of Pediatrics.

Outside of medicine, Putnam was a leader in the woman suffrage movement. She retired in 1935, living a secluded life in her home in Providence, Rhode Island. She died on February 3, 1951, of intestinal obstruction and arteriosclerotic heart disease.

See also Jacobi, Mary Corinna Putnam; Zakrzewska, Marie Elizabeth

Selected Additional Achievements

Vice president (1894, 1897) and president (1908), American Academy of Medicine; member and honorary fellow, American Association for the Advancement of Science; member, American Public Health Association and American Medical Association; Board of Directors, American Association for the Study and Prevention of Infant Mortality, International Union for the Protection of Infants, the Playground Association of America, and the American School Hygiene Association; chair, National Education Association's Committee on Racial Well-Being; secretary, Summer Playgrounds and Vacation School Committee (1893–1900). The Helen Putnam fellowship for advanced research was established at Radcliffe College in 1944.

References

Carey, Charles W. 1999. "Putnam, Helen Cordelia." In *American National Biography*, edited by J.A. Garraty and M.C. Carnes. New York: Oxford University Press.

Leonard, John William, ed. 1914. *Woman's Who's Who of America*. New York: American Commonwealth.

Link, Eugene P. 1977. "Putnam, Helen Cordelia." In *The Dictionary of American Biography, Supplement V, 1951–1955*, edited by J.A. Garraty. New York: Charles Scribner's Sons.

"Obituary." 1951. *Journal of the American Medical Association* (April 21):1280.

Putnam, Helen Cordelia. Deceased Alumnae Files, Special Collections on Women in Medicine, Archives and Special Collections, MCP Hahnemann University, Philadelphia.

Putnam, Helen Cordelia. 1893. *Supervision of School Gymnastics by Medical Specialists*. Providence, R.I.: Snow and Farnham.

JSB

R

Reinders, Agnes Shoemaker [Sister M. Theophane]
(1913–1993)
Nurse-midwife

Agnes Reinders was a pioneer in the field of nurse-midwifery who developed a nurse-midwifery service and educational program in Santa Fe, New Mexico, and helped to found the American College of Nurse-Midwifery. She was born on August 27, 1913, at her grandparents' farm near Owensboro, Kentucky. She was the second of nine children in a deeply religious farming family. After graduating from high school, she became a nun and received the name Sister M. Theophane.

Reinders chose nursing because of her desire to help others and through the influence of an aunt who was a nurse. Her Roman Catholic order, the Medical Mission Sisters, sent Reinders to the Catholic University of America in Washington, D.C., where she earned a B.S. in nursing in 1941. After graduating, she was head nurse at a local hospital for about six months and then an obstetrical supervisor of a maternity unit. Reinders soon learned that the archbishop of Santa Fe, New Mexico, and a public health doctor there wanted the Medical Mission Sisters to establish a nurse-midwifery service in the area. Consequently, in 1943, Reinders earned a nurse-midwifery certificate from the Mater-

nity Center Association in New York City and then moved to Santa Fe.

In Santa Fe Reinders helped to found and became director of the Catholic Maternity Institute (CMI). CMI nurse-midwives delivered babies in mothers' homes and, after its opening in 1951, at La Casita, the first free-standing birth center in the country. Reinders began planning a nurse-midwifery education program to be affiliated with Catholic University soon after arriving in Santa Fe. The school opened in 1945 and was the first school of nurse-midwifery associated with a university. She took time off from CMI to earn a master's degree in administration from Catholic University in 1946 and then resumed her position as director. In 1948, the CMI school was the first to offer a master's-level program in nurse-midwifery through its affiliation with Catholic University, and Reinders was made assistant professor in maternal and newborn nursing.

In addition to her work with CMI, Reinders was a key player in the movement to form a nurse-midwifery professional organization. Nurse-midwives had a section within the National Organization for Public Health Nursing but lost it when that organization was combined with two others to form the National League for Nursing. Reinders later said that she and other nurse-midwives "were convinced that unless nurse-midwives spoke with one voice [they] would never be recognized by organized medicine and organized nursing, . . . would never have uniform educational standards, no accrediting possibilities, and no forum from which to speak" (quoted in Tom, p. 108). Thus, Reinders wrote to leaders in nursing and nurse-midwifery to gain support for an organization and chaired a committee that established the American College of Nurse-Midwifery (ACNM). The ACNM was incorporated in 1955 and became the American College of Nurse-Midwives in 1969. Reinders was the first editor of the ACNM publication, *Bulletin of the American College of Nurse-Midwifery* (until 1959) and was the ACNM's second president (1957–1959).

After leaving the Catholic Maternity Institute in 1958, Reinders became an administrator at the Holy Family Hospital in Atlanta, Georgia. In 1964 and 1965, she took a sab-

batical and left the religious order, resuming the name Agnes Shoemaker. She then taught at Marquette University College of Nursing in Milwaukee, Wisconsin, until retiring in 1978. While in Milwaukee, she met Henry Reinders, whom she married in 1970.

Reinders died on September 28, 1993, after suffering a ruptured cerebral aneurysm.

Selected Additional Achievements

History of Nurse-Midwifery in the United States (1984; originally her master's thesis, 1947). Hattie Hemschemeyer Award, American College of Nurse-Midwives (1980); Hall of Fame, Marquette University College of Nursing (1984); fellow, American College of Nurse-Midwives (1993).

References

Tom, Sally Austen. 1978. "With Loving Hands: The Life Stories of Four Nurse-Midwives." Master's thesis, University of Utah.

VandeVusse, Leona, and Lisa Hanson. 2000. "Agnes Shoemaker Reinders (Sister M. Theophane)." In *American Nursing: A Biographical Dictionary*, edited by V.L. Bullough and L. Sentz. New York: Springer.

LS

Reiter, Frances Ursula (1904–1977)
Nurse

As a nursing educator, Frances Reiter advocated that the primary function of nurses was clinical practice, the "personal services carried out at the patient's side—in contact with and in behalf of him and his family" (quoted in "Frances Reiter, Prominent Nursing Educator," p. 349). She coined the term "nurse clinician" and recommended that following the completion of their education, nurses should specialize in a specific aspect of care, either through advanced education or clinical experience. She was born in Smithton, Pennsylvania, on June 13, 1904.

In 1931, Reiter graduated from Johns Hopkins Hospital Training School for Nurses in Baltimore and started working as a nurse at Johns Hopkins Hospital that same year. She left that institution in 1934, having

held the position of head nurse supervisor. She worked as a private-duty nurse until 1936, when she moved to the Montefiore Hospital in Pittsburgh to be assistant director of nursing service and nursing education. She again worked as a private-duty nurse from 1941 to 1942, while attending Teachers College at Columbia University in New York City. There she earned a B.A. in nursing education in 1941 and an M.A. in teaching biological sciences in 1942. She also began teaching nursing at Johns Hopkins, Boston University, and Massachusetts General Hospital during this time. She became an instructor at Teachers College in 1945 and eventually was promoted to professor. She left Teachers College in 1960 to become the first dean of the Graduate School of Nursing,

New York Medical College, which later became the Lienhard School of Nursing at Pace University. She married Harry Kreuter in 1951.

Reiter is best remembered for the 1965 American Nurses Association (ANA) paper "Educational Preparation for Nurse Practitioners and Assistants to Nurses: A Position Paper." She chaired the ANA Committee on Education, the group responsible for the paper. The committee recommended that all licensed nurses should be trained in institutions of higher education at the baccalaureate level. The associate's degree would be appropriate for technical nursing practice. Additionally, the paper advocated vocational education for nurses' assistants. The paper did not meet with much support when originally presented. At the time, hospital schools of nursing educated most nurses.

Reiter was among the first nurses who also became researchers. She published numerous articles in the professional literature and served on the first editorial board of *Nursing Research*, the first journal for nurses to publish findings of clinical studies.

Reiter retired in 1969 as dean emerita. She died on January 18, 1977, in Cherry, Illinois.

Selected Additional Achievements

Study for the U.S. Public Health Service, "Establishing Criteria for the Quality of Hospital Nursing" (1950–1954); numerous additional studies for various agencies. American Nurses Association honorary membership; American Nurses Association Hall of Fame (1984); Florence Nightingale Award of the International Red Cross; honorary fellow of the American Academy of Nursing.

References

American Nurses Association. *The Hall of Fame Inductees: Frances Reiter.* Online. http://nursingworld.org/hof/reitfx.htm. 30 March 2001.
"Frances Reiter—1931." 1968. *Alumnae Magazine* 67 (5):102–103.
"Frances Reiter, Prominent Nursing Educator, Dies." 1977. *American Journal of Nursing* 77 (March):349, 486.
Friedman, Alice Howell. 1988. "Reiter, Frances Ursula." In *Dictionary of American Nursing Biography*, edited by M. Kaufman. New York: Greenwood Press.

DTW

Richards, Linda Ann Judson (1841–1930)
Nurse

Linda Richards was one of the first trained nurses in the United States. She was born on July 27, 1841, near Potsdam, New York, the youngest of four daughters of Sanford and Betsy (Sinclair) Richards. As a child, she lived in Wisconsin and later in Vermont, where she received her early education. Both of Richards' parents died before she was an adult, and for a short time she lived at the home of a local physician. To support herself, Richards worked at the Union Straw Works in Foxboro, Massachusetts, in the 1860s. She always prided herself on being a "born nurse" and cared for ill neighbors in her spare time.

In her autobiography, *Reminiscences of Linda Richards* (1911), Richards wrote that her "desire to become a nurse grew out of what [she] heard of the need of nurses in the Civil War" (p. 5). In 1870, she began working at Boston City Hospital as an assistant nurse, a position that she later described as more like that of a maid than a nurse. She believed that the untrained nurses at the hospital were ignorant and heartless, and she remained there only three months.

In the meantime, Richards learned of a nurse training school to be organized by Dr. Susan Dimock at New England Hospital for Women and Children. It was one of the first such schools in the United States. Richards was the first of five students who enrolled for classes in September 1872. The course was one year and included training in medical,

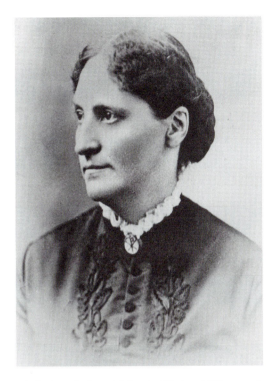

Linda Ann Judson Richards. National Library of Medicine.

surgical, and obstetrical nursing. There were no textbooks and, no entrance or final examinations, and the student nurses were not permitted to know the names of medicines that they administered to patients. Richards received her diploma in 1873. Although she is often considered America's first trained nurse, she actually graduated several years after lesser-known nurse Harriet Phillips was trained at Woman's Hospital in Philadelphia.

After graduating, Richards spent one year as night superintendent at Bellevue Training School in New York City, the first school in the United States organized on famed English nurse Florence Nightingale's model of nurse training. In November 1874, she returned to Boston and became superintendent of the Training School at Massachusetts General Hospital, where she initiated a program of regular classroom instruction. In the spring of 1877, she resigned and went to England to study Florence Nightingale's system of nursing. She met Nightingale, who

arranged for her to visit St. Thomas' Hospital School of Nursing and King's College Hospital, both in London, and the Edinburgh Royal Infirmary.

In 1878, Richards returned to the United States and worked with the superintendent of Boston City Hospital to develop a nurse training school as an integral part of the hospital. Their model was quickly imitated by other hospitals. It placed authority with medical and administrative personnel of hospitals, rather than with nurse-educators, and future nursing leaders would have to fight to reform the system. Due to ill health, Richards was on leave from the hospital from August 1879 to September 1881.

In late 1885, Richards sailed to Japan to organize the country's first nurse training school and to serve as a missionary. She spent five years in Japan and toured France before returning to the United States. For the remainder of her career, she held a succession of administrative positions in hospitals around the country. She was unable to stay long in any one job, because of her poor health.

Richards retired to a farm near Lowell, Massachusetts, in 1911. After suffering a stroke, she spent the last five years of her life at New England Hospital in Boston. Richards died there on April 16, 1930.

See also Dimock, Susan; Phillips, Harriet Newton

Selected Additional Achievements

First president, American Society of Superintendents of Training Schools for Nurses (1894). Purchased the first share of stock of the *American Journal of Nursing* (1900). American Nurses Association Hall of Fame (1976).

References

Bullough, Vern L. 1988. "Linda Ann Judson Richards." In *American Nursing: A Biographical Dictionary*, edited by V.L. Bullough, O.M. Church, and A.P. Stein. New York: Garland.

Goostray, Stella. 1971. "Richards, Linda." In *Notable American Women, 1607–1950: A Biographical Dictionary*, edited by E. T. James, J.W. James, and P.S. Boyer. Cambridge: Belknap Press of Harvard University Press.

Richards, Linda. 1911. *Reminiscences of Linda Richards: America's First Trained Nurse.* Boston: Whitcomb and Barrows.

Richards, Linda. 1915. "Early Days in the First American Training School for Nurses." *American Journal of Nursing* 16 (December):174–179.

LS

Richardson, Luba Lyons (1949–   )
Midwife, Nurse

Luba Lyons Richardson is a Victoria, British Columbia, midwife who has been instrumental in the development of midwifery regulation in that province. She was born on March 15, 1949, in New York City, the middle of three children of Jules and Florence Eisenberg. She grew up on Long Island, New York, and later studied elementary education at Nassau Community College in Hempstead, New York (1967–1969), and psychology at the State University of New York at Stonybrook (1969–1970). In 1971, she moved to British Columbia, Canada, where she married Jim Richardson. The birth of her three children, which she called a "life transforming experience," motivated her to become a midwife (Richardson, 2001).

Richardson began her training in midwifery in 1976, soon after having her second child. She completed her midwifery preceptorship in Nanaimo, British Columbia, under midwife Raven Lang. She then practiced midwifery for a short time in Parksville, British Columbia (1976–1979), before moving to Victoria, where she has practiced ever since. Today, she and two other women run the Victoria Midwifery Group. Richardson's philosophy of midwifery is based on the British Columbia model of midwifery as established by the College of Midwives of British Columbia (CMBC), which includes continuity of care, informed choice, and choice of birthplace. In 1990, Richardson completed her education as a registered nurse at Camosun College in Victoria. She then completed postgraduate courses in obstetrics at the British Columbia Institute of Technology and became a licensed midwife in the state of Washington (1994) and in the province of British Columbia (1998).

In 1995, the Ministry of Health of British Columbia established the CMBC, a regulatory body to oversee the practice of midwifery in that province. Richardson served as chair of the first board to begin the work of developing standards of practice, registration requirements, and continuing education for midwives. The CMBC implemented a rigorous registration process that included two written examinations, a daylong practical examination, and a weeklong orientation to the provincial health system. New registrants had to have completed a recognized midwifery program and demonstrated competence in both home and hospital births. Protecting choice of birthplace, including home birth, was especially important for Richardson. She sat on the advisory committee of the Home Birth Demonstration Project, established to integrate home births into the regulated system. She completed a lecture tour of hospitals to assist in the integration of the practice of home births in different communities around the province, as British Columbia midwives are required to offer both home and hospital births to their clients. She also lobbied successfully to ensure that home births were publicly funded, as are all maternity services in British Columbia.

Richardson continues to serve as president of the CMBC and is currently the chief of the Department of Midwifery for the Capital Health Region in Victoria. She has been a guest speaker at many midwifery conferences and workshops and has written several articles for *Island Parent Magazine*. She is currently raising her grandson, Max.

See also Lang, Raven

Selected Additional Achievements

Member, Midwives Association of British Columbia (1980–   ), Registered Nurses Association of British Columbia (1990–); board member, British Columbia Reproductive Care Program; Woman of Distinction Award in the area of Health, YM-YWCA of Greater Victoria (1988).

References

"Midwifery in British Columbia." September 1998. *Policy and Perspective* (4). Online. http://www.moh.hnet.bc.ca/msp/general/polper/polper4.html. 15 April 2001.

Richardson, Luba Lyons. April 12, 2001. Interview with author via E-mail. 12 April 2001.

Richardson, Luba Lyons. N.d. Curriculum Vitae.

Victoria Midwife Group. *Luba Lyons Richardson.* Online. http://www.midwiferygroup.com/luba.html. 15 April 2001.

JSB

Robb, Isabel Adams Hampton (1860–1910)
Nurse

Isabel Hampton Robb was a leader in American nursing and throughout her career strove to raise educational standards of nurses. To promote such standards on a national level, she was instrumental in the creation of the country's first two nursing organizations. She was born on August 26, 1860, in Welland, Ontario, Canada, the fourth of seven children of Samuel James and Sarah Mary (Lay) Hampton. She received her early education in a local school and later earned a teaching certificate from the Collegiate Institute in St. Catherine's, Ontario. For the next few years, she taught at a rural school in Merritton, Ontario.

In 1881, Robb emigrated to New York City to attend the Bellevue Hospital Training School for Nurses. She graduated in 1883 and took an appointment as supervising nurse at New York Women's Hospital. She then went to Rome, Italy, where she worked at St. Paul's House for Trained Nurses and also cared for private patients.

Robb returned to the United States in 1885 and in June of the following year took a position as the superintendent of nurses at Illinois Training School for Nurses in Chicago. At the training school Robb began her efforts to raise educational standards in nursing. Her first act in this direction was to establish the school's systematic, graded course for nurses, the first of its kind in the country. She also convinced Presbyterian Hospital to allow her students to care for patients there, thus broadening their clinical experience. This was one of the first affiliations of its kind in the United States. Perhaps the most pioneering change that Robb made was to abolish the practice of assigning students to private-duty work. This was a common custom among nursing schools, in which the money earned from these assignments went back to the school.

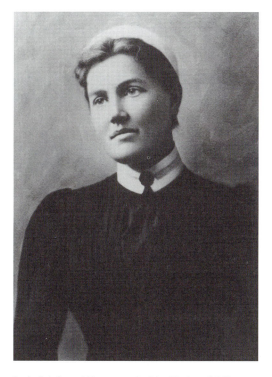

Isabel Adams Hampton Robb. National Library of Medicine.

Robb's commitment to the profession earned her the position of founding principal and superintendent of nurses at the new Johns Hopkins Training School for Nurses in 1889. She continued the graded curriculum that she had begun in Illinois and implemented a hospital affiliation with Mt. Wilson Sanatorium for Infants. She also instituted high entrance requirements and a one-month probationary period. As her assistant, she appointed nurse pioneer Lavinia Dock.

Continuing her efforts to professionalize nursing, Robb began a campaign for the establishment of a nursing organization devoted to implementing educational standards in the field. As chair of the subsection on nursing for the Conference of Charities, Correction, and Philanthropy (World's Fair, Chicago, 1893), she was determined to use the meeting as an opportunity to establish such an organization. She led a discussion between other nursing superintendents, and out of this meeting came the American Society of Superintendents of Training Schools for Nurses of the United States and Canada. This was the first national nursing organization in the United States, and it continues to exist today as the National League for Nursing.

One year after publishing her first book, *Nursing: Its Principles and Practice* (1893), she left Johns Hopkins to marry Dr. Hunter Robb. The couple settled in Cleveland, Ohio, and had two sons, Hampton and Philip. Although Robb never worked again as a nurse, she continued to be a great influence in the field through volunteer activities. In 1895, she spoke at the Society of Superintendents, proposing that all nursing schools establish a three-year graded course, an eight-hour workday for student nurses, and the universal abolition of private-duty assignments. Additionally, she taught at Cleveland's Lakeside Hospital Training School for Nurses and served as a member of its Board of Lady Managers. She was also on the Board of Directors of the Cleveland Visiting Nurse Association and established a teaching affili-ation between the association and local nursing schools.

Robb was an important force in the establishment of the second national nursing organization, the Nurses' Associated Alumnae of the United States and Canada (from 1911, the American Nurses Association). As first president of the Associated Alumnae (1897–1901), she and Adelaide Nutting, her Johns Hopkins successor, laid plans for the implementation of a course in hospital economics at Teachers College, Columbia University in New York. The course was eventually expanded to become the college's Department of Nursing Education. Robb was also active on the committee, chaired by Mary E. P. Davis, that established the *American Journal of Nursing*. The publication, which continues to be a major nursing journal, published its first volume in October 1900. The same year, she published her second book, *Nursing Ethics*.

Robb was involved in the 1900 formation of the International Council of Nurses to pursue nursing issues on an international level. At the council's 1909 meeting, she was named chair of a committee to achieve an international educational standard. In 1908 she became president of the Society of Superintendents.

On April 15, 1910, Robb was killed in a streetcar accident in Cleveland. After her death, the Isabel Hampton Robb scholarship fund was formed. The scholarship eventually became the Nurses Educational Funds, a private foundation devoted to assist nurses earning advanced degrees.

See also Davis, Mary E.P.; Dock, Lavinia Lloyd; Nutting, [Mary] Adelaide

References

Moody, Selma. 1938. "Isabel Hampton Robb: Her Contribution to Nursing Education." *American Journal of Nursing* 38 (10):1131–1138.

Noel, Nancy. 1988. "Isabel Adams Hampton Robb." In *American Nursing: A Biographical Dictionary*, edited by V.L. Bullough, O.M. Church, and A.P. Stein. New York: Garland.

Noel, Nancy. 1999. "Robb, Isabel Hampton." In

American National Biography, edited by J.A. Garraty and M.C. Carnes. New York: Oxford University Press.

Rodabaugh, Mary Jane. 1971. "Robb, Isabel Adams Hampton." In *Notable American Women*,

1607–1950: A Biographical Dictionary, edited by E.T. James, J.W. James, and P.S. Boyer. Cambridge: Belknap Press of Harvard University Press.

JSB

Roberts, Mary May (1877–1959)
Nurse

Mary Roberts was a leader in nursing best known for her nearly 30-year career as editor of the *American Journal of Nursing*. She was born on January 30, 1877, in Duncan City, Michigan (now part of Cheboygan), the oldest of four children of Henry W. and Elizabeth Scott (Elliot) Roberts. She graduated from high school in Cheboygan in 1895 and decided to become a nurse, despite her father's objection.

Roberts was accepted at the Jewish Hospital School of Nursing in Cincinnati, Ohio, and graduated in 1899. She then worked as a clinic nurse at Baroness Erlanger Hospital in Chattanooga, Tennessee, as the superintendent of nurses at Savannah Hospital in Georgia (1900–1903), as the assistant superintendent of nurses at Jewish Hospital School in Cincinnati (1904–1906), and as a private-duty and obstetric nurse in Evanston, Illinois. In 1908, she was made superintendent of nurses at Christian R. Holmes Hospital in Cincinnati. While in Ohio, she worked for passage of the state's nurse practice act and was a member of the Ohio nursing board. In 1917, with the United States' entry into World War I, she became director of the American Red Cross' Lake Division Bureau of Nursing, and in 1918, she became chief nurse and director of the Army School of Nursing at Camp Sherman, Ohio.

After her discharge in September 1919, Roberts decided to further her education at Teachers College, Columbia University. She graduated two years later with a bachelor of science degree and a diploma in the administration of nursing schools. She was then chosen by the editorial board of the *American Journal of Nursing (AJN)*, the official journal of the American Nurses Association (ANA), to succeed Sophia Palmer as editor. Soon after assuming her post, Roberts moved the *Journal* offices from Rochester, New York to New York City, the site of ANA headquarters. Roberts addressed many issues in the journal and was particularly interested in maintaining high educational and professional standards. She also broadened the journal's scope to include the clinical aspects of nursing and significantly enlarged its business and editorial staff. Under her direction, respect for the journal grew, and circulation went from 20,000 to 100,000. From 1934 to 1948, she was also in charge of the ANA's Nursing Information Bureau, an administrative unit of the *AJN* that was designed to disseminate information to the public on nursing.

In addition to her involvement with the *AJN*, Roberts was active in nursing organizations. In 1932, she sponsored a plan to make the National League of Nursing Education the education department of the ANA, which helped to clarify the relationship between the two organizations. She was also one of two nurses on the Committee on Costs of Medical Care, was a consultant to the Committee on the Grading of Nursing Schools, and was on the National Committee on Red Cross Nursing Service. She supported the International Council of Nurses and served as vice president and a member of its Ethics and Publications Committees. In 1930 and 1931, she traveled to Europe to visit nursing centers for the Rockefeller Foundation.

In 1949 Roberts retired from the *AJN* with the title editor emerita. During her later years, she contributed editorials, biographical essays, and reviews to the journal and wrote two books, *American Nursing: History and Interpretation* (1954) and *The Army Nurse Corps—Yesterday and Today* (1957). She suffered a stroke while working on an editorial in the *AJN* office and died soon after, on January 11, 1959.

See also Palmer, Sophia French

Selected Additional Achievements

Numerous articles and editorials in the *AJN* and other nursing journals. President, Ohio State Association of Graduate Nurses (1915–1917); chair, Florence Nightingale International Foundation (1934–1945). Bronze Medal, Ministry of Social Welfare, France (1933); Army Certificate of Appreciation (1949); Florence Nightingale Medal, International Red Cross (1949); honorary fellow, American College of Hospital Administrators (1949); Mary Adelaide Nutting Medal, National League of Nursing Education (1949); Mary M. Roberts Fellowship in Journalism established in her honor by the *AJN* (1950); ANA Hall of Fame (1984).

References

Hawkins, Joellen Watson. 1988. "Roberts, Mary May." In *Dictionary of American Nursing Biography*, edited by M. Kaufman. New York: Greenwood Press.

"Mary M. Roberts Retires as Editor." 1949. *American Journal of Nursing* 49 (5):261–271.

"Mary M. Roberts: January 31, 1877–January 11, 1959." 1959. *Nursing Outlook* 7 (2):72–73.

Tomes, Nancy. 1980. "Roberts, Mary May." In *Notable American Women: The Modern Period: A Biographical Dictionary*, edited by B. Sicherman and C.H. Green. Cambridge: Belknap Press of Harvard University Press.

LS

Robertson, Jennie Smillie (1878–1981)
Physician

Jennie Smillie Robertson was the first female surgeon in Canada. Barred from performing surgery in Toronto's male-dominated hospitals, she was inspired to establish an all-female Women's College Hospital in Toronto. She was born in rural Huron County, Ontario, Canada, on February 10, 1878, to farmers of Irish and Scottish decent. She was the third of seven children and was educated in the local area schools.

From a very young age Robertson dreamed of becoming a doctor. To pay for her medical education, she obtained a teaching certificate at the age of 18 and taught school in Huron County. Finally, when she was 25, she became one of three women in the last class to attend the Ontario Medical College for Women in Toronto. In 1906, the college closed its doors and was absorbed by the University of Toronto Faculty of Medicine, where Robertson completed the remainder of her medical education.

Graduating in 1909, Robertson found little opportunity for an internship in Toronto and consequently interned at the hospital associated with the Woman's Medical College of Pennsylvania in Philadelphia. She returned to Toronto in 1910 and began a private practice. The scarcity of female physicians in Toronto kept her well occupied, and it soon became evident to her that there was a specific need for women surgeons there. She tried to obtain specialized training in surgery in Toronto, but she could find no one who would accept a female surgical intern. As a result, she returned to Philadelphia for six months of study with the chief surgeon at the Woman's Medical College of Pennsylvania.

When she returned to Toronto, Robertson was not permitted to work as a surgeon in the local hospitals, despite her training. She performed her first operation, the removal of a diseased ovary, on a kitchen table in a private home. This experience made her realize the acute necessity for a facility in Toronto where women could act as, and train to become, surgeons. As a result, she and the few women physicians of Toronto gathered their resources, collected funding from friends, and founded Women's College Hospital. The hospital, staffed entirely by women, gave female physicians full privileges and provided new female graduates a place to receive training in surgery and other specialty branches of medicine.

Robertson practiced at Women's College Hospital for 40 years and was the chief of the Department of Gynecology for part of her tenure. At the 1924 meeting of the Canadian Medical Association in Ottawa, she joined Maude Abbott, Helen MacMurchy, and Elizabeth Bagshaw to establish the Federation of Medical Women of Canada. When she was 70, Robertson retired from medicine and married a childhood friend, Alex Robertson. She died in Toronto on February 26, 1981.

See also Abbott, Maude Elizabeth Seymour; Bagshaw, Elizabeth; MacMurchy, Helen

References

Hacker, Carlotta. 1974. *The Indomitable Lady Doctors.* Toronto: Clarke, Irwin.
Hellstedt, Leone McGregor. 1978. *Women Physicians of the World: Autobiographies of Medical Pioneers.* Washington, D.C.: Hemisphere.
"Obituary." 1982. *Macleans* 94:4.

CMB

Rogers, Martha Elizabeth (1914–1994)
Nurse

Martha E. Rogers developed an innovative theory of nursing, the science of unitary human beings, also referred to as "Rogerian science." She was born on May 12, 1914, in Dallas, Texas, the eldest of four children of Bruce Taylor Rogers and Lucy Mulholland Keener Rogers. The family moved to Knoxville, Tennessee, before she was one year old. She was unsure what career path to follow but had a great desire to help people; she considered law before enrolling in the science-medicine course of study at the University of Tennessee (1931–1933) in Knoxville. Because her parents disapproved of women physicians, however, Rogers enrolled at Knoxville General Hospital School of Nursing in 1933.

Rogers graduated with a diploma in nursing in 1936, but her desire for more education led her to George Peabody College in Nashville. There she earned a bachelor's degree in public health nursing (1937). From 1937 to 1939, she worked in Clare, Michigan, as a rural public health nurse. Next, she decided to further her education at Teachers College, Columbia University. She attended the college full-time in the summers and part-time the rest of the year, when she worked in Hartford, Connecticut, at the Visiting Nurse Association. From 1940 to 1945, she advanced from staff nurse to the acting director of education at the association. In 1945, she finished her master's degree in public health nursing and became executive director of the Phoenix, Arizona, Visiting Nurse Association. She then returned to school and earned a master's degree in public health (1952) and a doctor of science degree (1954) from Johns Hopkins University in Baltimore.

In 1954, Rogers was appointed head of the nursing division at New York University (NYU). She reformed the nursing curriculum there; among her innovations were the introduction of theory-based learning and the creation of a five-year undergraduate nursing program. During her time at NYU, Rogers contributed many articles to the nursing literature, as well as the books *Education Revolution in Nursing* (1961), *Reveille in Nursing* (1964), and *Introduction to the Theoretical Basis of Nursing* (1970). Her theory of the science of unitary human beings was first presented in the latter book, of which she said, "It had to be written. There had to be a book to teach nursing as a science, something for the students to learn in *nursing* or there was no point in having students" (quoted in Hektor, p. 70). The theory incorporates ideas from many disciplines, including anthropology, psychology, philosophy, literature, and physics. It "postulates that human beings are dynamic energy fields integral with environmental fields. Both human and environmental fields are identified by pattern and characterized by a universe of open systems" (Tomey and Alligood, p. 209). From Rogers' model, other nursing theorists have generated theories and new treatment modalities, such as therapeutic touch.

In 1974, Rogers helped to found SAIN, the Society for Advancement in Nursing. SAIN was organized as an advocacy group for nurses who had a baccalaureate education and believed in nursing as a learned profession. Although Rogers stepped down as head of NYU's nursing division in 1975, she continued to teach. She retired from the university in 1979 but continued to refine her theory; among other things, she was concerned with the problems and issues that will be faced by nursing when humans someday live in space.

Rogers died on March 13, 1994, in Phoenix of pulmonary failure, complicated by emphysema. The Martha E. Rogers Center at NYU was established in 1995 to honor her and to continue her work.

Selected Additional Achievements

Editor, *Nursing Science* (1963–1965); consultant to the surgeon general of the air force (1969–1973). American Nurses Association Hall of Fame (1996); numerous honorary doctorates.

References

American Nurses Association. *The Hall of Fame Inductees: Martha Elizabeth Rogers.* Online. http://www.nursingworld.org/hof/rogeme. htm. 23 July 2001.

Hektor, Lynne M. 1989. "Martha E. Rogers: A Life History." *Nursing Science Quarterly* 2 (2): 63–73.

Malinski, Violet M., Elizabeth Ann Manhart Barrett, and John R. Phillips, eds. 1994. *Martha E. Rogers: Her Life and Her Work.* Philadelphia: F.A. Davis.

Safier, Gwendolyn. 1977. *Contemporary American Leaders in Nursing: An Oral History.* New York: McGraw-Hill.

Tomasson, Robert E. 1994. "Martha Rogers, 79, an Author of Books on Nursing Theory (obituary)." *New York Times Biographical Service* 25 (3):401.

Tomey, Ann Marriner, and Martha Raile Alligood. 1998. *Nursing Theorists and Their Work.* 4th ed. St. Louis: Mosby-Year Book.

LS

Ross, Charlotte Whitehead (1843–1916)
Physician

Charlotte Whitehead Ross was the first woman physician to practice in Montreal and in the Canadian West. She was born on July 15, 1843, in Darlington, England, to Isabella and Joseph Whitehead. In 1848, her family moved to a farm in Huron County, Canada, and Ross began school in nearby Clinton. Later she attended Sacred Heart Academy, a finishing school in Montreal, and graduated in 1861. She then returned home and met David Ross, a railroad associate of her father. They married a few months later and relocated to Montreal.

Ross' husband was frequently absent while working on the construction of the western railway, but she remained in Montreal and devoted her time to caring for her two young children and an invalid sister. Her desire to learn more about her sister's illness motivated her to become a doctor. Her husband supported the idea as he wanted his family to settle in the Canadian wilderness, where it would be advantageous if his wife had the skills to treat illnesses and accidents.

Ross had three more children before she enrolled at the Woman's Medical College of Pennsylvania (now MCP Hahnemann University) in Philadelphia in 1870. Her thesis was on the diagnosis and treatment of miscarriage during the first four months of pregnancy. This topic was of great interest to her because she endured several miscarriages in addition to eight successful pregnancies. She graduated on March 11, 1875, and the following year returned to Montreal, where she established a medical practice that focused on the treatment of women. However, she was not registered with the College of Physicians and Surgeons in Quebec or licensed to practice medicine.

In 1881 Ross and her children made the move west, to Whitemouth, Manitoba, where her husband had built a sawmill and a log cabin. Initially, she had no intention of practicing medicine. As the only trained physician in the region, however, the volume of logging- and barroom-related injuries brought to her was too large to ignore. At first, her patients were predominantly men whose respect and trust were difficult to win. The locals were finally convinced of her ability the night when she was summoned to a barroom and proficiently sewed up a large neck wound on a drunken woodsman using only a household needle and thread. She practiced in Whitemouth for the next 30 years.

In 1887 Ross filed an application that would allow her to practice medicine, surgery, and midwifery in Manitoba. Although her request did not pass the legislature, and her medical practice was never legally recognized, she continued to practice medicine and became an active member of the Manitoba Medical Association. In 1912, after her husband died, she retired and moved to Winnipeg, where her daughter, Minnie, lived. Minnie's daughter, Edith, graduated from Manitoba Medical College in 1913 and went on to become the first female anesthesiologist at Winnipeg General Hospital.

Ross died on February 21, 1916, in Winnipeg of arteriosclerosis. Edith kept her grandmother's memory alive by establishing an award in Ross' name for the top student in obstetrics and gynecology at Manitoba Medical College.

References

Angel, Barbara, and Michael Angel. 1982. *Charlotte Whitehead Ross*. Winnipeg: Peguis.

Hacker, Carlotta. 1974. *The Indomitable Lady Doctors*. Toronto: Clarke, Irwin.

McGinnis, Janice P. Dickin, and Mary Percy Jackson. 1995. *Suitable for the Wilds: Letters from Northern Alberta, 1929–1931*. Toronto: University of Toronto Press.

Nicholson, Anna Mary, ed. 1949. *100 Years of Medicine, 1849–1949*. Saskatoon, Saskatchewan: Modern Press.

"Obituary." 1916. *Journal of the American Medical Association* 66 (18):1401.

Ross, Charlotte Whitehead. Deceased Alumnae Files, Special Collections on Women in Medicine, Archives and Special Collections, MCP Hahnemann University, Philadelphia.

CMB

Ross, Marie-Henriette LeJeune (1762–1860)
Midwife

Marie-Henriette LeJeune Ross, widely known as "Granny" Ross, attained near-legendary status through her long career as midwife and healer. She was born in Rochefort, France, in 1762 to Acadian farmers Joseph LeJeune and Martine Roy. Her family moved back and forth between France and Canada during most of her youth.

When she was about 16, Ross married her first husband, Joseph Comeau, who drowned in 1783. In 1786, she married a cousin, Bernard LeJeune, who also died. She married her third husband, James Ross, a disbanded British soldier, in 1793. They settled in the Bras d'Or region of Cape Breton Island and had four children, only two of whom lived to adulthood.

Ross became known in the area as a skillful midwife and healer who often employed homeopathic techniques. Her talents became more widely recognized when a smallpox epidemic swept through the region in the early 1800s. She quarantined the afflicted patients and used an inoculation procedure employed in Turkey in which unaffected patients were scratched with a needle that had been dipped into a smallpox blister or a fresh smallpox scab. She had the foresight to preserve a sample of vaccine, and over 70 years later her grandson, Thomas, used it to protect himself and others during another smallpox outbreak.

In 1802 Ross and her family moved 80 miles northwest to Northeast Margaree River, where she was both the first Caucasian woman to settle there and the only person with medical skills. In Margaree she continued to attend births and treat the ill, even after becoming blind, until her death in 1860.

References

Dennis, Clara. 1943. *Cape Breton Over.* Toronto: Ryerson Press.

Jackson, Elva E. 1971. *Cape Breton and the Jackson Kith and Kin.* Windsor, Nova Scotia: Lancelot Press.

Kernaghan, Lois Kathleen. 1985. "LeJeune, Marie-Henriette." In *Dictionary of Canadian Biography: Volume 8, 1851–1860*, edited by F.G. Halpenny. Toronto: University of Toronto Press.

MacDougall, J.L. 1972. *History of Inverness County, Nova Scotia, Canadiana Reprint Series, no. 43.* Belleville, Ont.: Mika.

Merritt, Susan E. 1995. *Her Story II: Women from Canada's Past.* St. Catherines, Ont.: Vanwell.

CMB

Roys-Gavitt, Elmina M. (1828–1898)
Physician

Elmina Roys-Gavitt was the creator and first editor of the *Woman's Medical Journal.* She was born on September 8, 1828, in Fletcher, Vermont, the second of eight children. At age 14, she moved with her family to Woonsocket, Rhode Island. She received her early education at home and in local schools.

During the Civil War, Roys-Gavitt assisted her brother in his work as a military surgeon in charge of Maryland hospitals. In 1863, she enrolled at the Woman's Medical College of Pennsylvania in Philadelphia (now MCP Hahnemann University). She wrote her thesis, "Chronic Disease," and graduated in 1867. After a two-year internship at the Clifton Springs Sanitarium in New York, she relocated to Rochester, Minnesota, and established a medical practice.

In 1871, Roys-Gavitt moved to Toledo, Ohio, and is considered to be the first woman physician of that city. She settled there permanently and married the Reverend F. C. Gavitt in 1876. In celebration of the state's first centennial, the Ohio governor asked her to compile a history of women physicians of that state. During the course of the project, she realized the necessity of a communication tool for women doctors and created the *Woman's Medical Journal* (later, the *Medical Woman's Journal*). The journal published its first issue in January 1893 with Roys-Gavitt as its first editor. She described its purpose in the "Salutatory" of that issue: "[I]t will be a purely regular journal, and will print news and notes of interest to the masculine as well as the feminine part of the profession. We shall do all in our power to reflect the sentiment of women practitioners, and shall enhance their interests so far as it lies in the power of journalism to do it" (reprinted in Mason-Hohl, p. 13).

Roys-Gavitt continued as editor until her death on August 25, 1898. The journal published its last issue in July 1952, yet it continues to serve as an invaluable record of the accomplishments of many medical women.

References

Lovejoy, Esther P. 1956. "Looking Backward." *Journal of the American Medical Women's Association* (April):137–139.

Mason-Hohl, Elizabeth. 1943. "Editorial." *Medical Woman's Journal* (January):13–20.

Special Collections on Women in Medicine, Archives and Special Collections, MCP Hahnemann University, Philadelphia.

JSB

Rutherford, Frances Armstrong (1842–1922)
Physician

Frances Rutherford was the first woman graduate of a mainstream medical school to practice in Grand Rapids, Michigan. She was born on October 8, 1842, in Bath, New York, and later received her academic education at Elmira College in Elmira, New York (1855–1856).

In 1863, Rutherford began a one-year study of medicine in Elmira, New York, under Dr. Rachel Gleason, co-owner of the Elmira Water Cure. In 1868, she graduated from the Woman's Medical College of Pennsylvania in Philadelphia (now MCP Hahnemann University). Afterward, she completed a short internship under Elizabeth and Emily Blackwell at the New York Infirmary for Women and Children. Additional medical education included study at New York Woman's Hospital (1873) and at hospitals and clinics in London and Berlin (1882–1883).

In 1868, Rutherford established a private medical practice in Grand Rapids, Michigan, becoming the first woman graduate of a mainstream medical school to work as a physician in that city. During her first year in Grand Rapids, she taught classes in physiology, hygiene, and chemistry at a local high school to make professional contacts.

Only one year after Rutherford's arrival, the city council appointed her as the country's first female city physician. She must have made a great impression on the city, for her salary is reported to have been twice that of her predecessor's, and she was offered the appointment again in 1871. She refused the offer, however, because the city charter did not allow her to serve a second term. She achieved another first in 1872, when the Michigan State Medical Society elected her as its first woman member. She served as the society's vice president the following year, making her the first woman officer of a state medical society.

Rutherford is also notable for the organization and founding of Grand Rapid's first training school for nurses at Union Benevolent Association Hospital (later, Blodgett Memorial Hospital), where she also served as visiting gynecologist. She maintained her practice in general medicine for the rest of her life, specializing somewhat in electric therapeutics. She was married for a short while to a lawyer. She died suddenly on May 24, 1922.

See also Blackwell, Elizabeth; Blackwell, Emily; Gleason, Rachel Brooks

Selected Additional Achievements

Second woman delegate, American Medical Association; cofounder (1893) and associate editor (1894–1901), *Medical Woman's Journal.*

References

"Death of a Pioneer Woman Physician." 1922. *Medical Woman's Journal* (June): 117.

Degree information provided by the Alumni Relations Office of Elmira College, Elmira, N.Y.

Pernick, M. 1984. "Rutherford, Frances Armstrong." In *Dictionary of American Medical Biography*, edited by M. Kaufman, S. Galishoff, and T.L. Savitt. Westport, Conn.: Greenwood Press.

Rutherford, Frances Armstrong. Deceased Alumnae Files, Special Collections on Women in Medicine, Archives and Special Collections, MCP Hahnemann University, Philadelphia.

Selmon, Bertha. 1947. "Pioneer Women in Medicine Spread to the States prior to 1900." *Medical Woman's Journal* (November): 40–44, 68.

JSB

S

Sabin, Florence Rena (1871–1953)
Physician

Florence Sabin was one of the best-known women scientists of her era and the first woman to teach at Johns Hopkins Medical School. She was born in Central City, Colorado, on November 9, 1871, the second of two surviving children of George Kimball Sabin and Serena (Miner) Sabin. Sabin and her sister, Mary, spent their early childhood in Colorado mining communities, where their father worked as an engineer. After her mother's death, Sabin lived with relatives in Chicago and Vermont, where she attended the Vermont Academy.

In 1889, Sabin entered Smith College in Massachusetts, where she developed an interest in biology and mathematics. She decided to study medicine by the time she earned her B.S. degree in 1893 and wished to enter Johns Hopkins University Medical School, which had opened the same year with a policy of accepting women. In order to earn money to pay for medical school, she taught mathematics in a Denver, Colorado, school and then worked at the Smith College zoology department. In 1896, she joined the fourth class to enter the Johns Hopkins Medical School. While there, she completed a research project under Dr. Franklin P. Mall in which she constructed a model of the mid-

and lower brain of a newborn. The model was manufactured and became a standard study aid in medical schools and was published as *An Atlas of the Medulla and Midbrain, a Laboratory Manual* (1901).

After graduating in 1900, Sabin began a prestigious one-year internship at Johns Hopkins. Afterward, Mall recommended that she be appointed as an assistant in his anatomy department, but his request was refused because she was a woman. Mall succeeded in getting her a fellowship in his department, where her research finally earned her an appointment as assistant (1903–1905), along with the distinction of being the first woman on the Johns Hopkins medical staff. By 1905, she was assistant professor, and in 1917, she rose to full professor, the first woman to achieve that rank at Johns Hopkins. During her early years of teaching, her most notable research addressed the origins of blood cells and the lymphatics, and her work discredited earlier theory about their development. Her research was published as a chapter in the important *Manual of Human Embryology* (Mall and Keibel, 1910–1912) and won an award for the "best scientific thesis written by a woman embodying new observations and conclusions based on

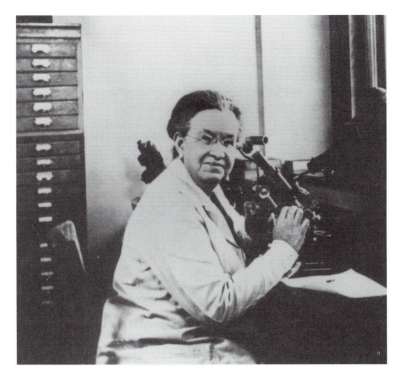

Florence Rena Sabin. Courtesy, Colorado Historical Society.

independent laboratory research" (quoted in Andriole, p. 326).

This success was followed by other important research projects in the area of lymphatics and blood vessels. However, Sabin was passed over by one of her students for Mall's post as chair of the anatomy department when he died in 1917. Regardless, her achievements were noted by her election as the first woman president of the American Association of Anatomists (1924) and as the first female member of the National Academy of Sciences (1925). She taught at Johns Hopkins until 1925, and many of her students went on to make important contributions in medicine. In 1925, she accepted a research appointment with the Rockefeller Institute in New York and was the first female member of the institute. She worked there for the next 13 years, leading research on the cellular aspects of immunity. Her research in this area was considered a major contribution to the understanding of tuberculosis.

In 1938, Sabin retired to Colorado to live with her sister. In 1944, at the request of the governor of Colorado, she studied the state's health needs as a member of its Post-War Planning Committee. She determined that Colorado suffered from a poorly run and inefficient public health system and embarked upon a speaking tour of the state, advocating public health reforms. Her work led to the successful passage of a series of health laws, also known as the Sabin Program. Between 1947 and 1951, she was chair of the Interim Board of Health and Hospitals of Denver.

Sabin died in Denver following a heart attack on October 3, 1953. For her achievements, the city of Denver named a public school after Sabin and her sister, a teacher. The University of Colorado dedicated Sabin Hall on her 80th birthday, and a bronze statue of her stands in the U.S. Capitol in Washington, D.C.

Selected Additional Achievements

Author of many scientific publications and the biography *Franklin Paine Mall: The Story of a*

Mind (1934); vice president, American Association of Anatomists (1909–1910); president, western branch of the American Public Health Association (1948); president, Denver Board of Health; National Achievement Award (1932); honorary life member, New York Academy of Sciences (1944); Trudeau Medal, National Tuberculosis Association (1945); honorary fellow, American Public Health Association (1947); Lasker Award (1951); Elizabeth Blackwell Citation, New York Infirmary (1953); recipient of numerous honorary degrees.

References

Andriole, Vincent T. 1959. "Florence Rena Sabin—Teacher, Scientist, Citizen." *Journal of the History of Medicine and the Allied Sciences* 14 (3):320–347.

Brieger, Gert H. 1980. "Sabin, Florence Rena." In *Notable American Women: The Modern Period: A Biographical Dictionary*, edited by B. Sicherman and C.H. Green. Cambridge: Belknap Press of Harvard University Press.

Corner, George W. 1977. "Sabin, Florence Rena." In *The Dictionary of American Biography, Supplement V, 1951–1955*, edited by J.A. Garraty. New York: Charles Scribner's Sons.

Morantz-Sanchez, Regina. 1999. "Sabin, Florence Rena." In *American National Biography*, edited by J.A. Garraty and M.C. Carnes. New York: Oxford University Press.

JSB

Safford, Mary Jane (1834–1891)
Physician, Civil War nurse

Mary Jane Safford began her healing career as a volunteer nurse during the Civil War. Afterward she practiced and taught medicine and was an advocate for women's health. She was born in Hyde Park, Vermont, on December 31, 1834, one of at least four children of Joseph Warren and Diantha (Little) Safford. The family moved to Crete, Illinois, when Safford was three or four years old. After the death of her parents, she lived with her brother, Alfred Boardman Safford. In 1854, the siblings moved to Shawneetown, Illinois, where Alfred Safford established and operated a public school.

Safford's life turned to healing after she and her brother opened a school in Cairo, Illinois. At the outbreak of the Civil War, Cairo was chosen as the base camp for General Grant's Union army. Safford cared for the Cairo soldiers and in 1861 was joined by Mary Bickerdyke, another volunteer nurse. Bickerdyke trained Safford in nursing, and the two established a camp hospital and kitchen. After the Battle of Belmont (November 1861), Safford, with her handkerchief tied to a stick, ventured past enemy lines to search and care for soldiers. Following the Battle of Fort Donelson (winter 1862), she and Bickerdyke made five trips on the hospital transport ship *City of Memphis*, accompanying wounded soldiers to hospitals in Cairo. Safford worked on the hospital ship *Hazel Dell* after the Battle of Shiloh (April 1862).

Safford's health suffered under the strain of her work, and in 1862 she began a five-year tour of Europe. In Paris, she underwent an operation for a back injury sustained during the war. Despite her need for rest, she visited many European hospitals and nursed the wounded after the Austro-Prussian War and during the Italian unification war.

Safford returned to the United States and enrolled in the New York Medical College and Hospital for Women (Homeopathic), founded by Dr. Clemence Lozier in 1863. Safford graduated in 1869 and returned to Europe for additional training at the University of Vienna and at other major German hospitals. She was the first woman to perform an ovariotomy at the University of Breslau in Prussia.

Safford returned to the United States about 1872, established a medical practice in Chicago, and married James Blake (whom she may have divorced around 1880). The couple moved to Boston in 1873. The same year, Safford joined the faculty of the newly organized homeopathic Boston University School of Medicine as professor of women's diseases and later as professor of gynecology (1879). She was admitted to the Massachusetts Homeopathic Medical Society, established a private practice, and was on the staff of Massachusetts Homeopathic Hospital.

Safford joined Boston University the same year as Caroline Eliza Hastings, another pioneering woman physician. The two women participated in a lecture series promoting women's dress reform. Safford decried tight corsets, which not only inhibited movement but also deformed and displaced the vital organs. She considered dress reform necessary for women's economic independence and argued that young women in comfortable clothing were more likely to "earn a much more healthful and quite remunerative a living by tilling the soils, or by entering the trades or professions" (quoted in Woolson, p. 27). An 1872 article in *The Woman's Journal* described Safford's own style of dress: "Her dress was . . . without a hint of flounce, overskirt, or bustle . . . compressing [her figure] in no part. Her boots . . . shaped to *her* feet, rather than compressing them to . . . arbitrary proportions" (*Woman's Journal*, May 18, p. 155).

In 1887, ill health prompted Safford to move to Tarpon Springs, Florida, with her two adopted daughters, Margarita and Gladys. She lived with her brother, Anson P.K. Safford, founder of the city and former governor of the Arizona Territory. She maintained a medical practice there until her death from typhoid fever on December 8, 1891.

See also Bickerdyke, Mary Ann Ball; Hastings, Caroline Eliza; Lozier, Clemence Sophia Harned

Selected Additional Achievements

Pre-Natal Influence (under the name Mary Blake, 1874); *Health and Strength for Girls* (under the name Mary Safford, 1884, with Mary E. Allen).

References

Biographical information is contained in *The Woman's Journal*, May 18, 1872, to December 19, 1891.

Fischer, Le Roy H. 1971. "Safford, Mary Jane." In *Notable American Women, 1607–1950: A Biographical Dictionary*, edited by E.T. James, J.W. James, and P.S. Boyer. Cambridge: Belknap Press of Harvard University Press.

Gordon, Sarah H. 1999. "Safford, Mary Jane." In *American National Biography*, edited by J.A. Garraty and M.C. Carnes. New York: Oxford University Press.

Woolson, Abba Goold, ed. 1874. *Dress-reform: A Series of Lectures, Delivered in Boston, on Dress as It Affects the Health of Women*. Boston: Roberts Brothers. (Five lectures given in the spring of 1874 by Mary J. Safford-Blake, Caroline E. Hastings, Mercy B. Jackson, Arvilla B. Haynes, and Abba Goold Woolson.)

JSB

Sanger, Margaret Louise Higgins (1879–1966)
Nurse

Margaret Sanger was at the forefront of the American campaign for birth control. Her fervent belief in a woman's right to control her reproductive function led her to break the law in order to make contraceptive information available to women. She was born on September 14, 1879, in Corning, New York, the 6th of 11 children of Anne (Purcell) and Michael Hennessey Higgins, a stonemason. She placed much of the blame for her mother's death at the age of 49 on the stress of bearing and raising 11 children. Sanger's early education was in the local Corning public schools and at Claverack College and Hudson River Institute (1895–1898), a boarding school in the Catskill Mountains of New York.

In 1898, Sanger took a teaching position in Little Falls, New Jersey, but decided she was not temperamentally suited for such work. In 1900, she enrolled at the nursing school of White Plains (New York) Hospital. She did well in school and was appointed head nurse of a women's ward, but her stud-

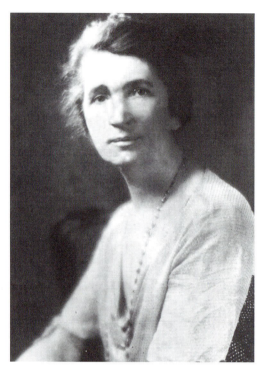

Margaret Louise Higgins Sanger. Library of Congress.

ies were interrupted by an operation to remove tubercular glands. To make up credits missed, she took courses at the Manhattan Eye and Ear Infirmary in New York City. While in New York, she met William Sanger, an architect and artist, whom she married on August 18, 1902. Married women were not permitted in nursing school; thus, she was prevented from completing her third year of training.

The Sangers settled in Westchester County and had three children, Grant (1903), Stuart (1908), and Margaret (1910). The increasingly estranged couple moved to New York City in 1910, where Sanger began working part-time as a nurse for Lillian Wald's Henry Street Visiting Nurse Service and became involved in the radical labor movement. As a nurse, she witnessed the economic and physical suffering of women who found themselves with unwanted pregnancies. In 1912, she began writing a column on sex education and health, "What Every Girl Should Know," for the socialist paper *The Call.*

A 1913 column was deemed unmailable by the U.S. Post Office under the Comstock Act of 1873. The act severely hindered efforts to distribute information on birth control, as it defined such information as obscene.

In March 1914, Sanger founded *The Woman Rebel*, a magazine intended to directly challenge the Comstock Act. In the first issue, she wrote: "The aim of this paper will be to stimulate working women to think for themselves and to build up a conscious fighting character" and "to advocate the prevention of conception and to impart such knowledge in the columns of this paper" (p. 1). The magazine was confiscated by the Post Office, and she was arrested in August. In the six weeks that she was given to prepare for trial, she instead compiled a pamphlet, *Family Limitation*, which listed detailed methods of birth control. She fled to Europe in October 1914 to avoid trial; en route, she wired confidants to distribute *Family Limitation*.

Sanger spent much of the next year in England. She became acquainted with Havelock Ellis, the author of numerous works exploring the nature of human sexuality, and began having an affair with him (she would go on to have affairs with several other prominent intellectual men of the time). Ellis' theories on the importance of female sexuality led her to begin thinking of birth control as important not just for socioeconomic reasons but because it allowed women to take pleasure in sex without fear of pregnancy. In the meantime, her husband had been tricked into selling a copy of *Family Limitation* to an undercover vice agent and was arrested. His case generated much sympathy for the cause, and Sanger returned to New York in October 1915, to a society more eager to hear her message on birth control. Her daughter's death in November 1915 generated more sympathy for Sanger, and the government dropped all charges against her the next February. She then went on a nationwide publicity campaign to promote birth control.

On October 16, 1916, Sanger and her sister Ethel Byrne, a registered nurse, opened the first birth control clinic in the United States, in the Brownsville section of Brooklyn, New York. In the 10 days that it was open, more than 400 women received contraceptive advice. Sanger was quickly arrested and admitted that she was providing information on birth control in violation of obscenity laws. She was found guilty and chose to serve 30 days in prison rather than to pay a fine. A 1918 appeal's court ruling upheld her conviction but also expanded physicians' rights to prescribe contraception. As a result, she began lobbying for birth control clinics staffed by physicians.

In 1922 Sanger, divorced from William since 1920, married the wealthy J. Noah Slee, who funded her efforts. She organized the American Birth Control League (ABCL) in 1921 in order to disseminate birth control information, foster the development of other birth control leagues and clinics, and lobby for birth control legislation. In 1923, she opened the Clinical Research Bureau, the first legal birth control clinic in the country. She resigned from the ABCL in 1928 and took full control of the Clinical Research Bureau, renaming it the Birth Control Clinical Research Bureau (BCCRB). A 1936 court case, *U.S. v. One Package*, involving Dr. Hannah Stone, medical director of Sanger's BCCRB, finally overturned the Comstock Act's ban on birth control information. In 1939, the ABCL and BCCRB were merged to form the Birth Control Federation of America, renamed the Planned Parenthood Federation of America (PPFA) in 1942. After 1939, Sanger's role in the organization diminished; the federation would not be led again by a woman until Faye Wattleton took the helm in 1978.

Sanger was also active in promoting birth control internationally. In 1952, she helped found the International Planned Parenthood Federation and served as its first president (1952–1959). She died in Tucson, Arizona on September 6, 1966, of congestive heart failure, one year after the U.S. Supreme Court ruled birth control legal for married couples (striking down an 1879 Connecticut law prohibiting the use of contraceptives).

See also Stone, Hannah Mayer; Wald, Lillian D.; Wattleton, [Alyce] Faye

Selected Additional Achievements

Woman and the New Race (1920); *The Pivot of Civilization* (1922); *Happiness in Marriage* (1926); *Motherhood in Bondage* (1928); *My Fight for Birth Control* (1931); *Margaret Sanger: An Autobiography* (1938). Periodicals: *Birth Control Review* (1917–1940), *Human Fertility* (1940–1948). Medal of Achievement, American Women's Association (1931); honorary L.L.D. degree, Smith College (1949); Gold Medal, Japan (1962); Albert and Mary Lasker Foundation Award (1950); Margaret Sanger Medallion created in her honor, PPFA (1966); honorary L.L.D., University of Arizona (1966); American Nurses Association Hall of Fame (1976).

References

Chesler, Ellen. 1992. *Woman of Valor: Margaret Sanger and the Birth Control Movement in America*. New York: Simon and Schuster.

Hawkins, Joellen Watson. 1988. "Sanger, Margaret Louise." In *Dictionary of American Nursing Biography*, edited by M. Kaufman. New York: Greenwood Press.

Katz, Esther. 1999. "Sanger, Margaret." In *American National Biography*, edited by J.A. Garraty and M.C. Carnes. New York: Oxford University Press.

New York University Department of History. *Margaret Sanger Papers Project*. Online. http://www.nyu.edu/projects/sanger/. 26 May 2001.

Reed, James. 1980. "Sanger, Margaret." In *Notable American Women: The Modern Period: A Biographical Dictionary*, edited by B. Sicherman and C.H. Green. Cambridge: Belknap Press of Harvard University Press.

Sanger, Margaret. 1914. "The Aim." *The Woman Rebel* 1 (1):1. Online. *Margaret Sanger Papers Electronic Edition*. http://adh.sc.edu. 26 May 2001.

LS

Schlotfeldt, Rozella May (1914–   )
Nurse

As dean of the school of nursing at Case Western Reserve University, Rozella Schlotfeldt increased opportunities for learning and research for both students and faculty. She was born on June 29, 1914, in DeWitt, Iowa, one of two daughters of John William and Clara Cecelia (Doering) Schlotfeldt. Her father died when Schlotfeldt was four, and her mother supported the family as a private-duty nurse. Since childhood, Schlotfeldt wanted to be a nurse, and after receiving her early education in local public schools, she earned a B.A. in liberal arts and nursing from the State University of Iowa in Iowa City (1935).

After graduation, Schlotfeldt was maternity nurse at the University of Iowa Hospital (1935–1936) and at the Veterans Administration Center in Des Moines (1936–1938). She then completed postgraduate studies in maternity nursing at New York Hospital and went on to serve as instructor and supervisor of maternity nursing at University of Iowa Hospital. After spending two years during World War II (1944–1946) in Europe with the United States Army Nurse Corps, she returned to the United States and earned an M.S. in nursing education and administration in 1947 from the University of Chicago. After serving as assistant professor at the University of Colorado School of Nursing (1947–1948), she joined the faculty of the Wayne State College of Nursing in Detroit. At Wayne State, she advanced from associate professor to full professor and associate dean (1948–1960). She also found time to earn a Ph.D. from the University of Chicago in 1956.

In 1960 Schlotfeldt became professor and dean of the Frances Payne Bolton School of Nursing at Western Reserve University (later, Case Western Reserve University). As dean, she replaced the two old houses that made up the nursing school with larger, modern facilities and modified the undergraduate program to serve the needs of students from various backgrounds. She recruited nationally prominent nursing specialists to head new master's programs in psychiatric, pediatric, and maternity nursing. To improve clinical training, she modeled the nursing department similarly to medical departments. That is, her faculty held joint appointments as nursing department heads at the university hospitals and were responsible for teaching, as well as patient care and research. A Ph.D. program was developed and approved under Schlotfeldt, although it was not implemented until after her retirement. She later wrote that her contributions to nursing were guided by her "firm conviction that nursing is an essential human service that must become a uniformly beneficial, consequential, and respected profession whose practitioners have mastered vast amounts of professional knowledge" (Schlotfeldt, p. 301).

Over the course of her career, Schlotfeldt has been a member of numerous committees devoted to exploring the role of nursing. Some of these include membership on the subcommittee of nursing for the National Institute of Mental Health (1957–1961), the advisory committee on nursing for the Office of the U.S. Surgeon General (1961–1963), the U.S. Public Health Service's nursing research study (1962–1966), and the Advisory Council on Nursing for the U.S. Veterans Administration. By 1982, she had published more than 100 publications on nursing, including articles, monographs, book chapters, and research reports.

Schlotfeldt resigned as dean from the School of Nursing in 1972 but continued as professor until her retirement in 1982. In the latter year, a scholarship and lectureship were established in her name at the Frances Payne Bolton School of Nursing.

Selected Additional Achievements

Schlotfeldt's numerous memberships in nursing organizations include the presidency of the Ohio State Board of Nursing Education and Nurse Registration (1971–1972). Centennial Award, Wayne State University (1968); Involved Nurse of 1969

Award, Ohio Nurses Association; Honorary Recognition Award, American Nurses Association (1970); Honorary Recognition Award, Cleveland Area League of Nursing (1972); Distinguished Service Award, University of Iowa (1973); honorary doctorate, Georgetown University (1972).

References

Bullough, Vern. 1992. "Rozella May Schlotfeldt." In *American Nursing: A Biographical Dictionary*, edited by V.L. Bullough, L. Sentz, and A.P. Stein. New York: Garland.

The Frances Payne Bolton School of Nursing. Online. http:/www.cwru.edu/pubs/crumag/fal1998/features/nursing/fpb75_7.shtml. 14 May 2000.

The National Cyclopaedia of American Biography. 1978. Vol. M. New York: James T. White.

Schlotfeldt, Rozella M. 1988. "Rozella M. Schlotfeldt." In *Making Choices, Taking Chances: Nurse Leaders Tell Their Stories*, edited by T.M. Schorr and A. Zimmerman. St. Louis: C.V. Mosby.

JSB

Sessions, Patty Bartlett (1795–1892)
Midwife

Patty Bartlett Sessions is considered to be the mother of all Mormon midwives. She was born on February 4, 1795, in Bethel, Maine, the first of nine children of Enoch and Anna (Hall) Bartlett. She learned to read and write at her father's shoemaking shop, which for a time doubled as a classroom. In 1812, against her parents' wishes, she married David Sessions and moved to his parents' home in Ketcham, Maine.

David Sessions' mother was a midwife, and one day, not long after her son's marriage, she was called to attend a birth. Ill health prevented her from getting there in time, and Patty Sessions took her place as the attendant. All went well; the local physician congratulated her and urged her to become a midwife, which she agreed to do. She learned her craft through experience and from her assisting her mother-in-law; she may have learned from a local Indian midwife as well. She also read about the subject and owned *Aristotle's Works: Containing the Masterpiece, Direction for Midwives, and Counsel and Advice to Child-Bearing Women* (1840). She delivered nearly 4,000 children during her career.

In 1814, the Sessions had a son and moved to Andover West Surplus, Maine. They eventually had seven more children. Sessions was a deeply spiritual woman who found the Mormon faith appealing; in July 1834 she was baptized into the religion, and her husband was baptized the next year. In June 1837, the Sessions family joined the Mormons' westward trek, arriving in Far West, Missouri, that November. The religious group was forced to leave there in 1839 and eventually settled in the valley of the Great Salt Lake, in what would later become the state of Utah, in 1847. Throughout the arduous westward journey, Sessions was kept busy as a midwife; not long after arriving in Utah, she delivered the first Mormon baby born there.

In keeping with early Mormon practice, David Sessions took two other wives. A year after David's death in 1850, Sessions married John Parry, who also took a second wife. In 1848, Sessions was a charter member of the Council of Health, an organization created to instruct members in midwifery, the care of children, handling of diseases, and other health-related topics. She was later president of the council. She was also a member of a select group of women who prayed together, spoke in tongues, and participated in faith healings. In addition to practicing midwifery, Sessions was an excellent gardener and developed a business selling fruits, seedlings, and seeds.

Sessions died on December 14, 1892.

References

Noall, Claire. 1974. *Guardians of Health: Utah's Pioneer Midwives and Women Doctors.* Bountiful, Utah: Horizon.
Smart, Donna Toland. 1996. "Patty Bartlett Sessions: Pioneer Midwife." In *Worth Their Salt: Notable but Often Unnoted Women of Utah,* edited by C. Whitley. Logan: Utah State University Press.
Smart, Donna Toland, ed. 1997. *Mormon Midwife: The 1846–1888 Diaries of Patty Bartlett Sessions.* Logan: Utah State University Press.

LS

Seton, Elizabeth Ann Bayley (1774–1821)
Nurse

Mother Elizabeth Seton started the first U.S. community of the Sisters of Charity of St. Vincent Paul, an order of nuns that originated in France, where they were well known for their hospital work. She was born on August 28, 1774, in New York City, the second child of Richard and Catherine Bayley. Her father was a prominent physician and professor of anatomy at King's College and served as the first city health officer in New York City.

On January 25, 1794, she married William Magee Seton, whose family owned a prosperous shipping firm. Five children were born to the couple. The family was forced into bankruptcy when the shipping business failed, and soon thereafter, William Seton's health began to decline due to tuberculosis. Following a voyage to Italy, he died on December 27, 1803. Elizabeth Seton remained in Italy for several months, staying in the home of Catholic friends. In 1805, the year following her return to the United States, she converted to Catholicism. Most of her friends and family were opposed to her conversion and withdrew their financial support. She attempted to support her family by teaching, but the anti-Catholic sentiment in New York at the time made it difficult for her to be successful.

In 1807, Seton was invited by Father William DuBourg to establish a girl's school in Baltimore. She arrived in Baltimore in 1808 and shortly afterward opened a school next to St. Mary's Seminary. On March 25, 1809, she took her first vows of the Sisters of Charity, the first American Catholic sisterhood. In June of that year, Seton, along with other young women that had joined in her work, moved to Emmitsburg, Maryland, to open a school for poor girls. The Sisters of Charity flourished here under Seton's leadership. Though their primary charge was education, the nuns were often called upon to nurse the sick and poor, especially during the epidemics of yellow fever, whooping cough, and tuberculosis common during the period. The Sisters of Charity were asked to tend to the poor and sick in other areas as well, eventually opening homes in New York, Cincinnati, Halifax, and other locations.

Seton died January 4, 1821, from tuberculosis. In 1823, the Sisters of Charity were asked to establish a nursing service for an infirmary associated with a medical school. The original order grew to provide nursing service throughout the early period of nursing's development. Seton's Sisters of Charity has grown into a comprehensive health care provider, with a number of health care facilities concentrated in the Staten Island, New York, area, including the Bayley Seton Hospital.

Seton became the first native-born American to be canonized by the Catholic Church, on September 14, 1975.

References

Allen, Stephen J. 1975. "Sainthood for Blessed Elizabeth Seton." *Hospital Progress* 56 (9):36–37, 40, 44.
Earley, Mary Elizabeth. 1997. *The Sisters of Charity of New York: 1960–1996.* Vol. 5. Bronx, N.Y.: Sisters of Charity of New York Press.
National Women's Hall of Fame. *Elizabeth Bayley Seton 1774–1821.* Online. http://www.

greatwomen.org/profs/seton_e.php. 15 February 2001.

Sabin, Linda. 1988. "Mother Elizabeth Ann Bayley Seton." In *American Nursing: A Biograph-* *ical Dictionary*, edited by V.L. Bullough, O.M. Church, and A.P. Stein. New York: Garland.

DTW

Sewall, Lucy Ellen (1837–1890)
Physician

Lucy Sewall was one of the earliest formally trained women physicians in the United States. She was born in April 1837 in Roxbury, Massachusetts, the older of two daughters of Samuel E. Sewall and Louisa Maria (Winslow) Sewall. She became interested in medicine in 1856 after she developed a friendship with Dr. Marie Zakrzewska of the New York Infirmary for Women and Children. In 1859, Zakrzewska relocated to Boston to teach at the New England Female Medical College. Shortly after, Sewall enrolled at the college and became Zakrzewska's assistant.

After her graduation in 1862, Sewall traveled to London and Paris for clinical study and practical training. She returned to Boston the following year and became resident physician (1863–1869) at New England Hospital for Women and Children, opened the previous year by Zakrzewska. In addition to the care of patients, Sewall was responsible for the instruction of students and for administrative duties. She resigned from her position as resident physician in 1869 to become one of the hospital's two attending physicians. Throughout her career, she also managed a successful private practice and earned a positive reputation for her obstetrics skills. She was also instrumental in founding the Massachusetts Infant Asylum, the first institution in Massachusetts devoted to caring for orphaned and unwanted babies. Fittingly, the maternity ward at New England Hospital was named after her.

Sewall resigned her position as attending physician in 1887, but she continued to serve in an advisory role. However, a heart condition, which had left her a semi-invalid for the last few years of her life, forced her to relinquish these duties completely in 1888. She died in Boston on February 13, 1890.

See also Zakrzewska, Marie Elizabeth

References

"Dr. Lucy Sewall." 1937. *Medical Woman's Journal* 44 (2): 49.

Ingebritsen, Shirley Phillips. 1971. "Sewall, Lucy Ellen." In *Notable American Women, 1607–1950: A Biographical Dictionary*, edited by E.T. James, J.W. James, and P.S. Boyer. Cambridge: Belknap Press of Harvard University Press.

Withington, Alfreda B. 1928. "Sewall, Lucy." In *Dictionary of American Medical Biography: Lives of Eminent Physicians of the United States and Canada, from the Earliest Times*, edited by H.A. Kelly and W.L. Burrage. New York: D. Appleton.

JSB

Sharpless, Amy Mildred (1909–1998)
Nurse, Midwife

Amy Mildred Sharpless' work as a midwife in Maryland and West Virginia is illustrative of the ways in which women's careers in the healing professions have been shaped by chance and by economic necessity. She was born on September 11, 1909, in Blaine, West Virginia, the daughter of Otha and Anna (Beckman) Sharpless. She graduated from Kitzmiller (Maryland) High School in 1927 and from Memorial Hospital School of

Nursing in Cumberland, Maryland, in 1930. She did postgraduate work at Western Reserve University in Cleveland, Ohio.

Sharpless had been planning on a career in hospital nursing but returned to her hometown to help her father in his funeral and ambulance businesses instead. She was the attending nurse in the ambulance when it went out on emergencies. Her midwifery career began in the early morning hours of November 9, 1937, when she was called to attend a laboring woman who was unable to get to a hospital. Not long after, she was called to a second and a third emergency birth, prompting her to earn midwifery certificates from the states of West Virginia and Maryland. She delivered a total of 784 babies, the last one in 1968.

Sharpless made sterile birthing pads from bleached feed sacks that she baked in her oven and then lined with newspaper. She insisted that any pregnant woman who came to her before her delivery date see a doctor for a prenatal examination. When called to a case, she quickly assessed the situation and strongly encouraged the woman to go to the nearest hospital if she believed there would be complications. She was dedicated to helping women in need and traveled through severe weather and over dangerous, unpaved mountain roads to assist at births. She provided postpartum care on the third and seventh days following delivery, which included checking the woman's uterus to ensure that it was properly contracting, bathing the mother and baby, and taking their vital signs. Her fee ranged from $10 to $25 over the course of her career, although she was not paid anything for many cases.

In addition to practicing midwifery, Sharpless was postmaster in Blaine for 10 years. Except for the occasional emergency birth, she ceased being a midwife in late 1950s, after her father died; she ran his funeral home for 17 years before retiring in 1972. She died in Oakland, Maryland, on March 9, 1998.

References

"A. Mildred Sharpless." 1998. *Cumberland Times-News.* Online. http://www.times-news.com/obits/s98/s0398008.htm. 2 February 2001.

Beckman, I. Lynn. 1990. "Mountaintop Midwife." *The Glades Star* 6 (September):444–447,449–450.

Beckman, I. Lynn. 1993. "Home Delivery: Amy Mildred Sharpless, Mountaintop Midwife." *Goldenseal* 19 (Winter):55–60.

Riechmann, Deb. 1995. "Former Midwife, Funeral Director Recalls Work." *Charleston Gazette* (September 7):1C.

LS

Shaw, Flora Madeline (1864–1927)
Nurse

Flora Shaw was the first director of the McGill School for Graduate Nurses in Montreal and was a leader in nursing in Canada and internationally. She was born on January 15, 1864, in Perth, Ontario, the daughter of Henry Dowsley Shaw, a businessman, and Flora Madeline (Matheson) Shaw. Her early education was at a private school in Perth and at Mrs. Mercer's Academy in Montreal.

In 1894, Shaw entered the Montreal General Hospital Training School for Nurses and graduated two years later. She was assistant superintendent at the school from 1896 to 1903, except for a short stint (1899–1900) as superintendent of nurses at Boston's Women's Charity Club Hospital. In 1903, she enrolled in Teachers College, Columbia University to study hospital economics, and she received a diploma in 1906. While in New York, she was matron of the nurses' home of Presbyterian Hospital and was an instructor of dietetics there.

Shaw returned to Montreal General (1906–1909) when Nora Livingston, the school's superintendent, instituted the first preliminary class in Canada there and named

Shaw the course's instructor. During this time, Shaw became active in professional nursing organizations and was the first secretary-treasurer of the Canadian Nurses Association in 1908. The next year, she was forced to resign her position at Montreal General, due to poor health. For the next six years, she recuperated at sanatoriums in New York and in Quebec. After a 1914 trip to England, she returned to Canada and worked as a volunteer social worker at the Montreal branch of the Canadian Patriotic Fund during World War I.

In 1920, Shaw became director of the newly founded McGill School for Graduate Nurses in Montreal. The school was the first in Canada to offer graduate courses in teaching, supervision, and administration in schools of nursing. The school grew to be a highly respected unit of McGill University under Shaw's leadership. In addition to her efforts at McGill, she worked for the passage of amendments to the Registration Act for Nurses in Quebec and was a member of the National Executive Committee of the Victorian Order of Nurses. She was also a popular guest lecturer and a frequent contributor to the nursing literature.

From 1922 to 1924, Shaw was president of the Canadian Association of Nursing Ed-ucation and was also president of the Association of Registered Nurses of the Province of Quebec (1922–1926). In 1926, she became president of the Canadian Nurses Association, but her tenure as president ended due to her untimely death in Liverpool, England, from a pulmonary embolism on August 27, 1927. She had been attending a conference of the International Council of Nurses.

See also Livingston, Nora G. E. [Gertrude Elizabeth]

Selected Additional Achievements

Memorial tablet in her honor unveiled, Montreal General Hospital (1934); Flora Madeline Shaw Chair of Nursing established at McGill University (1957).

References

"In Memoriam: Flora Madeline Shaw, R.N." 1927. *British Journal of Nursing* (September): 206.
Murphy, Sharon C. 2000. "Flora Madeline Shaw." In *American Nursing: A Biographical Dictionary*, edited by V.L. Bullough and L. Sentz. New York: Springer.
Slattery, Anne. 1929. *Pioneers of Nursing in Canada*. Montreal: Gazette Printing.

LS

Sheahan, Marion Winifred (1892–1994)
Nurse

Marion Sheahan was a public health administrator who oversaw the transformation of public health nursing during the 1930s and 1940s. She was born on September 5, 1892, in New York City, the second of four children of James C. and Catherine (Nolan) Sheahan. The family moved to Albany, New York, in 1901, where Sheahan graduated from Albany High School and received a diploma from St. Peter's Hospital School of Nursing (1913). Though she never completed a college degree, she took courses at Syracuse University in Syracuse, New York, and Columbia University in New York City. She married Frank W. Bailey on March 17, 1935, who died in 1947.

Sheahan initially worked as a private-duty nurse in Albany and volunteered in a child welfare clinic, where her interest in public health began. In 1917 she began working for Lillian Wald's famed Henry Street Visiting Nurse Service, which provided in-home nursing care to the poor immigrant population of New York City. From 1917 until 1920, Sheahan held a number of positions. After being rejected for service during World War I due to health problems, she took a position with the Albany City Health Department. She accepted a temporary appointment with the New York State Department of Health to assist physicians in improving medical care. She also worked in tuberculosis clinics and distributed diphtheria immunizations. In Cohoes, New York, an area with a high infant mortality rate, she volunteered one summer to give physical examinations for infants, a program that was very successful. She also worked as a county tuberculosis nurse in Niagara County during this period.

In 1920, Sheahan began work at the New York State Department of Health. Her primary work in her early years at the agency was with communicable disease outbreaks and child health care. She became assistant director and then director (1932) of the Division of Public Health Nursing, a position that she held until her retirement in 1948. Public health nursing became more important during her tenure due to the Great Depression of the 1930s. Social Security was created in 1937, which increased the need for public health nurses. Sheahan took this opportunity to review the role of New York's public health nurses and to improve the care that they provided. She arranged for additional training for existing nurses and was able to increase the number of state public health nurses due to the additional funding provided by Social Security. These programs were highly successful and were used as a model for other programs around the country.

Following her retirement from the New York State Department of Health in 1948, Sheahan was a visiting professor of nursing at the University of California at Berkeley. In 1949, she began work directing the National Committee for the Improvement of Nursing Services, an organization formed by six national nursing organizations to improve nurs-

ing education and services. The committee began collecting and analyzing data on nursing schools, which eventually led to the accreditation process. In 1952, the National League for Nursing (NLN) was formed, and Sheahan moved into the director position of its Division of Nursing Services. She eventually became the deputy general director of the NLN, a position that she held until 1963.

In 1960, Sheahan was the first nurse to serve as president of the American Public Health Association (APHA). In 1969, she received the Sedgwick Award, the highest honor of the APHA. She died on March 17, 1994, in Albany, New York.

See also Wald, Lillian D.

Selected Additional Achievements

Author of several articles in professional journals. Chairman, National Advisory Committee of the American Red Cross; president, National Organization for Public Health Nursing (1947–1949); fellow, APHA; member, President's Commission to Study the Health Needs of the Nation (1952). First nonphysician to receive the Lasker Award, Lasker Foundation (1949); Hermann M. Biggs Award, New York State Public Health Association (1954); Florence Nightingale Medal, International Conference of Red Cross Societies (1957).

References

"Association News: Miss Sheahan—The New President." 1960. *American Journal of Public Health* 50 (11):1807–1808.

Pavri, Julie M. 1995. "Association News: In Memoriam: Marion W. Sheahan Bailey, 1893–1994." *American Journal of Public Health* 85 (12):1719–1720.

Pavri, Julie. 2000. "Marion Winifred Sheahan." In *American Nursing: A Biographical Dictionary*, edited by V.L. Bullough and L. Sentz. New York: Springer.

Safier, Gwendolyn. 1977. *Contemporary American Leaders in Nursing: An Oral History.* New York: McGraw-Hill.

DTW

Sherwood, Mary (1856–1935)
Physician

Mary Sherwood was a physician who spent most of her distinguished career in Baltimore. She was born on March 31, 1856, in Ballston Spa, New York, one of six children of Thomas Burr Sherwood, a lawyer and farmer, and Mary Frances (Beattie) Sherwood. After graduating from the State Normal School in Albany, New York, she enrolled at Vassar College in Poughkeepsie, New York. She graduated Phi Beta Kappa from Vassar in 1883 with an A.B. and then taught chemistry there (1883–1885) and astronomy and mathematics at the Packer Collegiate Institute in Brooklyn (1885–1886). While teaching, she decided to study medicine.

According to her lifelong friend and colleague Dr. Lilian Welsh, Sherwood chose to pursue her medical studies at the University of Zurich in Switzerland, which had been accepting female students since 1865, "to be sure that her opportunities were equal to any man's" (Welsh, p. 39). In Zurich Sherwood met Welsh, a graduate of the Woman's Medical College of Pennsylvania who was seeking advanced training. The two women had the opportunity to study with several distinguished professors and took one of the first bacteriology courses offered in the world.

Sherwood graduated in 1890 and moved to Baltimore, where she took postgraduate training in pathology at Johns Hopkins University (1890–1891). She and Dr. Alice Hall were offered residencies at Johns Hopkins Hospital under prominent physicians William Osler and Howard Kelly. When Hall married, however, the offer to both was revoked because married women were not permitted to be interns, and the hospital would not appoint a lone woman to the staff. Sherwood was disappointed, but that disappointment was tempered somewhat when Kelly offered her a position working with him privately. She accepted and assisted him for two years (1891–1893).

In 1892, Sherwood asked Lilian Welsh to join her in Baltimore, and the two women set up a joint practice. The first few years of the practice were lean, due to prejudice against women physicians. In 1893, the women became codirectors of Baltimore's Evening Dispensary for Working Women and Girls (founded in part by physician Kate Campbell Hurd-Mead two years earlier) and worked there until its close in 1910. Physicians of the dispensary emphasized prenatal and postnatal care, lectured on hygiene, developed a visiting nurse service, and distributed sterile milk. By the time of its closing, 52 women had served on the dispensary's staff, and 22,000 women and children had been provided medical care.

From 1893 to 1897, Sherwood traveled to Philadelphia once a week to lecture on pathology at the Woman's Medical College of Pennsylvania. In 1894, she became medical director at Bryn Mawr School for Girls, where she made significant progress in public health. She was a firm believer in prevention and became adept at detecting the early signs of infectious diseases. She was proud of the fact that the only time Bryn Mawr had to be closed due to illness on her watch was during the 1918 influenza epidemic. She was also director of physical education at the school, and she lectured on hygiene. She worked at Bryn Mawr up until the day she died.

In 1919, Sherwood organized and served as director (1919–1924) of the Baltimore Health Department's Bureau of Child Welfare, making her the first woman to head a municipal bureau in the city. The bureau provided women prenatal and maternal care. In addition to her medical work, she was active in the woman suffrage movement, and she and Welsh participated in suffrage marches. Sherwood died on May 24, 1935, in Baltimore of heart failure.

See also Hurd-Mead, Kate Campbell; Welsh, Lilian

Selected Additional Achievements

Sherwood's medical school thesis on polyneuritis recurrens was published in the German medical journal *Virchow's Archiv* in 1891. Vice president and first female officer, Medical and Chirurgical Faculty of Maryland (1898–1899); member, Babies' Milk Fund Association of Baltimore (1904–?); chair, Midwifery Committee, Medical and Chirurgical Faculty of Maryland (1908–1915); Board of Trustees, Thomas Wilson Sanitarium; Public Bath Commission; chair, Obstetrical Section, American Child Health Association.

References

Ettinger, Laura E. 1999. "Sherwood, Mary." In *American National Biography*, edited by J.A.

Garraty and M.C. Carnes. New York: Oxford University Press.

Koudelka, Janet Brock. 1971. "Sherwood, Mary." In *Notable American Women, 1607–1950: A Biographical Dictionary*, edited by E.T. James, J.W. James, and P.S. Boyer. Cambridge: Belknap Press of Harvard University Press.

Sabin, Florence R. 1935. "Doctor Mary Sherwood." *Goucher Alumnae Quarterly* 13 (July): 9–13.

Welsh, Lilian. 1925. *Reminiscences of Thirty Years in Baltimore*. Baltimore: The Norman Remington.

LS

Shipp, Ellis Reynolds (1847–1939)
Physician

The long and productive career of Ellis Shipp is one of the best recorded for women physicians from the pioneering days of the American West. She was born on January 20, 1847, in Davis County, Iowa, the first child of William Fletcher and Anna (Hawley) Reynolds. In 1851, her parents were baptized into the Mormon Church, and they and her maternal grandparents left Iowa to join the westward trek of Mormons to Utah. When Shipp was 18, she went to live with Mormon leader Brigham Young and his family in Salt Lake City, where she attended school.

On May 5, 1866, she married Milford Bard Shipp, 11 years her senior, and the couple settled in their own home in Salt Lake City. Between February 1867 and November 1875, the Shipp household expanded considerably as five children were born to them (two of whom died in infancy), and Milford took three more wives. Although she did not have much formal education, Shipp frequently rose at 4:00 A.M. to study on her own. During these years, she often wrote in her diary about the desire to improve her mind. On November 13, 1872, she recorded that she was tired of "cooking, washing dishes, and doing general housework," and

she believed that a woman "should have ample time and opportunity to study and improve her mind" (p. 110).

Around 1873, Brigham Young called for women to go East to study medicine. The thought of leaving home overwhelmed Shipp, but her will to learn, her desire to provide an income for her large family, and her religious faith gave her the strength to go to Philadelphia for medical school. She left her three small children in the care of her sister wives and arrived at the Woman's Medical College of Pennsylvania in November 1875. Early on, she expressed an interest in women's and children's health. After attending a clinic on obstetrics and diseases of children by Dr. Emeline Cleveland on April 22, 1876, she wrote, "To be able to treat these conditions and diseases successfully, I think there could be no greater accomplishment in the medical line" (p. 210).

In the summer between her first and second years, Shipp traveled back to Utah to see her family. She was pregnant when she returned to Philadelphia for her second year of school, and her sixth child, Olea, was born in Philadelphia in May 1877. Despite caring for an infant, missing her family deeply, and financial difficulties, she persevered through the remainder of two and a half years of school. She graduated with honors in the spring of 1878.

Upon returning home to Utah, Shipp opened a practice in Salt Lake City, specializing in obstetrics and diseases of women. She also founded a school for midwives, which lasted until 1935. After taking her classes, which were two terms of six months each, students were examined and certified by the Salt Lake City Board of Health. Shipp trained at least 500 women over the span of her career, including her sister wives Lizzie and Mary and her daughter Olea. Believing that her work was needed outside her home state, in 1899, Shipp went to Mexico to teach. Until 1916, she traveled throughout the West, teaching classes in Arizona, Colorado, Idaho, and Canada.

Shipp was also on the staff of Deseret Hospital in Salt Lake City from 1882 to 1890. The hospital was formed by a group of Mormon women concerned with the lack of medical facilities in the city. In addition, Shipp and her sister wife and fellow physician Maggie were both editors and contributors to their husband Milford's journal, the *Salt Lake Sanitarian*, begun in 1888. In an ongoing series in the journal called "Mother's Methods" (June–November 1888) Shipp gave practical advice on the feeding and care of infants and children.

Shipp practiced medicine for almost 60 years and delivered 6,000 babies. She died on January 31, 1939, in Salt Lake City.

See also Cleveland, Emeline Horton

Selected Additional Achievements

Delegate, International Council of Women (Washington, D.C., March 1888); oldest living graduate and gold medal, Woman's Medical College (1935); Utah's Hall of Famous Women (1938).

References

Bauman, H. 1984. "Shipp, Ellis Reynolds." In *Dictionary of American Medical Biography*, edited by M. Kaufman, S. Galishoff, and T.L. Savitt. Westport, Conn.: Greenwood Press.

Noall, Claire. 1974. *Guardians of Health: Utah's Pioneer Midwives and Women Doctors*. Bountiful, Utah: Horizon.

"Pioneer Women Doctors." 1958. In *Our Pioneer Heritage*, edited by K.B. Carter. Vol. 6. Salt Lake City: Daughters of Utah Pioneers.

Register of the Ellis Reynolds Shipp Collection. 1977. *Manuscript Collection B-4*. Salt Lake City: Utah State Historical Society.

Rose, Blanche E. 1942. "Early Utah Medical Practice." *Utah Historical Quarterly* 10:14–33.

Shipp, Ellis Reynolds. 1962. *The Early Autobiography and Diary of Ellis Reynolds Shipp, M.D.* Edited by E.S. Musser. Salt Lake City: Deseret News Press.

LS

Shortt, Elizabeth Smith (1859–1949)
Physician

Elizabeth Shortt was instrumental in the success of Canada's first medical program for women at Queen's University in Kingston, Ontario. She was born on January 18, 1859, the third child of Sylvester Smith, a Winona, Ontario, farmer, and Isabella (McGee) Smith. She received her early education with a governess, at the Winona School, and at Hamilton Collegiate Institute.

Shortt began her career as a teacher, but by 1877 she had decided to study medicine, although no woman had yet graduated from a Canadian medical school. Undaunted, she took the first step toward obtaining her medical education by sitting for the matriculation examination of the College of Physicians and Surgeons in Toronto in 1879. During the examination, Shortt learned that the Royal College of Physicians and Surgeons, affiliated with Queen's University in Kingston, Ontario, was prepared to start a women's class, but only if there were a sufficient number of applicants. Shortt passed the examination and returned home to begin a letter-writing and advertisement campaign to generate interest in the program and to increase the number of applicants to Queen's. Her efforts paid off and in the spring of 1880, she and two other women entered Canada's first medical program for women. In October 1881, the women joined the men's regular class, although the women had separate dissecting rooms and listened to certain lectures in adjacent rooms. Despite this, the men firmly opposed the women's presence and harassed their female classmates. During this trying period, Shortt wrote in her diary that "not a day not a lecture passes . . . but something makes me shrink something hurts me, hurts me cruelly" (Smith, p. 275). When the men threatened to transfer to rival Trinity Medical College, the staff at Queen's acquiesced, promising to admit no more women and to completely segregate those currently enrolled.

With financial support from Jenny Trout, the first woman licensed to practice medicine in Canada, Queen's University opened the Women's Medical College. Shortt enrolled in 1883 and graduated with the college's first class the following year. After her graduation, she established a private practice and married Queen's professor Adam Shortt in 1886. In 1888, she was appointed as lecturer in medical jurisprudence and sanitary science at the Women's Medical College. When the Women's College closed in 1893, its students were transferred to the Ontario Medical College for Women, but the staff, including Shortt, were not offered positions at the new school.

Other than offering medical advice to friends and family, Shortt never returned to the formal practice of medicine. She became an active social reformer and was soon considered one of the leading Canadian women of her day. In addition to raising three children, she worked tirelessly for causes affecting the health and welfare of women and children. In Kingston, she was president of Canada's first Young Women's Christian Association and started a Local Council of Women. In 1908, the family moved to Ottawa, where Shortt helped form the Victorian Order of Nurses and the Women's Canadian Club. As vice president of the Ontario Council of Women, she campaigned for a variety of health issues, including tuberculosis education, fly control, general sanitation, and the pasteurization of milk. She also worked for the council's Committee on Immigration and was instrumental in the formation of a hostel for women immigrants. In 1920, she was appointed vice chairman of the Ottawa Provincial Board of Mother's Allowances, which advocated government money for women and children in homes where the father was not present. She retained this position until her death on January 14, 1949.

See also Trout, Jenny Kidd

References

Hacker, Carlotta. 1974. *The Indomitable Lady Doctors.* Toronto: Clarke, Irwin.

Smith, Elizabeth. 1980. *A Woman with a Purpose: The Diaries of Elizabeth Smith, 1872–1884.* Edited by V. Strong-Boag. Toronto: University of Toronto Press.

JSB

Sirridge, Marjorie (1921–   )
Physician

Marjorie Sirridge is dean of the University of Missouri-Kansas City Medical School. In spite of her current success, she struggled during her early career to find ways to pursue medicine and have a family. She was born on October 6, 1921, in Kingman, Kansas. She decided to become a physician, although both her family and academic advisers discouraged her. Despite this lack of encouragement, she graduated from the premedical program at Kansas State University (1942) and from the medical school at the University of Kansas (1944).

She married William Sirridge, also a University of Kansas medical student, on the day before their graduation. Sirridge then completed an internship at Charity Hospital in New Orleans and began a fellowship in Cleveland, Ohio. By the time she arrived for her fellowship in 1945, she was pregnant with her first child. She spent several months doing laboratory work; however, after the birth, she was unable to complete the fellowship because the family could not afford child care.

Sirridge ultimately had four children, one closely following the other. Not until 1951 did she attempt to fulfill her residency requirement. Parental responsibilities limited her to part-time work, although no part-time residency programs existed. She finally settled on a nonapproved, half-time residency at Bethany Hospital in Kansas City and a second similar residency at the University of Kansas Medical Center. After completing the second residency, she hoped to continue working at the Medical Center, but the faculty considered her unqualified because of her unorthodox training. In the meantime, she served as assistant clinical professor at the University of Kansas (1958–1971) and was in private practice with her husband.

In 1971, Sirridge left the University of Kansas and became a founding faculty member at the University of Missouri-Kansas City Medical School (UMKC). UMKC Medical School is a six-year combined B.A./M.D. program accepting students directly out of high school. She believes that allowing women to enter medical school early is an important feature of the program, as many women who "might have become very good and happy physicians" do not continue on to medical school because they are discouraged during their premedical studies (quoted in Morantz-Sanchez, p. 168). She maintains that balancing a medical career and a family is still the most difficult problem for women physicians. "Dr. Marjorie," as she is known by her students, serves as a role model for her young female students by being "very professional but open and friendly" (Sirridge, 1998).

Selected Additional Achievements

Laboratory Evaluation of Homeostasis (1967; 2nd ed. 1974; 3rd ed. 1983); "The Docent System: An Alternate Approach to Medical Education," *Pharos* (1980); "The Mentor System in Medicine—How it Works for Women," *Journal of the American Medical Women's Association* (1985); "Daughters of Aesculapius: A Selected Bibliography of Autobiographies of Women Medical School Graduates 1849–1920," *Literature and Medicine* (with B.R. Pfannenstiel, 1996). Continuing consultant professor, Shanghai Second Medical College (1981); first woman Medical Alumnus of the Year, University of Kansas (1983); first woman president, Medical-Dental Staff, Truman Medical Center (1984–1985); second woman president, Metropolitan Medical Society (1989); fellow, American College of Physicians (1991); master, American College of Physicians (1994); Doctor of the Year Award, Metropolitan Medical Society Alliance (1995); Marjorie S. Sirridge Outstanding Women in Medicine annual lectureship at UMKC (1997).

References

Morantz-Sanchez, Regina Markell, Cynthia Stodola Pomerleau, and Carol Fenichel, eds. 1982. *In Her Own Words: Oral Histories of Women Physicians.* Westport, Conn.: Greenwood Press.

Sirridge, Marjorie. (N.d.). Curriculum Vitae.

Sirridge, Marjorie S. 1996. "Special Armor." In *Women in Medical Education: An Anthology of Experience*, edited by D. Wear. Albany: State University of New York Press.

Sirridge, Marjorie S. April 9, 1998. Interview with author via E-mail.

JSB

Smellie, Elizabeth Lawrie (1884–1968)
Nurse

Elizabeth Smellie was the chief superintendent of the Victorian Order of Nurses of Canada, a national visiting nursing service. During World War II, she supervised the organization of the Canadian Women's Army Corps and, as a result of her efforts, became the first Canadian woman promoted to colonel. She was born on March 22, 1884, in Port Arthur, Ontario, Canada, to Janet Eleanor Lawrie and Dr. Thomas Stewart Traill Smellie. She received her early education in Port Arthur schools and at St. Margaret's College in Toronto.

Smellie graduated from Johns Hopkins Training School for Nurses in Baltimore in 1909 and went on to Simmons College in Boston, for postgraduate studies in public health nursing. During World War I, she served as a nursing sister for the Canadian Army Medical Corps as well as matron of the Moore Barracks Hospital in England (1915–1918). For her efforts during the war, she was awarded the Royal Red Cross in 1917.

When Smellie returned to Canada, she became assistant matron-in-chief of the Canadian Nursing Service (1918–1920) and then assistant to the director of the McGill School of Graduate Nursing (1921–1924). While at McGill, she coordinated the field instruction of nursing students of the Montreal branch of the Victorian Order of Nurses (VON). She was then appointed chief superintendent of the VON in 1924 and retained the position until 1947. As chief superintendent, she brought together prominent academics and government experts to act as an advisory committee to the VON. She also secured representation for the VON on the governing boards of the Canadian Medical Association and the Canadian Nurses Association. In 1924, she brought VON delegates from each province to the Canadian Nurses Association general meeting. With this meeting she had begun to establish the VON as a strong, cohesive organization that was an integral part of nursing and medicine in Canada.

The government's recognition of the VON's importance was evident during the depression, when the VON continued to receive federal and provincial grants. Unfortunately, these grants were not sufficient to maintain the level of service given prior to the depression, but Smellie vowed to serve patients regardless of their ability to pay. In fact, under her supervision, the number of home visits made by the VON during the 1930s was greater than in previous years. In 1938, in recognition of her work, the Canadian Nurses Association awarded her the Mary Snively Memorial Medal. During the depression years she also acted as a consultant to the Ontario Provincial Department of Health in Ottawa, and in 1939, she was appointed vice president of the American Public Health Association.

During World War II, Smellie took an extended leave of absence from the VON to join the Royal Canadian Army Corps as matron-in-chief. In 1942, she supervised the organization of the Canadian Women's Army Corps and was promoted to lieutenant colonel. She was then promoted to colonel (1944), the first woman in Canada to hold that rank. During her tenure as colonel, she led an active recruiting campaign across Canada to attract women to the army. After the war, she returned to her civil post with the VON until 1947. She then acted as a nursing consultant to the Department of Veteran Affairs from 1947 to 1948.

Smellie died on March 5, 1968, in Toronto.

See also Snively, Mary Agnes

References

The Canadian Who's Who. 1957. Vol. 7. Toronto: Trans-Canada Press.

Penney, Sheila M. 1996. *A Century of Caring: 1897–1997: The History of the Victorian Order of Nurses for Canada.* Ottawa: VON Canada.

Robbins, John E., ed. 1958. *Encyclopedia Canadiana.* Ottawa: Canadiana.

The Victorian Order of Nurses. Online. http://

www.porcupineinfo.com/von/page14.html. 4 May 1998.

Wallace, W. Stewart, and W.A. McKay, eds. 1978.

The Macmillan Dictionary of Canadian Biography. 4th ed. Toronto: Macmillan.

CMB

Smith, Margaret Charles (1906–)
Midwife

The career of Margaret Charles Smith, an Alabama granny (lay) midwife, is representative of generations of women who have practiced this profession. She was born on September 12, 1906, in Green County, Alabama, to Beulah Sanders. She was raised by her grandmother, Margaret Charles, who had been a slave. Smith began her career in the early 1940s, when she helped a family member deliver a baby while waiting for the midwife to arrive. Afterward, she was trained by a local lay midwife. Smith's methods, like those of other granny midwives, differed very little from those of her ancestors. She used abdominal massage, herbs to induce contractions, and heat in the form of fire, hot tea, or a bath to promote healing and relaxation. After delivery, the placenta, believed to have a life force important for the mother's health, was salted down and buried near the mother's home.

In the 1940s, Alabama law required lay midwives to obtain permits through their local health departments. After almost a decade of successfully delivering babies, Smith received a permit to officially practice lay midwifery. Around the same time, she began a 28-year career providing prenatal care at the Green County Health Department. Health Department rules prohibited the use of certain methods traditionally used by the lay midwife. Since Health Department nurses made regular inspections of the midwives' bags, many midwives, including Smith, prepared two bags: one for inspection and one to carry to births, which contained illegal oils, herbs, teas, or roots. Eventually, fear of imprisonment forced Smith to discontinue the use of illegal birthing aids.

A 1976 law prohibited the issuance of new permits to lay midwives. Midwives with permits were allowed to practice until their permits expired or were revoked. In 1981 Smith delivered her last baby yet remained an important figure in her community. She received the keys to her hometown, the first African American to do so, and was honored at the first Black Women's Health Project Conference (Atlanta, 1983). Of her own work, Smith believes, "I'm worth millions of dollars for what I've done. I thought I was doing a big thing. I was proud of it" (p. 156).

Smith had two children, Houston (1922) and Spencer (1926), but remained unmarried until the late 1930s. She had one child, Herman (1943), with her husband, Randolph Smith. She continues to live at her home in Eutaw, Alabama.

References

Davis, Sheila P., and Cora A. Ingram. 1993. "Empowered Caretakers: A Historical Perspective of the Roles of Granny Midwives in Rural Alabama." In *Wings of Gauze: Women of Color and the Experience of Health and Illness*, edited by B. Bair and S. Cayleff. Detroit: Wayne State University Press.

Holmes, Linda. 1984. "Medical History: Alabama Granny Midwife." *Journal of the Medical Society of New Jersey* 81 (5):389–391.

Smith, Margaret Charles, and Linda Janet Holmes. 1996. *Listen to Me Good: The Life Story of an Alabama Midwife*. Columbus: Ohio State University Press.

JSB

Snively, Mary Agnes (1847–1933)
Nurse

Mary Agnes Snively was superintendent of nurses at Toronto General Hospital in Canada for 25 years and a leader in the establishment of professional nursing organizations in Canada and abroad. She was born to Martin and Susan M. (Copeland) Snively on November 12, 1847, in St. Catharines, Ontario. She graduated from high school and then taught in the local schools. Future nursing leader Isabel Hampton Robb, who lived and taught near Snively and was beginning her own nursing career, stirred Snively's interest in nursing.

In October 1882, Snively resigned her teaching position and went to New York City to study nursing at the Bellevue Hospital Training School. She graduated in 1884 and accepted a position as superintendent of nurses at Toronto General Hospital. As superintendent, she was responsible for the nurse training school as well the hospi-

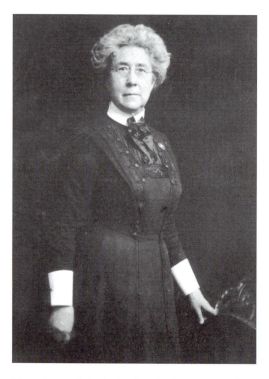

Mary Agnes Snively. National Library of Medicine.

tal's nursing service. When she began, the hospital and school were in disarray; there were no systematic course of study at the school, no written orders for the nurses, no patient history records, and no system of obtaining necessary ward supplies. The nurses had no place to live and slept wherever they found empty beds in the hospital. One of Snively's first acts was to appeal to the hospital administration for a nurses' residence, which opened in July 1887. Gradually, she was able to reform the hospital nursing service and the school.

Snively arranged for physicians and surgeons to teach classes in nursing and nursing ethics and introduced a written exam at the end of training. She also expanded the course of study to three years and instituted a required preliminary course of four months' training in domestic science, anatomy, physiology, and hygiene. Snively believed not only in practical training, which was the main method of instruction for nursing students of the day, but also in theoretical instruction, which she believed was "one of the chief factors in the development and advancement of a school for nurses" (Snively, p. 22). In addition to her educational reforms, she transferred housekeeping duties, such as dishwashing, from nurses to hospital maids.

Snively believed in state registration. She felt that a uniform educational policy was the first step toward this goal and served as chair of a committee to develop a two-year curriculum. In 1893, she helped found the American Society of Superintendents of Training Schools for Nurses of the United States and Canada (now the National League for Nursing) and was president of the organization in 1897. In 1899, she was instrumental in the formation of the International Council of Nurses and served as honorary treasurer for five years. In 1907, she was an organizer and president of the Canadian Superintendents Association. The next year, she helped found and was president of the Canadian National

Association of Trained Nurses, which became the Canadian Nurses Association in 1924. In 1909, she affiliated the Canadian National Association with the International Council of Nurses.

Snively retired from Toronto General in 1910 but remained active in nursing organizations and in missionary societies. She died on September 25, 1933. In 1934, the Canadian Nurses Association established a medal in her name.

See also Robb, Isabel Adams Hampton

Selected Additional Achievements

"A Nurse's Day in a Hospital," *Trained Nurse and Hospital Review* 13 (1894):8–12; "Graduation and First Case," in *How to Become a Trained Nurse: A Manual of Information in Detail*, edited by J. Hodson (New York: William Abbatt, 1898); "Organization and Legislation in Canada," in *Third International Congress of Nurses.* (Cleveland: J.B. Savage, [1901]; "What Manner of Women Ought Nurses to Be?" *American Journal of Nursing* 4 (August 1904):836–840; "The Toronto General Hospital Training School for Nurses," *Canadian Nurse* 1 (March 1905): 7–9; "Recollections," *ICN* 4 (July 1929):212–215.

References

Browne, Jean E. 1924. "A Daughter of Canada." *Canadian Nurse* 20 (October):617–620, (November):681–684, (December):734–736.

Browne, Jean E. 1933. "In Memoriam: Miss Mary Agnes Snively." *Canadian Nurse* 29 (November):567–570.

Mansell, D. 1999. "Profile of a Leader, Mary Agnes Snively: Realistic Optimist." *Canadian Journal of Nursing Leadership* 12 (1):27–29.

"Miss Snively and the Story of Nursing." 1910. *Nurses Journal of the Pacific Coast* 6 (April): 160–162.

Snively, Mary Agnes. 1905. "The Toronto General Hospital Training School for Nurses." *Canadian Nurse* 1 (June):21–24.

LS

Staupers, Mabel Keaton (1890–1989)
Nurse

Mabel Keaton Staupers led the integration of African American nurses into national nursing organizations and into the U.S. armed forces. Her astute leadership during the World War II era also led to professional recognition of black nurses by the major nursing associations. She was born in Barbados, West Indies, on February 27, 1890. She emigrated to the United States with her parents, Thomas and Pauline Doyle, in April 1903. Later that year, the family settled in the Harlem section of New York City, where she completed secondary school.

In 1914, Staupers moved to Washington, D.C., and enrolled in the Freedmen's Hospital School of Nursing (now Howard University College of Nursing). She graduated with honors in 1916 and married Dr. James Max Keaton the same year. The couple later divorced. In 1931 she married Fritz C. Staupers. Staupers began her nursing career by working as a private-duty nurse. This was typical of most nurses of the time, especially black nurses. Employment in hospitals or other traditional nursing positions was usually unattainable for blacks. In 1920, Staupers and African American physicians Louis T. Wright and James Wilson organized the Booker T. Washington Sanitarium, an inpatient hospital for black tuberculosis patients. The facility was the first in the Harlem area to allow black doctors to treat patients.

In 1921, Staupers received a fellowship at the Henry Phipps Institute of Tuberculosis in Philadelphia to work at the Jefferson Hospital Medical College. While there she observed the poor treatment of African Americans by college administrators and doctors. This experience heightened her awareness of the challenges faced by blacks. In 1922, the New York Tuberculosis and Health Association asked her to carry out a survey of health needs of blacks in Harlem. Her findings of inadequate response on the part of the city led to the establishment of the Harlem Committee of the New York Tuberculosis and Health Association. Staupers served as executive secretary of the organization for 12 years.

In 1934, Staupers was appointed executive secretary of the National Association of Colored Graduate Nurses (NACGN). The NACGN had been founded in 1908 through the efforts of black nurses Adah Thoms and Martha Franklin but had only moderate success in improving working conditions of African American nurses. Until 1934, NACGN lacked the funding to have a salaried official. After receiving grants from the General Education Board of the Rockefeller Foundation and the Julius Rosenwald Fund, the NACGN was able to hire Staupers as well as move into permanent headquarters at the Rockefeller Center in New York City, which also housed all of the major national nursing organizations.

With the outbreak of World War II, Staupers saw an opportunity to push for increased professional opportunities for black nurses. The United States Army set a quota of only 56 black nurses, while the navy would not allow any black nurses into the nurse corps. Staupers, along with other black leaders, lobbied to allow black nurses to serve. She contacted First Lady Eleanor Roosevelt, who took Staupers' case to the secretary of war and naval officials. Following an announcement in early 1945 by the surgeon general of the United States Army that a draft might possibly be enacted to meet the nursing shortage in the armed forces, Staupers launched a campaign to end discrimination against black nurses. After receiving a huge response from the public, the War Department declared an end to quotas in the Army Nurse Corps and struck down the naval exclusion on black nurses. Only weeks later, the first black nurse joined the Navy Nurse Corps.

In 1946, Staupers resigned her position with the NACGN, hoping to take a rest. However, she was soon back at work, lobbying the American Nurses Association for full membership for black nurses. In 1948, this goal was realized. Following this achievement, it was decided that the NACGN should be disbanded, having met its goals of eliminating segregation of nurses. Staupers was elected president of NACGN to oversee its legal dissolution. The NACGN officially disbanded in January 1951.

Staupers wrote a book recounting the fight to integrate nursing: *No Time for Prejudice*, published in 1961. She died on September 30, 1989.

See also Franklin, Martha Minerva; Thoms, Adah Belle Samuels

Selected Additional Achievements

Founder, National Council of Negro Women (1935); NAACP Spingarn Medal Recipient (1951); American Nurses Association Hall of Fame (1996); Alumni Award, Howard University.

References

Hine, Darlene Clark. 1982. "Mabel K. Staupers and the Integration of Black Nurses into the Armed Forces." In *Black Leaders of the Twentieth Century*, edited by J.H. Franklin and A. Meier. Urbana: University of Illinois Press.

Hine, Darlene Clark. 1988. "Mabel Keaton Staupers." In *American Nursing: A Biographical Dictionary*, edited by V.L. Bullough, O.M. Church, and A.P. Stein. New York: Garland.

Hine, Darlene Clark. 1993. "Staupers, Mabel Keaton." In *Black Women in America: An Historical Encyclopedia*, edited by D.C. Hine, E. Barkley, and R. Terborg-Penn. Brooklyn, N.Y.: Carlson.

"Mabel Keaton Staupers, R.N., 1890–." 1969. *Journal of the National Medical Association* 61 (2):198–199.

DTW

Stevenson, Sarah Ann Hackett (1841–1909)
Physician

Sarah Stevenson was a pioneer midwestern doctor who, in 1876, became the first female member of the American Medical Association. She was born on February 2, 1841, in Buffalo Grove, Illinois, the fourth of seven children of John Davis Stevenson, a farmer, and Sarah T. (Hackett) Stevenson. She attended Mount Carroll (Illinois) Seminary as well as the Illinois State Normal University, from which she graduated in 1863. After graduation, she taught school in Bloomington, Mount Morris, and Sterling, Illinois.

Around 1870, Stevenson went to Chicago, where she studied anatomy and physiology at Woman's Hospital Medical College. Physician Mary Harris Thompson cofounded the college the same year, which was affiliated with her Chicago Hospital for Women and Children. Stevenson left Chicago for London, England, around 1871 to study at the South Kensington Science School with noted biologist Thomas Huxley. Huxley's lectures were the inspiration and basis for a high school textbook that she wrote, *Boys and Girls in Biology* (1875). Following her studies abroad, Stevenson returned to Chicago to finish her medical education. She graduated from Woman's Hospital Medical College in 1874 as valedictorian. After graduation, she returned to Europe for postgraduate training at hospitals and clinics.

In 1875, Stevenson established a private practice in Chicago that would last until 1903. She also joined the faculty of her alma mater as professor of physiology and histology (1875–1880) and later as professor of obstetrics (1880–1894). In addition, she was consulting physician at Woman's and Provident Hospitals as well as attending physician at the Mary Thompson Hospital (formerly Chicago Hospital for Women and Children). She was the first woman to be appointed to the staff of Cook County Hospital in Chicago (1881) and the first woman to be appointed to the Illinois State Board of Health (1893). She also helped found the Illinois Training School for Nurses (1880), the

Home for Incurables, and the Chicago Maternity Hospital.

Stevenson is probably best known as the first woman member of the American Medical Association (AMA). In 1876, the Illinois State Medical Society chose her as an alternate delegate to the AMA annual convention in Philadelphia when another delegate became ill. Just five years earlier, female membership was such a hotly contested issue that the AMA had tabled the matter without a vote. In 1876, however, Dr. William H. Byford and another male colleague supported Stevenson's admission to the conference; they paid her fee and registered her under her full name to prevent accusations of disguising her gender. Opponents motioned to refer her registration to the Judicial Council, but the motion was quickly struck down and the AMA received Stevenson as a delegate from Illinois.

Stevenson wrote a popular book, *The Physiology of Woman: Embracing Girlhood, Maternity, and Mature Age* (1880), aimed at "the false teaching which women have received" about their bodies (p. 17). It contained plainly written essays on topics ranging from basic anatomy and skin care, to a description of the three stages of labor. Her feminist and reformist views are evident throughout the book, as when she states, "The whole *status* of the girl is made to depend, not upon what she is or does, but how she looks. . . . Looks, not books, are the murderers of American women" (p. 68). Stevenson also firmly believed in coeducation of the sexes in medicine. An appendix to the book is devoted to a carefully reasoned argument on not only why women should be educated as physicians but also why they should attend school with men.

In 1903, Stevenson suffered a stroke and retired from the practice of medicine. By 1906, she was debilitated to the point of hospitalization at St. Elizabeth's Hospital in Chicago. She died on August 14, 1909, at

St. Elizabeth's; her death was officially attributed to exhaustion.

See also Thompson, Mary Harris

Selected Additional Achievements

Read her paper, "A Study of Placenta Previa: Especially the Causes of Hemorrhage" before the Obstetrics Section, First Pan-American Medical Congress, Washington, D.C. (1893). Chair, Illinois State Medical Society's Committee on Progress in Physiology (1875–1876); first superintendent, Department of Hygiene, Woman's Christian Temperance Union (1881–1882).

References

Beatty, William K. 1982. "Sarah Hackett Stevenson—Concerned Practitioner and Social Activist." *Proceedings. Institute of Medicine of Chicago* 35:99–101.

Bonner, Thomas Neville. 1971. "Stevenson, Sarah Ann Hackett." In *Notable American Women, 1607–1950: A Biographical Dictionary*, edited by E.T. James, J.W. James, and P.S. Boyer. Cambridge: Belknap Press of Harvard University Press.

"Noted Woman Doctor Dead." 1909. *The Chicago Sunday Tribune* (August 15).

Stevenson, Sarah Hackett. 1882. *The Physiology of Woman, Embracing Girlhood, Maternity and Mature Age*. 4th ed. Chicago: Fairbanks Palmer.

LS

Stewart, Isabel Maitland (1878–1963)
Nurse

When Isabel Maitland Stewart entered nursing, nurse education consisted of training or apprenticeship programs that taught elementary, routine nursing procedures. She pointed out the weakness of such instruction and was instrumental in laying the groundwork for modern nursing education. She was born on January 14, 1878, in Ontario, Canada, the fourth of nine children of Francis Beattie and Elizabeth (Farguharson) Stewart. After receiving her early education, she taught at a rural school, later receiving her teaching certificate in 1895 from Manitoba Normal School. During the next four years, she taught at local schools and attended one year at the Winnipeg Collegiate Institute.

Dissatisfied with teaching, Stewart entered Winnipeg General Hospital Training School of Nursing in 1900. With her entrance into nursing school, she became aware of the need to improve nursing education, which was often given by head nurses of hospital wards rather than trained educators. In 1903, following her graduation, she practiced as a private-duty nurse, was a district nurse in Winnipeg, and served as head nurse at Winnipeg General Hospital. During this time, she also helped establish a visiting nurse association and an alumni association journal for her alma mater.

In 1907, Stewart read an article by Adelaide Nutting describing new educational opportunities available for graduate nurses at Teachers College, Columbia University in New York City. Stewart enrolled in the program and earned a B.S. in 1911 and an M.A in 1913. She also earned a special certificate in hospital economics in 1909 and a special diploma in hospital economics in 1910. She intended to earn a Ph.D. but never completed her doctoral work.

Stewart spent the rest of her career at Teachers College. There, she held the positions of instructor, assistant professor, and associate professor. In 1925, she succeeded Nutting as professor and director of the Department of Nursing Education. As director, Stewart developed the first course for the training of nursing educators. When the course was expanded into an entire program for preparation of nursing educators, it attracted nursing students from all over the world.

Most nurse training programs of the time focused on teaching nurses only the mechanical skills required of them. Stewart did not deny the importance of manual skills, but proposed a complete education that would develop the "creative imagination, the sensitive spirit, and the intelligent understanding lying back of these techniques and skills" (quoted in Donahue, 1983, p. 142). To this end, she was a founder of the Association of Collegiate Schools of Nursing, of which she served as the first secretary and president (1937–1941).

For several years Stewart worked with the Curriculum Committee of the National League of Nursing Education, first as its secretary (1914–1919) and then as chair (1920–1937). Three studies resulted from the work of this committee, which outlined plans for nursing education, including suggested courses and their content and objectives. The final study, *A Curriculum Guide for Schools of Nursing*, was considered the most ambitious effort up to that time on behalf of nursing education. In 1923, Stewart served as chair of a league committee to study methods for grading and classifying schools of nursing. As a result of the work, an independent Committee on the Grading of Nursing Schools was formed.

A prolific writer, Stewart published 123 articles and 17 pamphlets. Her books, *A Short History of Nursing* and *The Education of Nurses*, are now considered classics in nursing literature. She also published the *Nursing Education Bulletin*, perhaps the first journal devoted to nursing research. For her efforts in nursing research, the Isabel Maitland Stewart Research Professorship in Nursing Education was established at Teachers College in 1961.

During both world wars, Stewart was active in nurse recruitment efforts. She wrote much of the nurse recruitment material and chaired the curriculum committee of the Vassar College Training Camp during World War I. At the outbreak of World War II, she was instrumental in the formation of the National Nursing Council for National Defense. She was appointed chair of the Council's Committee on Educational Policies and Resources. She was also successful in obtaining federal funds that established the U.S. Cadet Nurse Corps for the training and selection of nurses for defense needs.

Stewart was active internationally as well. As early as 1918, she chaired a League Committee on International Affairs. For the International Council of Nurses, she chaired the program committee for its congress held in Finland in 1925. From 1925 to 1947, she chaired the Council's Committee on Education. She also completed a council study of postgraduate education in 1950.

After her retirement from Teachers College in 1947, Stewart remained active in the profession. She continued to write and served as chair of the National League of Nursing's committee on historical source material. She died of a heart attack on October 5, 1963, in Chatham, New Jersey.

See also Nutting, [Mary] Adelaide

Selected Additional Achievements

American Society of Superintendents of Training Schools for Nurses and the Associated Alumni of the United States and Canada, secretary (1915) and second vice president (1920); editor, department of nursing education, *American Journal of Nursing* (1916–1921); member of the Board of Directors, National League of Nursing Education (1925–1943); chair of the committee on education, International Council of Nurses (1925–1947); second vice president, American Council on Education (1944); editor, *Nursing Education Monographs*. Awards include: honorary membership, History of Nursing Society, McGill University (1928); Mary Adelaide Nutting Award, National League of Nursing Education (1947); Pro Benignetate Humana Medal, government of Finland (1949); Florence Nightingale Medal, International Committee of the Red Cross Society (1955); and honorary degrees from Western Reserve University (1948), Columbia University (1954), and the University of Manitoba (1956). *A Short History of Nursing* (with Lavinia Dock, 1920, 1925, 1931, 1938; 1938 ed. with Anne L. Austin published as *A History of Nursing*); *The Education of Nurses, Historical Foundations and Modern Trends* (1943); *A Century of Nursing* (with Agnes Gelinas, 1950).

References

Donahue, M. Patricia. 1983. "Isabel Maitland Stewart's Philosophy of Education." *Nursing Research* 32 (3):140–146.

Donahue, M. Patricia. 1988. "Isabel Maitland Stewart." In *American Nursing: A Biographical Dictionary*, edited by V.L. Bullough, O.M. Church, and A.P. Stein. New York: Garland.

Goostray, Stella. 1954. "Isabel Maitland Stewart: The Story of a National and International Leader in Nursing Education." *American Journal of Nursing* 54 (3):302–306.

Stewart, Isabel M. 1929. "The Science and Art in Nursing." *Nursing Education Bulletin* 11:1–4.

Stewart, Isabel M. 1931. "Trends in Nursing Education." *American Journal of Nursing* 31 (5): 601–611.

Taylor, Effie J. 1936. "Isabel Maitland Stewart—Educator." *American Journal of Nursing* 36 (1):38–44.

Yost, Edna. 1965. *American Women of Nursing.* Rev. ed. Philadelphia: J.B. Lippincott.

JSB

Stimson, Julia Catherine (1881–1948)
Nurse

Julia Stimson was the first woman to earn the rank of major in the United States Army. Her career as a prominent nursing leader spanned both world wars. She was born on May 26, 1881, in Worcester, Massachusetts, the second of seven children of Henry Albert Stimson and Alice Weaton (Bartlett) Stimson. She attended public schools in St. Louis, Missouri, and the Brearley School in New York City. She received her B.A. degree from Vassar in 1901 and afterward took a summer course at the Marine Biology Laboratory in Woods Hole, Massachusetts. The next fall, she began graduate studies in zoology at Columbia University. After two years at Columbia, she was a medical illustrator at Cornell University Medical College.

Stimson wanted to become a physician, but her parents strongly disapproved, arguing that it was an improper career for a woman. She decided on nursing after meeting Annie Goodrich, superintendent of the New York Hospital Training School for Nurses. In 1904, Stimson entered the New York Hospital Training School and graduated in 1908. Her first position was as superintendent of nurses at Harlem Hospital in New York City. During her short time there, she wrote *Nurses' Handbook of Drugs and Solutions* (1910) and assisted in the establishment of the Harlem Hospital Social Services Department.

In 1911, Stimson was appointed head of the Social Service Department at Washington University Hospitals in St. Louis, Missouri.

In 1913, she took on additional duties as superintendent of nurses at the university hospitals. Involved with the Red Cross since 1909, she organized St. Louis nurses for public health work in Hamilton, Ohio, during the Ohio Valley flood in 1913. At the outbreak of World War I, the Red Cross made her chief nurse for Hospital Base 21, established at Washington University. In May 1917, she learned she had to be ready for mobilization to Rouen, France. She wrote to her parents that the responsibility for preparing her nurses for deployment was overwhelming, yet "to be in the first group of women ever called out for duty with the United States Army . . . is all too much good fortune for any one person like me" (Stimson, 1927 reprint, p. 3). The letters that she sent home during the war were published in 1918 as *Finding Themselves*. Just after leaving for France, she was awarded a master's degree in sociology from Washington University.

On April 10, 1918, in addition to her army duties, Stimson became chief nurse of the American Red Cross service in France. On November 15 of the same year, the army promoted her to director of the Army Expeditionary Force's Nursing Service. Her wartime honors include the Distinguished Service Medal, the British Royal Red Cross, the French Médaille de la Renaissance Français, and the Médaille d'Hygiéne Publique.

In July 1919, Stimson went to Washington, D.C., to serve as dean of the Army

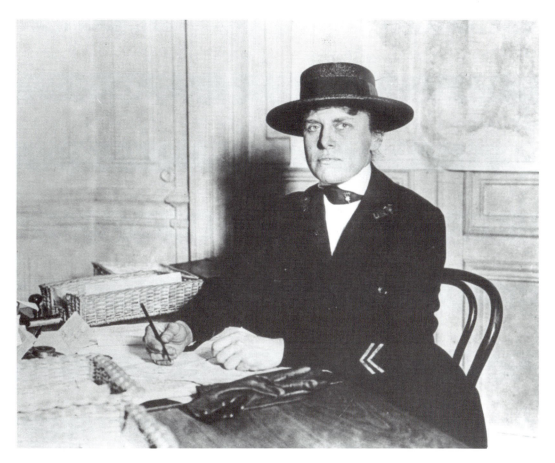

Julia Catherine Stimson. National Library of Medicine.

School of Nursing, a position that she held until the school closed in 1933. She was also acting superintendent of the Army Nurse Corps, a position that was made permanent on December 30. As superintendent, she increased nurses' opportunities for continuing education and membership in professional organizations, improved housing conditions, and increased retirement privileges. In 1920, Congress granted army nurses "relative" rank, which gave them more, but not equal, authority, status, and pay as their male counterparts. Stimson earned the relative rank of major, the first woman to achieve that rank in the United States Army. She served as major and superintendent until her retirement from the Army Nurse Corps in 1937. On the occasion of her retirement, the United States Army surgeon general declared that Stimson had "secured for the members of [the] Corps a recognition in the Army second to none of the various Services" (Surgeon General, p. 5).

Stimson remained active as president of the American Nurses Association from 1938 to 1944. In 1941, she organized the Nursing Council on National Defense to meet the nursing requirements of World War II. In 1942, when Stimson was 60 years old, the army recalled her services for six months to recruit nurses for World War II. In 1947, nurses finally received full commissioned rank, equal to that of men. In August 1948, Stimson was appointed to Colonel just six weeks before her death in Poughkeepsie, New York, on September 29. In 1955, the Stimson Library of the Army Medical School at Brooke Army Medical Center was dedicated to her memory.

See also Goodrich, Annie Warburton

Selected Additional Achievements

"Compulsory Health Insurance" (master's thesis, Washington University 1917), *Women Nurses with the Union Forces during the Civil War* (1928), *History and Manual of the Army Nurse Corps* (1937), and several articles in nursing and military journals. She received an honorary doctor of science degree, Mount Holyoke College (1921) and the Florence Nightingale Medal of the International Red Cross (1929).

References

Goostray, Stella. 1971. "Stimson, Julia Catherine." In *Notable American Women, 1607–1950: A Biographical Dictionary*, edited by E.T. James, J.W. James, and P.S. Boyer. Cambridge, Mass.: Belknap Press of Harvard University Press.

Hunt, Marion. 1999. "Stimson, Julia Catherine." In *American National Biography*, edited by J.A. Garraty and M.C. Carnes. New York: Oxford University Press.

The National Cyclopaedia of American Biography. 1927. Current Volume B. New York: James T. White.

Sabin, Linda E. 1988. "Julia Catherine Stimson." In *American Nursing: A Biographical Dictionary*, edited by V.L. Bullough, O.M. Church, and A.P. Stein. New York: Garland.

Sarnecky, Mary T. 1993. "Julia Catherine Stimson: Nurse and Feminist." *Image Journal of Nursing Scholarship* 25 (3):113–119.

Stimson, Julia Catherine. 1927. *Finding Themselves: The Letters of an American Army Chief Nurse in a British Hospital in France.* Reprint ed. New York: Macmillan.

Surgeon General, Department of the Army. 1958. *Highlights in the History of the Army Nurse Corps.* Washington, D.C.: Government Printing Office.

JSB

Stone, Hannah Mayer (1893–1941)
Physician

Hannah Stone was an early advocate for the legal availability of contraception for her female patients. She was born on October 15, 1893, in New York City, the daughter of Max, a pharmacist, and Golda (Rinaldo) Mayer. She received a pharmacy degree from Brooklyn College of Pharmacy in 1912. She later attended Columbia University (1914–1916) and earned a medical degree from the New York Medical College (1920).

In 1920 Stone became associated with Lying-In and St. Marks Hospitals of New York. Her contact with female patients made her realize "the urgent and pressing need for the dissemination of adequate birth control information, information which would enable these mothers to space the birth of their children, to regain their health between their successive child bearings, and to afford better care for the children they had already born [sic]" ("Stone"). This interest led to her association with the Clinical Research Bureau. The bureau was founded by Margaret Sanger in 1923 and was the first legal birth control clinic in the country. Stone served as medical director of the bureau from 1925 until her death.

Renamed the Birth Control Clinical Research Bureau in 1928, the institution grew to become the nation's foremost birth control testing and research facility. During the 1930s, Stone and her staff provided contraceptive instruction and devices to over 10,000 patients every year. The clinic also offered a range of gynecological services and served as a training facility for physicians and students. Although the clinic leaders attempted to operate within the constraints of New York law, the bureau's legal existence was often challenged. In April 1929 Stone and four other staff members were arrested when police raided the clinic and seized patient records. Stone and her colleagues were charged with illegally disseminating contraceptive information. The raid prompted public sympathy, most importantly from the medical community, which condemned the police action and called for the return of patient records. A judge dismissed the case, citing insufficient evidence.

In 1933 Stone became the center of another legal battle. Sanger arranged to have birth control devices sent to Stone from Japan. The package was seized by customs officials, citing violation of the Tariff Act of 1930, and the *United States v. One Package* trial resulted. After three years of trials and appeals, the U.S. Circuit Court of Appeals ruled in favor of Stone, arguing that the law was not designed "to prevent the importation, sale or carriage by mail of things which might intelligently be employed by conscientious and competent physicians for the purpose of saving life or promoting the well-being of patients" (quoted in "Obituary," *New York Times*).

In addition to her work with the bureau, Stone was director of the New Jersey Birth Control League and maintained a private gynecological practice. With her husband, Dr. Abraham Stone, she wrote *A Marriage Manual: A Practical Guide-Book to Sex and Marriage*. The couple also founded a marriage consultation service at the Labor Temple in New York City (1930) and a second such service at the Community Church of New York (1933).

Throughout her career, Stone wrote several medical articles and made many presentations on the benefits and practice of contraception. She died in New York City on July 10, 1941.

See also Sanger, Margaret Louise Higgins

References

The National Cyclopaedia of American Biography. 1943. Vol. 30. New York: James T. White.
New York University Department of History. *Margaret Sanger Papers Project.* Online. http://www.nyu.edu/projects/sanger/. 5 July 1999.
"Obituary." 1941. *The Nation* 153:63.
"Obituary." 1941. *New York Times* (July 11):15.
"Stone, Hannah M." Vertical file. Special Collections on Women in Medicine, Archives and Special Collections, MCP Hahnemann University, Philadelphia.

JSB

Stowe, Emily Jennings (1831–1903)
Physician

Emily Stowe is considered the first Canadian woman to practice medicine in Canada. She was born in Norwich, Ontario, on May 1, 1831, the first of seven children of Hannah (Howard) and Solomon Jennings. The Jennings provided all their children with a comprehensive home education, and of the six daughters, three went on to become physicians.

Before studying medicine, Stowe became a teacher in 1847. Desirous of a formal education, she applied to Victoria College in Coburg, Ontario, but was refused admission because women were not yet eligible to attend. She continued to teach and furthered her education by attending the provincial normal school in Toronto. In 1854 she graduated with a first class teacher's certificate and was subsequently appointed as the principal of the public school in Brantford, Ontario. She thus became the first woman principal in Canada, albeit at half the salary of that of her male colleagues.

In 1856, she married John Stowe and left teaching, as few school boards would allow teachers to remain after marriage. Stowe was not resentful, however, since she believed the occupation of homemaker to have important and far-reaching effects on humanity. The couple settled in Mount Pleasant, Ontario, and had three children, including Augusta, who would become the first woman physician educated in Canada. In 1863, Stowe's husband contracted tuberculosis, and to support the family she took a teaching position at the Nelles Academy in Mount Pleasant. At the same time, she began her struggle to become a physician, in part to help her husband through his recovery.

No medical school in Canada had yet begun accepting women students. Stowe therefore left Canada to study at the New York Medical College and Hospital for Women (Homeopathic), founded by woman physician Clemence Lozier. She graduated in 1867, and after a brief apprenticeship in London, Ontario, with a homeopathic practitioner, she moved her family to Toronto to establish a medical practice specializing in the treatment of women and children. She thus became the first Canadian woman to practice medicine in Canada, even though she was not yet licensed to practice legally in Ontario. To become licensed, it was necessary for physicians trained in the United States to take a course at an Ontario medical school and to pass an examination given by the Council of the College of Physicians and Surgeons. This proved problematic because the medical schools in Ontario remained closed to women. Stowe ignored the law and practiced unlicensed, but she was subsequently fined and threatened with a jail sentence. To avoid further complications, Stowe continued to apply to medical school and finally, in the early 1870s, her application was accepted. The Toronto Faculty of Medicine allowed Stowe and Jenny Kidd Trout, who would later become Canada's first licensed female physician, to enroll in a course if they made no objections to "whatever happened." The women agreed to the terms and endured the rude behavior of their classmates and instructors.

Despite taking the course, Stowe did not become licensed until 1880. It is not known whether she took the required examination and failed, if she was barred from taking it, or if she refused to take it. It is speculated that she was given her license without taking the examination, after proving her competence during a malpractice trial in 1879. She was accused of being involved in the death of a young woman who was thought to have died of an attempted abortion. The young woman had gone to Stowe for assistance and threatened to drown herself if Stowe did not help her. Anxious to be rid of the pregnant, unmarried, unemployed woman, Stowe prescribed a harmless tonic. Her actions were judged to be in accordance with the law and current medical protocol, and Stowe was cleared of all charges. Stowe also won support from liberal male physicians who had spoken on her behalf during the trial. In 1880, several of these physicians were elected to serve on the Ontario Medical Council, and on the fourth day of their first annual meeting, the council granted Stowe her license to practice.

After her own long struggle to become a licensed physician in Canada, Stowe worked to gain the right for women to study medicine in Canada. Originally, she worked with Jenny Kidd Trout to establish a women's college in Toronto. Stowe held a public meeting with the Toronto Women's Suffrage Association on June 13, 1883, to discuss the establishment of a medical college for women. In attendance were many prominent doctors, lawyers, and judges. The plan for the college was met with much enthusiasm, and the Woman's Medical College opened its doors in October 1883, the same month as the Women's Medical College at Queen's University in Kingston. In 1895, the two colleges joined in Toronto to become the Ontario Medical College for Women. Ultimately, in 1906, the students and staff were absorbed into the University of Toronto's Faculty of Medicine.

In addition to practicing medicine, Stowe was an ardent supporter of women's rights. In 1877 she helped found, and acted as president of, the Toronto Women's Literary Club. Despite its name, the club met to discuss women's education, women in the professions, and the conditions of women in the workforce. Stowe retired from medical practice in 1893 after suffering a hip fracture. She continued, however, to be active with the suffragist movement. In 1896, Stowe, her daughter Augusta Stowe Gullen, and the Dominion Women's Enfranchisement Association staged a mock parliament to raise public awareness of the cause of women's rights. In 1898, Stowe moved to Muskoka, north of Toronto. She died on April 30, 1903, following a short illness.

See also Gullen, Augusta Stowe; Lozier, Clemence Sophia Harned; Trout, Jenny Kidd

References

"Acquittal of Emily Stowe, M.D." 1879–1880. *Canada Lancet* 12:61–62.
Duffin, Jacalyn. 1992. "The Death of Sarah Lovell and the Constrained Feminism of Emily Stowe." *Canadian Medical Association Journal* 146 (6): 881–888.
Fryer, Mary Beacock. 1990. *Emily Stowe: Doctor*

and Suffragist. Toronto: Hannah Institute and Dundurn Press.
National Library of Canada. *Women's Exhibition— Emily Jennings Stowe and Augusta Stowe Gullen.* Online. http://www.nlc-bnc.ca/digiproj/women/ewomen1f.htm. 15 December 1997.
Ray, Janet. 1978. *Emily Stowe.* Don Mills, Ont.: Fitzhenry and Whiteside.
Waxman, Sydell. 1995. *Changing the Pattern: The Story of Emily Stowe.* Toronto: Napoleon.

CMB

Sturgis, Katharine Rosenbaum Boucot (1903–1987)
Physician

Katharine Sturgis was an American physician noted for her work in the prevention of tuberculosis and lung cancer. She was born in Philadelphia on September 3, 1903, the seventh of eight children of Morris Rosenbaum. After graduating from William Penn High School in 1921, she began premedical studies at the University of Pennsylvania. Before finishing her course work, she eloped with Arthur Guest in 1922.

For the following 11 years, Sturgis abandoned her medical education to care for her children, Arthur and Nancy. Around 1932, she took a position as secretary to Dr. Isidor Ravdin, an experience that reignited her medical interests. Sturgis and Guest divorced soon after, and in 1934 she entered Pennsylvania State University to complete her premedical studies. The following year, she matriculated at the Woman's Medical College of Pennsylvania in Philadelphia (now MCP Hahnemann University). The pressure of medical school and single motherhood took its toll on her health. In 1938, a bout with tuberculosis forced her to put her education on hold for three years.

In 1940, Sturgis returned to the Woman's Medical College, seeking part-time status because of her fragile health. Although the faculty fought rigidly against it, Sturgis was successful in becoming the college's first part-time student. She graduated later the same year and afterward finished an internship at Woman's Medical College Hospital.

From 1944 to 1945, she completed a tuberculosis residency at Herman Kiefer Hospital in Detroit in which she surveyed tuberculosis patients in that city. In 1945, she married Joseph Boucot, who died in 1962.

After Sturgis completed the residency, Dr. Herman Hilleboe, head of tuberculosis control for the U.S. Public Health Service, asked her to direct a mass chest X-ray survey in Philadelphia. She felt compelled to take the position because she realized that "however devotedly [she] worked on [her] patients at Herman Keifer, as soon as one was discharged there was another to take the bed" (quoted in Morantz-Sanchez et al., p. 64). She interviewed any patients with abnormal X-rays and then referred them to further medical care. She and Dr. David Cooper, director of tuberculosis control for Philadelphia, studied the relationship between diabetes and tuberculosis (1945–1947). In 1951, the two physicians established the Philadelphia Pulmonary Neoplasm Research Project to study lung cancer. She included a smoking history in the questionnaire filled out by patients and soon determined a relationship between lung cancer and smoking. Realizing that regular screenings did little to help the spread of the disease, she advocated prevention over cure. She campaigned against smoking, often admonishing total strangers to quit the habit.

In addition to her work with lung cancer, Sturgis held positions at the Veterans Administration (1953–1968), the Landis State Hospital (1963–1968), the National Cancer Institute (1957–1962) and the Milton S. Hershey Medical Center of Pennsylvania State University (1963–1968). She also served as visiting chief of the Chronic Chest Disease Service at Philadelphia General Hospital for several years. She began teaching at Woman's Medical College in 1943 and in 1952 was named chair of the Department of Preventive Medicine and clinical professor of medicine. She also taught radiology and internal medicine at the University of Pennsylvania (1947–1963). She found time to earn a master's of public health (1954) from Johns Hopkins in Baltimore and in 1955 was certified by the American Board of Preventive Medicine. In 1960, she was appointed as the first female chief editor (1960–1971) of the American Medical Association's *Archives of Environmental Health*, a then-floundering journal. Under her leadership, the journal attained its largest circulation up to that point. In November 1969, she became the first woman president of the American College of Preventive Medicine.

In 1964, Sturgis married Dr. Samuel Booth Sturgis. The couple was married until Samuel's death in 1983. She died on March 28, 1987, from complications resulting from valvular heart disease.

Selected Additional Achievements

Sturgis published more than 100 scientific papers on pulmonary disease. She was the first woman president, College of Physicians of Phila-delphia, the Pennsylvania Thoracic Society, the Philadelphia County Medical Society, and the Laennec Society of Philadelphia; first woman vice president, American Thoracic Society; and first woman appointed to the Council of the National Institutes of Environmental Health Sciences; board member, Philadelphia Division of the American Cancer Society; fellow, American College of Physicians; officer, American College of Chest Physicians; president, Delaware Valley Citizen's Council for Clean Air; member, Mayor's Advisory Committee on Tuberculosis; professor emerita of preventive medicine, Woman's Medical College of Pennsylvania (1968). Awards include the Trudeau Medal of the National Tuberculosis and Respiratory Disease Association (1969); the Strittmatter Award, Philadelphia County Medical Society; the Elizabeth Blackwell Citation and six honorary doctorates.

References

Chapman, John S. 1995. "A Perspective: *Archives at 50 Years.*" *Archives of Environmental Health* (July 17):261.

Morantz-Sanchez, Regina Markell, Cynthia Stodola Pomerleau, and Carol Fenichel, eds. 1982. *In Her Own Words: Oral Histories of Women Physicians.* Westport, Conn.: Greenwood Press.

Sturgis, Katharine Boucot. Manuscript Collection MS-146, Special Collections on Women in Medicine, Archives and Special Collections, MCP Hahnemann University, Philadelphia.

Sturgis, Katharine Boucot. 1970. "Great Programs Born in the 1960s." *Newsletter of the American College of Preventive Medicine* 11 (3): 1–2.

Weiss, William. 1987. "Editorial." *Philadelphia Medicine* 83 (6):219–221.

JSB

Sutliffe, Irene H. (1850–1936)
Nurse

Irene Sutliffe was an admired and respected nursing education administrator. While at the New York Hospital School of Nursing, she taught some of the best-known nurses of the early twentieth century, including Mary Beard, Lillian Wald, and Annie Goodrich. Sutliffe was born in Albany, New York, on November 12, 1850, to George Washington and Charlotte (Ramsey) Sutliffe. She attended Cathedral School in Albany and entered the New York Hospital School of Nursing in 1878.

Following graduation in 1880, Sutliffe was asked to establish a school of nursing at the Hamot Hospital in Erie, Pennsylvania, an impressive accomplishment for a newly graduated nurse. She returned to New York in 1886 to establish the Long Island Hospital School of Nursing in Brooklyn. Later that year she was appointed director of the New York Hospital School of Nursing, where she worked until 1902. In 1898, during the Spanish-American War, she also served as head of the nursing service at Camp Black, Hempstead, Long Island. When an outbreak of polio swept New York City in 1916, she organized and directed an emergency hospital.

During her tenure as a nursing educator, Sutliffe faced challenges such as an absence of nursing textbooks, the lack of a structured nursing curriculum, and nursing techniques that varied widely in how they were practiced. She participated in the Conference of Charities, Correction, and Philanthropy held as part of the World's Fair in 1893 in Chicago. She presented a paper at this meeting to encourage the organization of the profession, thus leading to higher, more uniform standards. This meeting eventually led to the formation of the American Society of Superintendents of Training Schools for Nurses of the United States and Canada (now the National League for Nursing).

As director of the New York Hospital School of Nursing, Sutliffe worked with only one assistant, despite her poor health. She often faced opposition from the medical professionals of New York Hospital, who felt that student nurse education was of secondary importance. She created an arrangement for students to study at Sloane Maternity Hospital, citing a need for nurses to have experience in maternal care. By creating one of the earliest diet kitchens in the country that provided nutritious meals for poor residents who were ill, she emphasized the role of nutrition in good health.

Sutliffe was named dean emerita of the New York Hospital School of Nursing in 1932. She was given an apartment in the nurses' residence in the new quarters of the hospital. She remained there until her death on December 30, 1936.

See also Beard, Mary; Goodrich, Annie Warburton; Wald, Lillian D.

References

Bullough, Vern L. 1992. "Irene H. Sutliffe." In *American Nursing: A Biographical Dictionary*, edited by V.L. Bullough, L. Sentz, and A.P. Stein. New York: Garland.

Higgins, Loretta P. 1988. "Sutliffe, Irene H." In *Dictionary of American Nursing Biography*, edited by M. Kaufman. New York: Greenwood Press.

"Obituaries, Irene H. Sutliffe." 1937. *American Journal of Nursing* 37 (2):215–218.

Pennock, Meta Rutter, ed. 1940. *Makers of Nursing History; Portraits and Pen Sketches of One Hundred and Nine Prominent Women*. New York: Lakeside.

DTW

T

Taussig, Helen Brooke (1898–1986)
Physician

Helen Brooke Taussig was the first woman to achieve the rank of full professor at Johns Hopkins University School of Medicine in Baltimore. She was born in Cambridge, Massachusetts, on May 24, 1898, the youngest of four children of Frank and Edith (Guild) Taussig. Although a combination of dyslexia and tuberculosis made her early education difficult, she graduated from the Cambridge School for Girls in 1917.

Taussig began her undergraduate education at Radcliffe in Cambridge in 1917 but transferred in 1919 to the University of California at Berkeley to complete her degree (1921). After a year abroad, she returned to Cambridge to study medicine. Harvard had not yet begun to accept women medical students, but she was allowed to enroll in a histology course there, the only female in the class. She was required to sit apart from the men during lectures, and her laboratory sessions were taken alone. In 1922 she enrolled at Boston University, where she was allowed to take a greater number of courses and where she began her lifelong study of cardiology. In 1924 she was accepted to medical school at Johns Hopkins. Throughout medical school she investigated heart muscle physiology at the Johns Hopkins Heart Clinic. She graduated in 1927 with three scholarly articles to her credit.

After graduation, Taussig continued her work at the Heart Clinic for another year and then interned in the newly established Children's Heart Clinic at the Harriet Lane Home of Johns Hopkins University Hospital. She was appointed head of the clinic in 1930, the same year that she began to experience a marked loss of hearing of unknown origin. Undaunted, she learned to lip-read, wore hearing aids, and used an amplified stethoscope. She also taught herself to feel a child's heart murmur with the tips of her fingers.

At the clinic Taussig encountered many cyanotic, or blue, babies. She discovered that blue babies suffered from a lack of oxygen due to a defect in their heart that prevented adequate circulation through the lungs. She designed an operation where blood would bypass the heart obstruction, flow freely to the lungs, and pick up enough oxygen to revitalize the child and restore pink color to the skin. However, as she was not a surgeon, she needed one to develop and test the technique. She recruited Alfred Blalock, and together they spent several years perfecting the operation. Following 200 favorable operations in dogs, Blalock performed a successful operation on a 15-month-old girl in 1944. Following two more positive attempts, they published their results in the *Journal of the American Medical Association* in 1945. Although the landmark paper had immediate impact internationally and resulted in saving the lives of tens of thousands of children, Taussig was not promoted to full professor at Johns Hopkins until 1959, nor was she elected to the National Academy of Sciences, one of America's most prestigious groups, until 1973. In contrast, Blalock received a full professorship upon arrival at Johns Hopkins in 1941 and was elected to the academy in 1945.

In 1961 Taussig traveled to Europe to study the origin of unusual birth defects occurring in Germany. After touring pediatric clinics in Germany and Britain, she determined the malformations to be caused by the sleeping pill thalidomide. As a result, thalidomide, which had induced approximately 10,000 birth defects before it was removed from the world market in 1962, was never sold in the United States.

Taussig retired from Johns Hopkins in 1963. During her retirement she published 41 of her 129 scientific articles. In 1965 she was elected president of the American Heart Association, becoming not only the first female president of the association but also the first pediatrician. She died on May 21, 1986, as a result of injuries sustained in an automobile accident.

Selected Additional Achievements

Taussig's *Congenital Malformations of the Heart* (1947) describes the methods of identifying congenital heart malformations and provides the basis by which pediatric cardiology was established. She received many international awards and honors, including the Elizabeth Blackwell Centennial Award (1949); Honorary Medal, American College of Chest Physicians (1953); American Heart Association Award of Merit (1957); the American College of Cardiology Honorary Fellow-

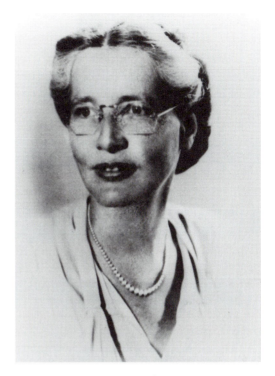

Helen Brooke Taussig. National Library of Medicine.

ship (1960); and the Medal of Freedom of the United States (1964). The Cardiac Clinic at Johns Hopkins was renamed the Helen B. Taussig Children's Pediatric Cardiac Center (1970). She was also awarded over 20 honorary degrees, including one from Harvard (1959).

References

Baldwin, Joyce. 1992. *To Heal the Heart of a Child: Helen Taussig, M.D.* New York: Walker and Co.

Gilbert, Lynn, and Gaylen Moore. 1981. *Particular Passions: Talks with Women Who Have Shaped Our Times.* New York: Clarkson N. Potter.

"Medicine's Living History: Dr. Taussig Remembers the First Blue Baby Operation." 1972. *Medical World News* 13 (4):38–47.

"Pediatrician with a Heart: Dr. Helen Taussig." 1965. *Medical World News* 6 (39): 94–106.

CMB

Taylor, Euphemia Jane [Effie] (1874–1970)
Nurse

Effie Taylor was an international nursing leader as well as a respected psychiatric nurse. She was born in Hamilton, Ontario, Canada, on April 18, 1874, the first of nine children of Irish immigrant parents. Her father was a progressive man who believed in providing exceptional educational opportunities to his daughters as well as his sons. Taylor graduated from the Hamilton (Ontario) Collegiate Institute and went on to spend two years at the Wesleyan Ladies College in Hamilton, studying literature and drama. She chose a career in nursing, however, after feeling helpless while her father suffered through a lengthy and eventually fatal illness.

In March 1904, Taylor moved to Baltimore to attend the Johns Hopkins School of Nursing. After completing a six-month course, she worked as a student nurse. She received a diploma from Johns Hopkins in 1907 and then worked as head nurse of the private wards in Johns Hopkins Hospital. In 1908 she began course work at Teachers College, Columbia University in New York City. She returned to the Johns Hopkins School of Nursing in 1909 to serve as a junior instructor. In 1912, she became director of the nursing service at the newly organized Henry Phipps Psychiatric Clinic at the Johns Hopkins Hospital. She remained there until 1918, when, during World War I, she served as director of a unit at the Army School of Nursing and chief nurse at Camp Meade, Maryland.

After Taylor returned to Johns Hopkins Hospital in 1919, she was associate principal of the School of Nursing until 1922, when she was appointed the first executive secretary of the National League of Nursing Education, headquartered in New York City. She stayed in this position only briefly, however, as she was asked to assist Annie Goodrich in the establishment of a school of nursing at Yale University in 1923. The Yale School of Nursing was considered an experiment in nursing education and was the first

institution in the country to grant a bachelor's degree in nursing. Taylor initially served as an associate professor at Yale. In 1926 she received a B.S. degree from Teachers College, and the following year, she was named the first professor of psychiatric nursing at Yale. In 1934, she became dean of the Yale School of Nursing, a position that she held until 1944.

As an active member of the international nursing community, Taylor served as president of the National League of Nursing Education from 1932 to 1946 and held the same position with the International Council of Nurses (ICN) from 1937 to 1947. Her leadership of the ICN during World War II included moving the headquarters of the organization to her home in New Haven, Connecticut, from war-torn London. Following her tenure as president of the ICN, she acted as the ICN representative to the United Nations.

Taylor was among the early advocates in the nursing field for equal work for equal pay. She felt that this was a leading reason for poor professional relations between men and women in hospitals. As a psychiatric nurse, Taylor saw the value of nurses viewing the patient as a whole, not just as a particular affliction or injury. She felt that all nurses, not just those specializing in psychiatric care, would benefit from training in mental health nursing.

Taylor died in Hamilton, Ontario, on May 20, 1970.

See also Goodrich, Annie Warburton

Selected Additional Achievements

Numerous articles in *American Journal of Nursing*. Florence Nightingale Medal, International Red Cross (1959); Mary Adelaide Nutting Award, National League of Nursing Education (1959); honorary master of arts degree, Yale University (1926); honorary doctor of humane letters degree, Keuka College, Keuka Park, New York (1944); American Nurses Association Hall of Fame (1986).

References

Friedman, Alice Howell. 1988. "Taylor, Euphemia Jane." In *Dictionary of American Nursing Biography*, edited by M. Kaufman. New York: Greenwood Press.

Pennock, Meta Rutter, ed. 1940. *Makers of Nursing History; Portraits and Pen Sketches of One Hundred and Nine Prominent Women.* New York: Lakeside.

Stewart, Isabel M. 1939. "Effie Jane Taylor, R.N." *American Journal of Nursing* 39 (7):733–737.

DTW

Thomas, Mary Frame Myers (1816–1888)
Physician

Mary Thomas was one of the first women in the United States to earn a medical degree. She was born on October 28, 1816, in Bucks County, Pennsylvania, the second of two daughters of a Quaker couple, Samuel and Mary (Frame) Myers. Soon after Thomas' birth, her mother died, and her father married Paulina Iden, with whom he had seven more children. Two of Thomas' sisters, Hannah Myers (later, Longshore) and Jane Viola Myers, would also become physicians.

In 1839, she married Owen Thomas, a physician. The couple lived the next 10 years in Salem, Ohio, where they had three daughters. In 1849, the Thomases moved to Ft. Wayne, Indiana, where Mary began studying medicine with her husband. In September 1853, Thomas left Ft. Wayne to enroll in the first session of the female department of Penn Medical University in Philadelphia. Her younger sister, Hannah Longshore, was demonstrator of anatomy at the school. Thomas' Philadelphia medical education was interrupted by the illness and death of her oldest daughter, but she was able to attend medical lectures (as a guest) at Western Reserve College in Cleveland through the winter of 1853–1854. In the spring of 1856 Thomas resumed her studies at Penn Medical University and graduated in July of that year.

After graduation, Thomas practiced medicine with her husband in Richmond, Indiana. During the Civil War, she worked with the U.S. Sanitary Commission, a private relief organization for soldiers and their families. She also worked with her husband, an army contract surgeon, in Nashville, Tennessee.

Although she provided medical service in Nashville, the army recognized her as a nurse rather than a physician. In Richmond after the war, her husband took up dentistry, while Thomas continued in medicine. Thomas served on the city board of public health in Richmond, and from 1867 until her death, she was a physician for the Home for Friendless Girls, an organization that she had helped to found.

Thomas supported women in medicine and helped secure the appointment of women physicians to state hospitals for the insane. She believed in the coeducation of female and male medical students and pointed out the irony of a sex-divided medical system in an 1883 address: "Many men physicians honestly deem it improper, if not positively indelicate to talk to mixed classes on the different organs of the body, and their functions in health and disease, and yet see no objections to being specialists in gynecology, and visiting women patients under any and all circumstances, that they think necessary as their professional advisors" (Thomas, p. 6).

In addition to her medical career, Thomas was a strong supporter of women's rights and held several positions in the burgeoning movement. In January 1859, she read a petition to the Indiana General Assembly requesting a married woman's property law and a woman suffrage amendment to the state constitution. She died in Richmond, Indiana, on August 19, 1888, of dysentery. At her request, six women were pallbearers at her funeral.

See also Longshore, Hannah E. Myers

Selected Additional Achievements

Vice president (1855) and president (1856), Indiana Women's Rights Society; member, Wayne County Medical Society (1875); president, Indiana state suffrage association (?–1875); first woman regularly admitted to the Indiana State Medical Society (1876); president, American Woman Suffrage Association (1880); editor of *Lily*, a women's rights newspaper.

References

Adkinson, Florence M. 1888. "The Mother of Women." *Woman's Journal* (September 29): 307–308.

Phillips, Clifton J. 1971. "Thomas, Mary Frame Myers." In *Notable American Women, 1607–1950: A Biographical Dictionary*, edited by E.T. James, J.W. James, and P.S. Boyer. Cambridge: Belknap Press of Harvard University Press.

Thomas, Mary F. 1979. "The Influence of the Medical Colleges of the Regular School, of Indianapolis, on the Medical Education of the Women of the State." *Indiana Medical History Quarterly* 5 (3):5–15. Reprinted from *Transactions of the Indiana State Medical Society*, 1883.

Waite, Frederick C. 1933. "The Three Myers Sisters—Pioneer Women Physicians." *Medical Review of Reviews* 39 (March):114–120.

LS

Thompson, Mary Harris (1829–1895)
Physician

Mary Harris Thompson founded the third hospital in the United States devoted exclusively to the care of women and children and cofounded a woman's medical college. She was also one of the first women in the United States to routinely perform major surgery. She was born on April 15, 1829, near Fort Ann, New York, the second child of John Harris Thompson, a partner in an iron mine, and Calista (Corbin) Thompson. At an early age, she taught herself Latin and mathematics. She attended Troy Conference Academy in West Poultney, Vermont, and Fort Edward Collegiate Institute in New York. At both schools she also acted as instructor in order to pay her way. She planned a career teaching physiology and anatomy and, in preparation, enrolled at the New England Female Medical College in Boston.

While attending medical school classes, however, Thompson's interest in medicine grew, and she decided to become a physician. After two lecture courses, in 1862 she went to Dr. Elizabeth and Dr. Emily Blackwell's New York Infirmary for Women and Children and served a yearlong internship. While in New York, she also attended clinical lectures at Bellevue Hospital. In 1863, she returned to the New England Female Medical College and received her M.D. As there were increasing numbers of women physicians on the East Coast, and she did not want to interfere with their practices, Thompson went west to Chicago to practice medicine.

Thompson arrived in Chicago in the midst of the Civil War on July 3, 1863, and soon became active with the U.S. Sanitary Commission, a private relief organization for soldiers and their families. Her work with the widows and children of soldiers led her to believe in the necessity of a women's and children's hospital in the city. At the time, Chicago had only three hospitals; none had women on staff, and one did not accept women as patients.

With the assistance of other interested citizens, Thompson opened Chicago Hospital for Women and Children on May 8, 1865. She was head of the medical and surgical staff there for the next 30 years and specialized in abdominal and pelvic surgery. In 1871, the hospital was destroyed by the great Chicago fire but was rebuilt in 1873 with the help of the Relief and Aid Society. Thompson was an innovative and creative surgeon who designed a surgical abdominal needle and used an early method of surgical sterilization before it was considered necessary.

Although Thompson had arrived in Chicago with a medical degree, she was not satisfied with her education from the New England Female Medical College and soon desired to add to her medical knowledge. She applied to Rush Medical College in Chicago but was denied entrance. Then Dr. William H. Byford, a faculty member at the Chicago Medical College, helped her and two other women students gain admission to Chicago Medical for the 1869–1870 academic year. Because of her previous medical study, Thompson received her diploma from the school in 1870, after one term of study. She was the first woman to be granted a degree from the college. After her graduation, the school reversed its policy and refused to admit women. Thompson's two women classmates, who were just beginning their medical studies, were not permitted to continue.

Byford then suggested to Thompson that they organize a women's medical college in Chicago to be associated with her Chicago Hospital for Women and Children. In 1870, the school opened as the Woman's Hospital Medical College, with Byford as director and Thompson as professor of hygiene and clinical obstetrics. Seventeen students registered the first year, and three women, including the two dismissed from Chicago Medical, received their degrees in 1871. Among the prominent women physicians who would graduate from the college were Sarah Stevenson and Marie Mergler. Two days after the school's second year had begun, it burned in the 1871 fire. Classes continued, however, and the school was rebuilt. A training school for nurses was added in 1874, and the college was reorganized in 1879 as Woman's Medical College. When the college became part of Northwestern University and was renamed Northwestern University Woman's Medical School in 1892, Thompson was appointed professor of clinical gynecology. The school was closed in 1902 after other Chicago medical colleges had begun to admit women.

Thompson died suddenly on May 21, 1895, after suffering a stroke. Following her death, Chicago Hospital for Women and Children was renamed Mary Thompson Hospital of Chicago, in her honor.

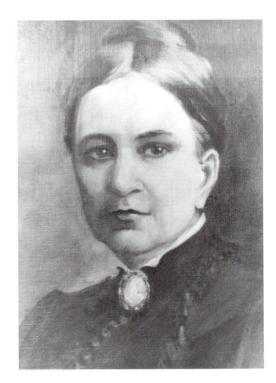

Mary Harris Thompson. Archives & Special Collections on Women in Medicine, MCP Hahnemann University.

See also Blackwell, Elizabeth; Blackwell, Emily; Mergler, Marie Josepha; Stevenson, Sarah Ann Hackett

Selected Additional Achievements

"A Case of Prolonged Gestation and Unusual Labor," *Medical and Surgical Reporter* 44 (May 21, 1881):561–565; "Two Interesting Cases of Ovariotomy," *American Journal of Obstetrics* 17 (October 1884):1040–1046. Presenter of "Why Diseases of Children Should Be Made a Special Study," 37th Annual Meeting (St. Louis, 1886), American Medical Association, section on Diseases of Children, printed in *Journal of the American Medical Association* 7 (October 1886): 399–402. Member (1873) and vice president (1881–1882), Chicago Medical Society, Illinois State Medical Society (1875), American Medical Association (1886), International Medical Society (1887).

References

Beatty, William K. 1981. "Mary Harris Thompson—Pioneer Surgeon and Hospital Founder."

Proceedings. Institute of Medicine of Chicago 34 (3):83–86.

"Biographical Sketches of the Life and Work of the Pioneer Women in Medicine: Mary Harris Thompson, M.D." 1901. *Woman's Medical Journal* 11 (September):333–334.

Bonner, Thomas Neville. 1971. "Thompson, Mary Harris." In *Notable American Women, 1607–1950: a Biographical Dictionary*, edited by E. T. James, J. W. James, and P. S. Boyer. Cambridge: Belknap Press of Harvard University Press.

Hast, Adele. 1999. "Thompson, Mary Harris." In *American National Biography*, edited by J. A. Garraty and M. C. Carnes. New York: Oxford University Press.

Ruud, Helga M. 1946. "The Women's Medical College of Chicago: Later Called the Northwestern University Woman's Medical College: 1870–1902." *Medical Woman's Journal* 53 (June):41–46, 64.

"Semi-Centennial Celebration of Mary Thompson Hospital of Chicago for Women and Children—1865–1915." 1915. *Woman's Medical Journal* 25 (December):280–283.

LS

Thoms, Adah Belle Samuels (ca. 1863–1943)
Nurse

Adah Thoms, an African American nurse, spent most of her career breaking down racial barriers in nursing, most notably in the United States Army. She also wrote the first book on the history of the African American nurse, *Pathfinders: A History of the Progress of Colored Graduate Nurses* (1929). She was born on January 13, probably in 1863, in Richmond, Virginia, one of at least two children of Harry and Melvina Samuels. She received her early education in local public and normal schools. After teaching for a short time in Richmond, she moved to New York City in 1890.

In 1893 Thoms entered the nursing program at the Woman's Infirmary and School of Therapeutic Massage. The only black student in a class of 30, she graduated in 1900. She then worked as a nurse in New York City before accepting a position as head nurse at St. Agnes Hospital in Raleigh, North Carolina. At this time, she was married for a short time to a Mr. Thoms, who may have been a physician.

Dissatisfied with the quality of her nursing education, Thoms enrolled in the Lincoln Hospital and Home School of Nursing in 1903. The school, formed in response to racial discrimination in nursing education, was 1 of only about 10 African American nursing schools in the country. During Thoms' second year as a student, she also served as head nurse of the Lincoln Hospital surgical ward. After her graduation in 1905, she continued at the hospital as operating room nurse and as supervisor in the surgical ward. The following year, she was promoted to assistant director of nurses and was occasionally appointed as acting director of the nurse training school.

Although Thoms ably carried out her duties as acting director, she was never officially appointed to the position because African Americans did not traditionally hold executive positions at the hospital. This setback did not stop her from leaving her mark. In 1917, while serving as interim director, she added a course in public health nursing to the program, making the school one of the first to offer such a course. The class, which Thoms herself attended, was taught by a staff member of the Henry Street Visiting Nurse Service, founded by Lillian Wald. Thoms also received further education at the New York School of Philanthropy (later, New York School of Social Work), at Hunter College, and at the New School for Social Research.

From the beginning of her career, Thoms was an advocate for the African American nurse. In 1908, as president of the Lincoln Hospital Alumnae, she organized a meeting of nurses that led to the formation of the National Association of Colored Graduate Nurses (NACGN). She was the NACGN's first treasurer and then president from 1916 until her retirement. The NACGN was formed to combat discrimination in the profession and to promote leadership among black nurses.

Thoms' most important act as president came in 1917, when the U.S. Congress declared war on Germany. She encouraged all black nurses to enroll in the American Red Cross Nursing Service, the only entryway into the United States Army Nurse Corps. However, when the nurses applied, their applications were rejected because of their race. Thoms began a rigorous letter-writing campaign to Jane Delano, chair of the National Committee on Red Cross Nursing Service, urging acceptance of her nurses into the corps. Delano informed Thoms that while the Red Cross was willing to accept the nurses, the surgeon general of the United States Army was not. In July 1918 the first African American nurse was accepted by the Red Cross, but the surgeon general acquiesced only after a major influenza epidemic depleted the supply of available nurses. In December 1918, when the war was over, 18 black nurses were finally allowed into the Army Nurse Corps. These nurses were assigned to camps in Illinois and Ohio, and although they were charged with the full range of duties, they lived in segregated facilities.

Still determined to make the nation aware of the value of the African American nurse in times of public need, she formed the Blue Circle of Nurses in 1917. These nurses were recruited by the Circle for Negro War Relief to work in local communities to teach poor, rural African Americans the role of hygiene and diet in health. In 1921, she approached President Warren G. Harding at an NACGN conference and requested that he acknowledge the existence of the NACGN as a body of trained nurses who were prepared whenever their country needed them. The same year, she was appointed by the assistant surgeon general to the Woman's Advisory Council on Venereal Diseases for U.S. Public Health Service.

While many in the NACGN felt that the association should merge with the National Medical Association, the African American doctors' organization, Thoms was convinced that it was important for nurses to maintain their identity as a profession. Instead, she encouraged a merger with the American Nurses Association and with the National Organization of Public Health Nurses. The NACGN was formally disbanded in 1951, three years after the American Nurses Association began admitting black women and eight years after Thoms' death.

Thoms' other important accomplishments included seeing the participation of black nurses in the International Council of Nurses. In 1916, she began working with the National Urban League and the National Association for the Advancement of Colored People to improve inadequate conditions in segregated nursing schools and hospitals. She also traveled often to address state and local African American nursing associations. After 1920, she encouraged black nurses to use their newly won right to suffrage and to urge their patients to do so as well.

In 1923, Thoms retired from Lincoln Hospital and from the NACGN. She then married Henry Smith, who died within the year. Diabetes led to failing sight in her later years and was a major contributor to her death from arteriosclerotic heart disease on February 21, 1943.

See also Delano, Jane Arminda; Wald, Lillian D.

Selected Additional Achievements

First recipient, Mary Mahoney Medal (1936); Harlem Committee, New York Tuberculosis and Health Association, National Negro Health Circle, New York State Nurses Association; American Nurses Association Hall of Fame (1976).

References

Davis, Althea. 1988. "Adah Belle Samuels Thoms." In *American Nursing: A Biographical Dictionary*, edited by V.L. Bullough, O.M. Church, and A.P. Stein. New York: Garland.

Hawkins, Joellen Watson. 1988. "Thoms, Adah B. (Samuels)." In *Dictionary of American Nursing Biography*, edited by M. Kaufman. New York: Greenwood Press.

Hine, Darlene Clark. 1993. "Thoms, Adah Belle Samuels." In *Black Women in America: An*

Historical Encyclopedia, edited by D.C. Hine, E. Barkley, and R. Terborg-Penn. Brooklyn, N.Y.: Carlson.

Staupers, Mabel Keaton. 1961. *No Time for Prejudice: A Story of the Integration of Negroes in Nursing in the United States.* New York: Macmillan.

Staupers, Mabel Keaton. 1971. "Thoms, Adah B. Samuels." In *Notable American Women, 1607–1950: A Biographical Dictionary*, edited by E.T. James, J.W. James, and P.S. Boyer. Cambridge: Belknap Press of Harvard University Press.

JSB

Titus, Shirley Carew (1892–1967)
Nurse

Shirley Carew Titus was a leader in nursing education, as well as an advocate for the professional rights of nurses, including collective bargaining and a 40-hour week. She was born on April 28, 1892, in Alameda, California, one of six children of Henry and Sarah (Simmons) Titus. She grew up in California and graduated from San Jose High School. She attended St. Luke's Hospital School of Nursing in San Francisco, serving as assistant director of nursing at the hospital while she was still a student and graduating in 1915.

Titus attended Teachers College at Columbia University in New York City, earning a B.S. in 1920 and a diploma in administration of schools of nursing. She was appointed director of nursing and principal of the nursing school at Columbia Hospital in Milwaukee and in 1925 became director of the nursing service and the nursing school at the University of Michigan in Ann Arbor. While in this position, she began advocating the hiring of graduate nurses in hospitals, rather than utilizing student nurses as the primary hospital employees. She felt that this would improve patient care as well as provide student nurses with additional study time. She recommended that the cost of professional nursing services be funded by an additional charge on hospital bills. Articles written by Titus on these proposals appeared in *American Journal of Nursing* during the 1920s.

In 1930, Titus earned a master's degree in philosophy from the University of Michigan. That same year, she was appointed professor of nursing education and dean of the new nursing school at Vanderbilt University in Nashville, Tennessee. The school was the first independent school of nursing at a university, eventually offering the baccalaureate degree in 1939. Titus advocated the inclusion of liberal arts studies in the nursing curriculum as well as an emphasis on public health nursing.

In 1942, Titus became executive director of the California Nurses' Association (CNA), which was responsible for initiating the first economic security program for nurses in the United States. In 1946, CNA negotiated a major contract with East Bay Hospitals, the first instance of collective bargaining for nurses. The following year the 40-hour workweek was introduced. The American Nurses Association House of Delegates endorsed the economic security plan in California and passed a resolution recognizing CNA and Titus.

Titus remained executive director of CNA until her retirement in 1956. She lived in Mill Valley, California, during her retirement years with her former Vanderbilt colleague, Mary Dodd Giles. She died on March 21, 1967, in San Francisco.

References

Conta, A. Lionne. 1988. "Shirley Carew Titus." In *American Nursing: A Biographical Dictionary*, edited by V.L. Bullough, O.M. Church, and A.P. Stein. New York: Garland.

Higgins, Loretta P. 1988. "Titus, Shirley Carew." In *Dictionary of American Nursing Biography*, edited by M. Kaufman. New York: Greenwood Press.

"Shirley C. Titus." 1967. *CNA Bulletin* 63 (April):2.

DTW

Tompkins, Sally Louisa (1833–1916)
Nurse

Sally Tompkins was a nurse for the Confederate army during the Civil War and the first American woman to be given a commission in the military. She was born on November 9, 1833, in Poplar Grove, Mathews County, Virginia. She was the youngest child of Christopher and Maria Boothe (Patterson) Tompkins, both from prominent Virginia families. When her father died shortly before the Civil War, she moved to Richmond.

In July 1861, after the first Battle of Manassas, casualties began streaming into Richmond, and hospitals were overflowing. Tompkins was one of many citizens who established a private hospital to care for the wounded. She opened Robertson Hospital on August 1, 1861, in the home of Judge John Robertson, whose family had fled to the country. Robertson Hospital held 25 beds and utilized four African American slaves, society women, and veterans as nurses. Tompkins' hospital quickly developed a reputation of providing excellent care. When the Confederate government ordered all private hospitals closed, President Jefferson Davis appointed Tompkins as a captain in the cavalry (September 9, 1861) in order to keep the facility open.

Tompkins refused government pay but received rations for her hospital. She also used her own money and gifts to keep the hospital running. Robertson Hospital treated a total of 1,333 patients, with only 73 succumbing to death. A primary reason for the low mortality rate was Tompkins' insistence on cleanliness. She also provided spiritual guidance and sent recovered soldiers back to the front with clean clothing and a prayer book. After Richmond fell to the Union army, Tompkins managed to keep the hospital open until June 13, 1865, to care for immobile patients.

In 1905, Tompkins accepted an offer to live at Richmond's Home for Confederate Women. She died there on July 25, 1916, and was buried in Mathews County with full military honors.

References

Coleman, Elizabeth Dabney. 1956. "The Captain Was a Lady." *Virginia Cavalcade* (Summer): 35–41.

Cunningham, H.H. 1971. "Tompkins, Sally Louisa." In *Notable American Women, 1607–1950: A Biographical Dictionary*, edited by E.T. James, J.W. James, and P.S. Boyer. Cambridge: Belknap Press of Harvard University Press.

"Death Claims Woman Officer of Confederacy." 1916. *Richmond Times-Dispatch* (July 26):3.

LS

Trout, Jenny Kidd (1841–1921)
Physician

Jenny Kidd Trout was the first woman licensed to practice medicine in Canada. She was also responsible for spearheading the establishment of medical colleges for women in Ontario. She was born in Kelso, Scotland, on April 21, 1841, to Andrew and Elizabeth Gowanlock. The family emigrated to Canada in 1847 and settled on a farm outside Stratford, Ontario. Trout attended local schools and the Ontario Normal School, where she studied to become a teacher. She obtained her teaching certificate in 1861 and taught in communities around Stratford until 1865, when she married Edward Trout, also a teacher.

The couple settled in Toronto, where Trout began to experience various ailments that were attributed to nervousness. A friend suggested that she try electrotherapeutics, the accepted treatment for her condition at the time. The treatments were successful, and Trout was inspired by her illness to pursue a career in medicine. While Edward Trout was establishing a publishing career, the couple lived with the family of Emily Stowe, the first Canadian woman to practice medicine in Canada. Stowe encouraged Trout, and together they attended the Toronto Faculty of Medicine. The women were allowed to attend lectures only if they agreed to never complain about any ill treatment that they might receive. They complied, but Trout found it difficult to complete her medical training in the antifemale climate at Toronto. Therefore, in 1872 she traveled to Philadelphia to study at the Woman's Medical College of Pennsylvania.

Trout graduated in 1875 and returned to Toronto to apply for registration with the College of Physicians and Surgeons. To be licensed to practice medicine in Canada, graduates from the United States were required to take a course at an Ontario medical school and pass an examination given by the Council of the College of Physicians and Surgeons. Since Trout had already completed a course at the University of Toronto before going to Philadelphia, all that was lacking for licensure was the examination. She sat for the oral examination and passed very capably.

Thus legally licensed to practice medicine in Toronto, Trout set out to treat women using the same therapies that she had been administered during her illness. In 1877, with monetary support from her husband, she established the Therapeutic and Electrical Institute. The institute was well equipped and had the capacity to house 60 patients. Additionally, Trout established branch offices in Hamilton and Brandtford, ran a free dispensary for the disadvantaged in Toronto, and traveled around Ontario giving lectures. Eventually, the strain of her many commitments plus the financial failure of the institute forced her retirement in 1882.

Trout did not remain idle in her retirement, however. She turned her attention to the establishment of a medical college for women in Ontario. Originally, she worked with Emily Stowe to found a women's college in Toronto, offering $10,000 seed money if the governing board and staff of the college included women. The medical community and academics of Toronto were not prepared to accept Trout's conditions, so she transferred her offer to Queen's University in Kingston. Queen's had been offering a summer medical course for women since 1880 and was very receptive to Trout's suggestions. The medical college in Kingston opened in the fall of 1883. Stowe continued to champion a women's medical college in Toronto, and the University of Toronto finally decided to open a women's college, also in October 1883. Both colleges included women on their staffs and governing boards. In 1895, the two colleges joined to become the Ontario Medical College for Women. Ultimately, in 1906, the students and staff were absorbed into the University of Toronto's Faculty of Medicine.

Trout was also an ardent suffragist, and in the late 1870s she served as the president of the Woman's Temperance Movement and as vice president of the Association for the Advancement of Women. In 1908, Trout and her husband moved to Los Angeles, where Trout spent her time in mission work and Bible study. She had no children of her own, but she adopted a grandniece and grandnephew, Helen and Edward Huntsman, after their mother died. Trout died in Los Angeles in 1921.

See also Stowe, Emily Jennings

References

Edwards, David. 1877. *Notabilities of Toronto in 1877*. Toronto: P. Gross.
Hacker, Carlotta. 1974. *The Indomitable Lady Doctors*. Toronto: Clarke, Irwin.
Morgan, Henry J., ed. 1912. *The Canadian Men and Women of the Time: A Handbook of Canadian Biography of Living Characters*. 2nd ed. Toronto: W. Briggs.
Trout, William H. 1916. *Trout Family History*. Milwaukee, Wis.: W.H. Trout.

CMB

V

Van Blarcom, Carolyn Conant (1879–1960)
Nurse-midwife

Carolyn Conant Van Blarcom was the first American nurse to become a registered midwife. She was born on June 12, 1879, in Alton, Illinois, to William Dixon and Fanny Emelie (Conant) Van Blarcom. By 1893, William had abandoned his family, leaving Fanny Van Blarcom to raise six children. At the age of six, Van Blarcom suffered from rheumatic fever and later from rheumatoid arthritis. Too weak to attend school, she was educated at home until age 14, when her mother died. Van Blarcom was sent to live with her grandfather and other relatives. Between 1896 and 1898, she attended the Hasbrouck Institute in Jersey City, New Jersey.

Against family opposition, Van Blarcom entered the Johns Hopkins Hospital Training School for Nurses in 1898. Ill health forced her to take an additional year to complete the three-year program. She graduated in 1901 and was appointed the school's instructor of obstetrics and assistant superintendent of nurses.

In 1905, Van Blarcom left Johns Hopkins for St. Louis, Missouri, to assist in the reorganization of the St. Luke's Hospital Training School for nurses. Worsening arthritis forced her to resign. Three years later, when her health improved, she became director of the Maryland Tuberculosis Sanatorium in Sibillisville. Afterward, she took a similar position at a sanatorium in New Bedford, Massachusetts. Her success in running the sanatorium led to her appointment as secretary of the New York State Committee for the Prevention of Blindness.

In this work, Van Blarcom found that a common eye infection, ophthalmia neonatorum, was the leading cause of blindness in newborns. She also learned that a 2 percent nitrate solution applied to the newborn's eyes prevented the disease. However, many midwives, who made up 50 percent of birth attendants, were unaware of this procedure. Van Blarcom was thus inspired to organize a study, funded by the Russell Sage Foundation, of midwifery practices in the United States, England, and 14 other countries. As a result of her findings, she wrote *The Midwife in England* (1913), in which she concluded that the United States was seriously lacking in its training and licensing of midwives.

This began Van Blarcom's career as a midwife education reformer and advocate for mother and infant health. She became the first American nurse to be licensed as a midwife and the first to complete a national survey of city and county midwifery laws. In addition to writing for medical and popular publications on midwifery, she assisted in the establishment of Bellevue School of Midwifery in New York City in 1911. By 1916, the Committee for the Prevention of Blindness had become a national organization with Van Blarcom as its secretary. She also organized and served as secretary (1916–1917) of the Illinois Society for the Prevention of Blindness.

During World War I, Van Blarcom served as director of the Atlantic Division of the American Red Cross Nursing Service. In this capacity, she assisted in the transfer of nursing equipment overseas. During 1917 and 1918, she completed a cross-country speaking tour recruiting nurses for the Red Cross.

After 1918, Van Blarcom resumed her efforts on behalf of mothers and infants. In 1922, she published *Obstetrical Nursing*, a textbook, which went into six editions. The same year, she published a layperson's version, *Getting Ready to Be a Mother*. This book, which went into four editions, was written as a health care manual for mothers during and after pregnancy. *Building the Baby*, an infant care manual, was published in 1929. Van Blarcom also wrote 12 educational pamphlets on pre- and postnatal care, which have been described by nursing historian Joellen Hawkins as Van Blarcom's most important work. The pamphlets, written in a concise and meaningful way, were distributed to thousands of mothers by state and county health departments.

The ill health that plagued Van Blarcom throughout her life forced her into retirement during the 1930s. She was, however, active during World War II as director of the nurses' aid training program of the Pasadena, California, chapter of the American Red Cross. During her retirement, she also chaired the Health and Sanitation Committee of the Women's Civil League and organized the Pasadena Committee for Maternal Welfare. She died in Arcadia, California, of bronchopneumonia in March 1960.

Selected Additional Achievements

Chair, Midwifery Committee, National Organization for Public Health Nursing; speaker, Third English-speaking Conference on Infant Welfare (London, England, 1924); honorary member of England's Midwives' Institute; speaker, Congress of the International Council of Nurses (Helsinki, 1925); speaker, Third Annual Conference of State Directors in Charge of Local Administration of the Maternity and Infancy Act (Washington, D.C., 1926); member, committee on nurses' scholarships and nursing recruitment, Huntington Hospital.

References

Hawkins, Joellen Watson. 1988. "Van Blarcom, Carolyn Conant." In *Dictionary of American Nursing Biography*, edited by M. Kaufman. New York: Greenwood Press.

Litoff, Judy Barrett. 1971. "Van Blarcom, Carolyn Conant." In *Notable American Women, 1607–1950: A Biographical Dictionary*, edited by E.T. James, J.W. James, and P.S. Boyer. Cambridge: Belknap Press of Harvard University Press.

Pennock, Meta Rutter, ed. 1940. *Makers of Nursing History; Portraits and Pen Sketches of One Hundred and Nine Prominent Women*. New York: Lakeside.

Perry, Marilyn Elizabeth. 1999. "Van Blarcom, Carolyn Conant." In *American National Biography*, edited by J.A. Garraty and M.C. Carnes. New York: Oxford University Press.

JSB

Van Hoosen, Bertha (1863–1952)
Physician

Bertha Van Hoosen was an outstanding American surgeon who devoted her career to the obstetrical and gynecological health of women. She was born on March 26, 1863, in Stony Creek, Michigan, the younger of two daughters of Joshua and Sarah Ann (Taylor) Van Hoosen. She graduated from Pontiac High School in 1880 and then entered the literary department of the University of Michigan. During her studies, she decided on a career in medicine and included science courses in her curriculum. In her autobiography, *Petticoat Surgeon* (1947), she described her reason for choosing medicine: "I was responding to a call of the woman in me—woman, preserver of the race—to mitigate suffering and save life" (1980 reprint, p. 55).

Van Hoosen earned a bachelor's degree in 1884 but was unable to immediately enroll in medical school; her father, unhappy with his daughter's career choice, refused to pay her tuition. To earn her way, she spent a year as a teacher of calisthenics and physiology at the Mary Institute in St. Louis, Missouri, where she also attended medical clinics. In St. Louis, she lived with Mary McLean, an 1883 graduate of the University of Michigan Medical School.

In the fall of 1885, Van Hoosen enrolled in the University of Michigan Medical School. In addition to her studies, she served as demonstrator of anatomy and was an obstetrical nurse. After graduating in 1888, she spent the next four years engaged in clinical studies at Woman's Hospital in Detroit and Kalamazoo State Hospital for the Insane. She also worked at the New England Hospital for Women and Children in Boston, founded by Marie Zakrzewska in 1862.

In 1892, Van Hoosen opened a private practice in Chicago and specialized in providing medical care to women "who were suffering—perhaps dying—because they could not force themselves to submit to an examination from a male physician" (Van Hoosen, p. 109). She developed a positive reputation among the women of the city, and soon her practice flourished. She was also an instructor of anatomy and embryology at the Woman's Medical School of Northwestern University (1892–1902) and gave public health lectures to various organizations.

In 1896, Van Hoosen began a one-year term as head of the obstetrical department at Chicago's Women and Children's Hospital. Afterward, she applied for the position of head of gynecology and obstetrics at her alma mater but was denied the position because she was a woman. She returned to Northwestern to assume the role of professor and head of gynecology. When the Woman's Medical School at Northwestern closed in 1902, she accepted a professorship in clinical gynecology at the Illinois University Medical School (1902–1912) despite strong opposition by some faculty and students to a woman professor. The first course that she taught was an elective, so that any student opposing a woman teacher would not be required to attend. The adjoining hospital, which normally provided postoperative care for patients used for clinical demonstration, refused to accept her patients. Undaunted, she bought and equipped her own charity hospital. Despite these obstacles, she performed well in the surgical amphitheater. She wrote in *Petticoat Surgeon*, "I was sure that with the knife in my hand I would be . . . oblivious to the crowd or to outside disturbance" (1980 reprint, p. 142). Her reputation grew, and by the end of the first term, the amphitheater was filled with students, sometimes from other colleges.

Along with her regular duties, Van Hoosen attended clinics at the Mayo Clinic every three months to observe the most advanced surgical techniques. She continued visiting the Mayo Clinic until her appointment in 1913 as head of the gynecological staff at Cook County hospital. Earning the position required taking a Civil Service Board examination. Van Hoosen, the only woman among 300 examinees, earned the highest score and was awarded the position. This achievement also won her the distinction of being the first female doctor to earn a civil service appointment. In 1920, she became head of the hospital's obstetrical staff. She also served as head and professor of obstetrics at Loyola University Medical School (1918–1937), becoming the first woman to head a medical department at a coeducational university.

Around 1904, Van Hoosen began using scopolamine-morphine for women in labor and became a pioneer in its use. Although this form of anesthetic was controversial among many American physicians, Van Hoosen considered it a great boon to twentieth-century women, whom she believed had the right to choose a painless delivery. She delivered 2,000 healthy babies using this method.

Van Hoosen was aware that in her position as a successful medical woman, she played an important role in helping other women advance in the profession. As a professor, she trained over 20 women surgeons, many of whom went on to become medical missionaries overseas. She assisted her female colleagues when called, often traveling out of state to give medical advice or perform surgeries for nonsurgically trained women physicians. The most important of her achievements on behalf of women was the formation of the American Medical Women's Association (AMWA) in 1915 and later the association's publication, the *Journal of the American Medical Women's Association*. Although women were entering the medical field in greater numbers, they were still barred from many male-established professional organizations. Van Hoosen, herself a skilled obstetrician, was denied membership in the Chicago Gynecological and Obstetrical Society. As the first president of the AMWA, she fought unsuccessfully for the right of women physicians to serve in the military during World War I. Not until 1943 did Margaret Craighill earn the distinction of being the first woman doctor to be a commissioned officer in the U.S. military.

Van Hoosen made other notable accomplishments, including the establishment of the first human breast milk bank in Chicago in 1930. She also founded a hospital where working-class women could give birth at an inexpensive flat rate and spoke for many years on sex education to the Committee on Social Purity of the Chicago Women's Club. She performed her last operation in 1951. She died of a stroke on June 7, 1952, at a convalescent home in Romeo, Michigan.

See also Craighill, Margaret; McLean, Mary Hancock; Zakrzewska, Marie Elizabeth

Selected Additional Achievements

"The New Movement in Obstetrics," *Medical Woman's Journal* (June 1915): 121–123, "Scopolamine Anesthesia in Obstetrics," *Current Research in Anesthesia and Analgesia* (May–June 1928): 151–154; *Scopolamine-Morphine Anaesthesia* (1915). Honorary M.A., Michigan University and honorary fellowship, International College of Surgeons. First and only woman to read a paper at the Sixteenth International Congress of Medicine (Budapest, 1909) and at the Pan-American International Association (Panama, 1930).

References

Chaff, S. L. 1984. "Van Hoosen, Bertha." In *Dictionary of American Medical Biography*, edited by M. Kaufman, S. Galishoff, and T.L. Savitt. Westport, Conn.: Greenwood Press.

McGovern, Constance M. 1999. "Van Hoosen, Bertha." In *American National Biography*, edited by J.A. Garraty and M.C. Carnes. New York: Oxford University Press.

Morantz, Regina Markell. 1980. "Van Hoosen, Bertha." In *Notable American Women: The Modern Period: A Biographical Dictionary*, edited by B. Sicherman and C.H. Green. Cambridge: Belknap Press of Harvard University Press.

Van Hoosen, Bertha. 1980. *Petticoat Surgeon*. Reprint ed. New York: Arno Press. Original ed. Chicago: Pellegrini and Cudahy, 1947.

JSB

Ventre, Fran (1941–   )
Nurse-midwife

Fran Ventre opened the first freestanding birth centers in Massachusetts and in Brooklyn, New York. Throughout her career as a lay midwife and a certified nurse-midwife, she has been a proponent of midwifery as an alternative to the depersonalization and institutionalization that often exist in the hospital birth setting. She was born on August 14,

1941, in Brooklyn, New York, the third child of Sonia and Fred Katz. After graduating from Abraham Lincoln High School in Brooklyn, she received a B.S. degree in education from the University of Wisconsin in 1962. The following year she married Robert Ventre, and the couple eventually had two sons and a daughter.

Ventre became a midwife during the early 1970s, after receiving certification by the American Society for Psychoprophylaxis in Obstetrics (now Lamaze International, Inc.). In 1975, she became licensed as a lay midwife in Maryland and was the only one to receive this certification after the enactment of licensing legislation in the 1920s. During the 1970s, she helped found the Home Oriented Maternity Experience (HOME), an organization that provides information to women interested in home births. Ventre earned a nursing degree from Montgomery College in Takoma Park, Maryland (1977), and graduated from the nurse-midwifery program at Georgetown University in Washington, D.C. (1978). The same year, she was instrumental in thwarting passage of a bill that threatened to end licensing of midwives in Maryland.

Ventre then relocated to Massachusetts, where state law made it illegal for her to assist in home births. However, she continued to attend women at home births while working with a private obstetrician. In 1980, she helped start the North Shore Birth Center as a pilot project approved by the Massachusetts Department of Health. The center was affiliated with Beverly Hospital near Boston, and she was its midwife director. The center was the state's first licensed, freestanding birthing facility and continues to exist today. Ventre also served on a special task force with the state's Department of Public Health to write birth center rules and regulations. She left the center in 1984 but continued as a nurse-midwife for the Harvard Community Health Plan and attended births at Brigham and Women's Hospital. She earned a master of public health degree from Boston University in 1991.

In 1999, Ventre returned to Brooklyn to open the Brooklyn Birthing Center, the borough's first and only freestanding birth facility. The atmosphere is purposefully homelike, with individual rooms painted in soothing colors. The center provides care before, during, and after pregnancy and birth, as well as overall well-woman health screenings, and is affiliated with three area hospitals in the event that acute care is needed.

Ventre was one of the founders of the Midwives' Alliance of North America in 1982 and served as the Massachusetts chapter's first regional representative (1982–1985). She also served twice as chair of the Massachusetts chapter of the American College of Nurse-Midwives. She has volunteered in Senegal, West Africa, and for migrant Mexican women in a birth center in Texas. Her devotion to midwifery is summed up in this conviction: "Midwifery is a vocation, a romance, an addiction, a religion. It isn't something you dabble in; there's a part of yourself, of your life, that you give away" (*Pregnancy, Birth and Beyond*). Presently, she is working in the Maternal Infant Health program with local midwives in Kosovo for Doctors of the World.

References

The Brooklyn Birthing Center. Online. http://www.brooklynbirthingcenter.com. 13 August 2000.

Brooks, Rolston. 1981. "Born Free: North Shore Birth Center." *Sojourner: The Women's Forum* 7 (4):9.

Chester, Penfield. 1997. *Sisters on a Journey: Portraits of American Midwives.* New Brunswick, N.J.: Rutgers University Press.

Katz, Nancie L. 1999. "Midwife's Opening Birth Center." *New York Daily News* (October 11, Suburban Section):1.

Pregnancy, Birth and Beyond. Online. http://www.monarch-design.com/baby/quotes.html. 12 August 2000.

Ventre, Fran, Peggy Garland Spindel, and Kate Bowland. 1995. "The Transition from Lay Midwife to Certified Midwife in the United States." *Journal of Nurse-Midwifery* 40 (5):428–437.

Ventre, Fran. March 29, May 20, 2001. Interview with author via E-mail.

JSB

W

Wald, Florence Schorske (1917–)
Nurse

Florence Schorske Wald, a former dean of the Yale University School of Nursing, is responsible for introducing the hospice concept to the United States. She was born on April 19, 1917, in New York City. Due to a chronic respiratory illness, she spent much of her youth in the hospital. Her interaction with nurses led her to choose nursing as a profession.

Wald earned a bachelor's degree at Mount Holyoke College in South Hadley, Massachusetts, in 1938 and a master's degree in nursing from Yale University in 1941. During World War II, she served in the United States Army Signal Corps as a research technician. After the war, she held positions as a staff nurse with the New York Visiting Nurse Service, as a research assistant at the College of Physicians and Surgeons in New York, and as a lecturer in psychiatric nursing at Rutgers University in New Brunswick, New Jersey. After earning a master's degree in mental health nursing at Yale, she was appointed assistant professor in psychiatric nursing in 1957. The following year, she became dean of the Yale School of Nursing. In 1959, she married Henry Wald.

In 1963, British physician Cicely Saunders spoke at Yale about St. Christopher's, a hospice in Sydenham, England. St. Christopher's was the first modern hospice in the world. Wald was very impressed by the promise of hospice care, which she characterized as "an interdisciplinary comfort-oriented care that allows terminally ill patients to die with dignity and humanity with as little pain as possible in an environment where they have mental and spiritual preparation for the natural process of dying" (quoted in Snodgrass, p. 275). Terminally ill patients who receive hospice care are included in the decision-making process regarding their treatment.

In 1967, Wald resigned from Yale and, with a committee of nurses, physicians, and clergy, began studying care given to terminally ill patients and their families. By 1974, her findings led to in-home hospice services in New Haven, Connecticut; in 1980, a building was completed for an inpatient facility. The hospice movement has gained great momentum, and it is estimated that there are now over 3,000 hospice services available in the United States. Wald continues her work with hospice care. In 1995, she began serving on the advisory committee of the National Prison Hospice Movement.

Wald currently resides in Branford, Connecticut.

Selected Additional Achievements

Distinguished Alumna Award, Yale University School of Nursing (1976); American Nurses Association Hall of Fame (1996); National Women's Hall of Fame (1998).

References

Beaudoin, Christina. 2000. "Florence Schorske Wald." In *American Nursing: A Biographical Dictionary*, edited by V.L. Bullough and L. Sentz. New York: Springer.

Friedrich, M.J. 1999. "Hospice Care in the United States: A Conversation with Florence S. Wald." *JAMA* 281 (18):1683–1685.

Snodgrass, Mary Ellen. 1999. *Historical Encyclopedia of Nursing*. Santa Barbara, Calif.: ABC-Clio.

DTW

Wald, Lillian D. (1867–1940)
Nurse

Lillian Wald founded a visiting nurse service and settlement house to provide much needed health care and, later, social services to immigrants living on New York City's Lower East Side. Her success with the Henry Street Visiting Nurse Service helped to define the field of public health nursing. She was born on March 10, 1867, in Cincinnati, Ohio, the third of four children of Max D. and Minnie (Schwarz) Wald. The family moved to Rochester, New York, when Wald was very young. Max Wald was a successful optical goods dealer, and Wald was able to attend a private school, Miss Cruttenden's English-French Boarding and Day School. When she was 16, Wald applied to Vassar College, but she was refused admission because of her young age. For the next several years she studied on her own and led an active social life, which she found increasingly dissatisfying. In 1889, she was visiting her expectant sister when a trained nurse was called to attend her; the woman sparked Wald's interest in the new profession of nursing.

In August of that year, she entered the New York Hospital School of Nursing, then under the direction of nurse Irene Sutliffe. She graduated two years later, in March 1891, and spent a year working at the Juvenile Asylum in New York City. Next, she enrolled at the Woman's Medical College of the New York Infirmary, founded by pioneering physician Elizabeth Blackwell in 1868. In 1893, Wald was asked to teach home nursing to immigrants on New York's Lower East Side. In March of that year, the young daughter of one of her students went to Wald and led her through the grimy streets to her mother, who had just given birth in a dilapidated tenement home. The shock of seeing such destitution and suffering had a profound effect on Wald, motivating her to do something practical for the people of the neighborhood.

Wald immediately left medical school and

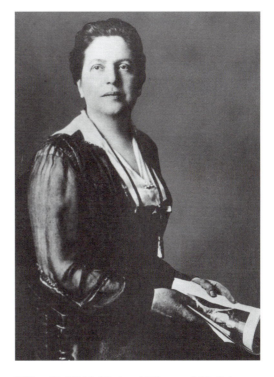

Lillian D. Wald. National Library of Medicine.

moved to the Lower East Side, where, in her words, she and nursing friend Mary Brewster "were to live in the neighborhood as nurses, identify ourselves with it socially, and, in brief, contribute to it our citizenship" (Wald, 1915, pp. 8–9). They founded the Nurses' Settlement, later called the Henry Street Settlement, and soon added a Visiting Nurse Service, based on Wald's belief that many of the sick could be treated effectively in their homes rather than in the hospital. In 1895, with financing from banker Jacob H. Schiff, Wald purchased a building on Henry Street that would be the basis for the Nurse Service and her home for nearly 40 years.

Nurses who shared Wald's vision, such as nursing leader Lavinia Dock, soon joined Wald at Henry Street, and the service quickly grew. By 1913, the Visiting Nurse Service consisted of seven houses on Henry Street and two uptown branches, with 92 nurses making 200,000 home visits annually. Wald divided the East Side neighborhoods into territories and then into districts, in order for her nurses to serve the community more efficiently. She insisted on autonomy for her nurses, despite initial reluctance of local physicians to accept nurses as independent health care providers. In addition to home nursing calls, the Henry Street nurses maintained first-aid stations and convalescent facilities. They also worked to control infectious diseases such as tuberculosis. Unlike other visiting nurse services, the Henry Street Visiting Nurse Service was available to people of all religions and races. Additionally, Wald charged patients a small fee, in order to maintain their dignity. The Henry Street Settlement and the Visiting Nurse Service were financed privately, and Wald was a very effective fund-raiser.

Many American and international nurses received practical training at Henry Street, and similar programs were set up around the country, resulting in the growth of public health nursing. Wald believed that the nurse was "an effective and indispensable educator, and that her profession [was] of community importance" (Wald, 1934, p. 74). In addition to her work at Henry Street, she helped start a school nurse program in New York City in 1902, the first such program in the United States. In 1909, she suggested a nursing program for Metropolitan Life Insurance policyholders, and in 1912, she was instrumental in getting the American Red Cross to set up the Town and County Nursing Service. In recognition of her efforts in public health nursing, a term that she originated, she was made first president of the National Organization for Public Health Nursing in 1912.

Wald's work at Henry Street led her to provide more than just health care to area residents. She is often remembered as a social worker, as well as a nurse, because the settlement provided vocational guidance, scholarships for children, housekeeping classes, and other social, cultural, and civic activities. In the 1920s, a Neighborhood Playhouse at Henry Street became a leading experimental theater in New York. Wald was also an advocate for social reforms; she was a member of numerous reform organizations and backed politicians who supported her views. She was particularly distressed by working children and supported child labor laws as well as the creation of a federal Children's Bureau. She also helped found the Women's Trade Union League (1903) to protect women from the dangers of sweatshops.

Wald was a pacifist; she marched against involvement in World War I and was president of the American Union against Militarism. Her views would later lead some to brand her as unpatriotic and impacted her fund-raising efforts. During the war, she was chair of the committee on home nursing of the Council of National Defense. She was also chair of the Red Cross Nurses' Emergency Council, Atlantic division, during the 1918 influenza epidemic and was responsible for recruiting volunteer nurses and coordinating nursing agencies.

By the mid-1920s, Wald began to suffer from heart trouble and anemia and was less involved in the everyday work at Henry Street. In 1933, she resigned her position as head worker and moved to Westport, Connecticut. She died there on September 1,

1940. The Henry Street Settlement and the Visiting Nurse Service of New York continue today.

See also Blackwell, Elizabeth; Dock, Lavinia Lloyd; Sutliffe, Irene H.

Selected Additional Achievements

Gold Medal, National Institute of Social Sciences (1913); honorary doctor of laws, Mount Holyoke College (1912); bronze bust placed in Hall of Fame for Great Americans, New York University (1971); American Nurses Association Hall of Fame (1976).

References

Bremner, Robert H. 1971. "Wald, Lillian D." In *Notable American Women, 1607–1950: A Biographical Dictionary*, edited by E.T. James, J.W. James, and P.S. Boyer. Cambridge: Belknap Press of Harvard University Press.

Daniels, Doris Groshen. 1989. *Always a Sister: The Feminism of Lillian D. Wald*. New York: Feminist Press at City University of New York.

Duffus, R.L. 1938. *Lillian Wald: Neighbor and Crusader*. New York: Macmillan.

Falk, Gerhard. 1988. "Lillian D. Wald." In *American Nursing: A Biographical Dictionary*, edited by V.L. Bullough, O.M. Church, and A.P. Stein. New York: Garland.

Wald, Lillian D. 1915. *The House on Henry Street*. New York: Henry Holt.

Wald, Lillian D. 1934. *Windows on Henry Street*. Boston: Little, Brown.

LS

Walker, Mary Edwards (1832–1919)
Physician

Mary Edwards Walker is the first and only woman to have earned the Congressional Medal of Honor. She was born in Oswego, New York, on November 26, 1832, one of six children of Vesta (Whitcomb) and Alvah Walker. Her interest in medicine was probably inspired by her father, who studied medicine in search of a cure for his lingering illness. Walker was educated at a local school run by her parents and later attended the Falley Seminary (1850–1852) in Fulton, New York. She graduated from Syracuse Medical College in 1855, only six years after Elizabeth Blackwell became the first woman in the United States to earn a medical degree. Walker maintained private practices in Ohio and New York during the 1850s and 1860s. She married classmate Dr. Albert Miller shortly after their graduation but separated from him in 1869.

At the outbreak of the Civil War Walker petitioned the Army Medical Department in Washington, D.C., for an appointment as an army surgeon. At that time, there had never been a woman officer in the army, and her application was rejected. In the meantime, she volunteered as assistant physician and surgeon at Indiana Hospital in the U.S. Patent Building. She volunteered because the surgeon general refused to appoint a woman as surgeon.

In 1862, Walker received a diploma from the Hygeio-Therapeutic College in New York. She then volunteered as a surgeon at battle sites where medical need was so great that her assistance, in spite of her sex, could not be turned away. Although not recognized as an official member of the military, she insisted on wearing a modified version of a Union officer's uniform. In 1863, she accepted a position with the 52nd Ohio Infantry as a contract assistant surgeon, despite opposition from other army personnel. In April 1864, she traveled into enemy territory en route to providing civilian medical care. She was captured as a prisoner of war and spent four months at a political prison in Virginia. After her release from prison, she was offered a civilian contract position as surgeon in charge at a Kentucky female prison. Opposition to her appointment by male hospital employees forced her to request a transfer. In 1865 she began her last wartime assignment as director of an orphan asylum in Tennessee. She requested her own discharge from the army later in the same year.

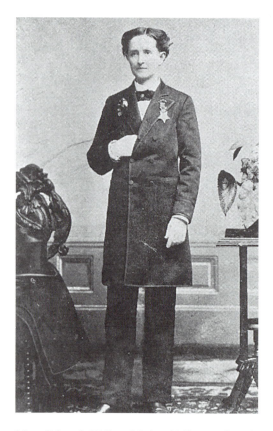

Mary Edwards Walker. National Library of Medicine.

Walker was disappointed to have never received the recognition of a commissioned army officer. She persistently complained to the government until President Andrew Johnson awarded her the Medal of Honor in 1866. Although the medal did not endow her with officer status, it was a physical token of her service, and she wore it proudly every day. Also in 1866, she sailed for Great Britain and France to visit hospitals and medical facilities to encourage the acceptance of women in medicine.

Walker, elected president of the National Dress Reform Association in 1866, was a passionate supporter of the issue. She considered contemporary women's dress unhealthy and warned that the stylish, yet tight-fitting, outfits of the day prevented freedom of motion and interfered with respiration and digestion.

She advocated clothing styled in the male fashion, and later in life, she donned full male attire. She was arrested many times for impersonating a man.

In 1917, a federal review board rescinded her Medal of Honor after determining that she had never actually served as an officer in the Union army. Later that year, Walker made an unsuccessful trip to Washington to urge the board to reconsider. While there, she slipped on the Capitol steps and never recovered from the fall. She died in 1919, at the age of 86. In 1977, a grandniece was able to persuade President James Earl Carter to restore the medal. She is still the only woman to have received this award. In 1982, the U.S. Postal Service issued a stamp in her likeness.

See also Blackwell, Elizabeth

Selected Additional Achievements

A Woman's Thoughts about Love and Marriage, Divorce, etc. (1871), *Hit* (1871), *Unmasked, or the Science of Immortality: To Gentlemen by a Woman Physician and Surgeon* (1878), *Isonomy* (1898), *Crowning Constitutional Argument of Mary E. Walker* (1907).

References

Binker, Mary Jo. 1995. "Feminism's Tinker, Tailor, Physician, Spy." *Insight on the News* 11 (28):27.

Filler, Louis. 1971. "Walker, Mary Edwards." In *Notable American Women, 1607–1950: A Biographical Dictionary*, edited by E.T. James, J.W. James, and P.S. Boyer. Cambridge: Belknap Press of Harvard University Press.

Leonard, Elizabeth D. 1994. *Yankee Women: Gender Battles in the Civil War*. New York: W.W. Norton.

The National Cyclopaedia of American Biography. 1906. Vol. 13. New York: James T. White.

Poynter, Lida. 1946. "Dr. Mary Walker, M.D.: Pioneer Woman Physician." *Medical Woman's Journal* 53 (10):43–51.

Spiegel, Allen D., and Peter B. Suskind. 1996. "Mary Edwards Walker, M.D.: A Feminist Physician a Century ahead of Her Time." *Journal of Community Health* 21 (3):211–235.

JSB

Warner, Estella Ford (1891–1974)
Physician

Estella Ford Warner was the first female commissioned officer in the U.S. Public Health Service. She was born on December 21, 1891, in Ironwood, Michigan, the daughter of Cortes Ford, a banker and judge, and Estella (Green) Ford. The family lived in Michigan and Wisconsin until 1899, when they moved to Skagway, Alaska. She received her early education in Skagway public schools and with private tutors. After eight years in Alaska, the family moved to Portland, Oregon, where Warner graduated from Allen Preparatory School.

In 1910, Warner matriculated at the University of California to prepare for a career as a concert pianist. However, she found her science courses more fulfilling and transferred to the premedical program after only three months. Next, she entered the University of Oregon School of Medicine. She earned her medical degree in 1918 and then completed an internship at Good Samaritan Hospital in Portland. In March 1918, she married medical school classmate Douglas Holmes Warner, a commissioned naval officer. He died of influenza in October the same year.

After her husband's death, Warner began working for the Young Women's Christian Association, supplying medical care to World War I refugees in England, France, and Archangel, Russia. While abroad, she also studied pediatrics in London. She returned to Oregon in 1920 and subsequently held a series of public health positions. She was director of the Division of Child Hygiene for the Portland Department of Health (1920–1922) and director of the Division of Maternal and Child Health for the Oregon State Department of Health (1922–1925). She then served as chief of medicine (1925–1928) and as director (1928–1930) of the Marion County Child Health Demonstration in Salem. During this time, she also maintained a private pediatrics practice and was medical adviser for women at Reed College in Portland.

In the early 1930s, Warner began working for the U.S. Public Health Service (USPHS) to improve medical services in the United States and abroad. She held many positions with the USPHS, including the directorship of the Division of Child Hygiene in Washington, D.C. (1931–1935). In 1936, she was admitted into the Public Health Service Commissioned Corps with the rank of surgeon, the first woman commissioned into the service; she was promoted to senior surgeon in 1942. As district medical officer for the USPHS Office of Indian Affairs in Albuquerque (1937–1942) and in San Francisco, (1942), she administered public health programs to American Indians. She was also medical director for the USPHS regional office in Kansas City, Missouri, and worked with food handlers in schools across seven states. In 1951, she traveled to Lebanon to establish a public health department at American University in Beirut. Around 1952, she went to India to head a U.S. medical assistance program. There she helped improve the water supply in rural villages, established hospitals and clinics, and trained midwives, physicians, and nurses.

In 1956, Warner retired to Albuquerque; she died there on September 10, 1974.

Selected Additional Achievements

Member, American Medical Association, American Public Health Association, National Organization for Public Health Nursing, American Academy of Pediatrics, and the National Research Council on Child Health and Development.

References

Bernard, Marcelle. 1951. "Estella Ford Warner, M.D." *Journal of the American Medical Women's Association* 6:284.

Brown, Mona. 1954. "Doctor to India." *New York Times Magazine* (May 16):44.

"Estella Ford Warner, M.D." 1945. *Medical Woman's Journal* 52 (10):50–51.

"Obituary." 1974. *New York Times* (September 13):40.

Scheele, Leonard A. 1956. "Estella Ford Warner." *Public Health Reports* 71 (4):375–376.

JSB

Wattleton, [Alyce] Faye (1943–   )
Nurse

Faye Wattleton is an African American reproductive rights advocate. For nearly 20 years, she served as president of the Planned Parenthood Federation of America, bringing the issue of reproductive freedom into the national spotlight. She was born in St. Louis, Missouri, on July 8, 1943, the only child of George Edward, a factory worker, and Ozie (Garrett) Wattleton, an itinerant minister for the Church of God. Because of her mother's ministry, Wattleton received her early education in various schools around the Midwest and South. Stories about her maternal grandmother, Ola, who struggled to care for at least nine children, influenced her opinion about the importance of family planning.

In 1960, Wattleton entered the Ohio State University Nursing School in Columbus. There, she decided to pursue an obstetrics specialty. After earning a degree in 1964, she taught maternity nursing at the Miami Valley Hospital School of Nursing in Dayton, Ohio.

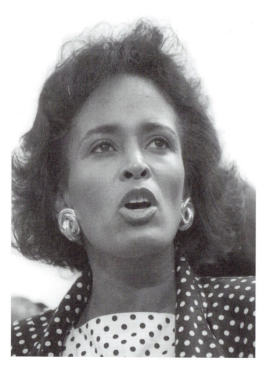

[Alyce] Faye Wattleton. AP/WIDE WORLD PHOTOS.

In 1966, she entered the maternal and infant health care program at Columbia University in New York City. At Columbia, she studied at Harlem Hospital, where she observed the fate of many female patients who received botched illegal abortions. After earning a master's degree and a midwifery certificate in 1967, she went on to serve as assistant director of the Montgomery County Combined Public Health District in Dayton.

After a year in that position, Wattleton joined the board of the Dayton affiliate of the Planned Parenthood Federation of America (PPFA) because she was interested in its efforts to prevent unwanted pregnancies. In 1970, she became executive director of the Dayton office, and over the next seven and a half years, she turned the small affiliate into one of the largest in the country. In 1973, she married Frank Gordon, whom she divorced in 1981. The couple had one daughter, Felicia, in 1975.

In 1978, Wattleton began her most notable work as the president of the PPFA, the nation's oldest and largest voluntary family-planning service. PPFA had been founded in 1921 (as the American Birth Control League) by Margaret Sanger. When Wattleton took the helm, she became the first woman to run the organization since Sanger resigned in 1928. Wattleton was also the first African American and the youngest person to hold this position. Her goals as president were to encourage the development of new contraceptives, reduce adolescent pregnancies, increase sex education, increase services to rural areas, and continue access to safe abortions.

Since 1973, when *Roe vs. Wade* made abortion legal, Planned Parenthood had become the focus of violence and demonstrations by opposition groups. In addition, some politicians who opposed abortion were proposing restrictions on government-funded family planning services. In an effort to keep reproductive freedom safe and legal, Wattleton made many speeches, appeared on television, and gave numerous interviews to rally the public around her cause. In 1981, she testified before the U.S. Senate to defend the use of Title X funding for family-planning services. Her work to maintain government funding stemmed from her desire to help poor "women whose health was weakened by the strain of bearing each new child, women whose families suffered the economic consequences of one more mouth to feed" (Wattleton, p. 11).

Wattleton's efforts were not limited to the United States. PPFA's international division, Family Planning International Assistance, relied on the federal government for many of its family-planning efforts. In 1984, when the U.S. government announced that it would no longer provide funds for international family-planning programs, Wattleton again found herself leading the efforts to maintain these programs.

By the time that Wattleton resigned in 1992, the number of PPFA donors had increased from 85,000 to 1 million. After leaving PPFA, she hosted a short-lived television talk show and in 1995 founded the Center for Gender Equality, a national policy center on women's issues. She lives in New York City and is a lecturer and consultant.

See also Sanger, Margaret Louise Higgins

Selected Additional Achievements

How to Talk with Your Child about Sexuality (1986). Chair, National Executive Director's Council, Planned Parented Federation (1975); American Humanist Award (1986); Women's Honors in Public Service (1986), American Nursing Association; Board of Directors, U.S. Commission for the United Nations Children's Education Fund (1986); Congressional Black Caucus Humanitarian Award (1989); Better World Population Medal (1989); Award of Excellence, American Public Health Association (1989); Margaret Sanger Woman of Valor Award, Planned Parenthood Federation (1992), National Women's Hall of Fame (1993); and 12 honorary doctoral degrees.

References

Cunningham, Carolyn, and Adrienne Lash Jones. 1992. "Faye Wattleton." In *Notable Black American Women*, edited by J.C. Smith. Detroit: Gale Research.
Johnson, Anne Janette. 1995. "Faye Wattleton." In *Contemporary Black Biography: Profiles from the International Black Community*, edited by L.M. Mabunda. Detroit: Gale Research.
Moritz, Charles, ed. 1991. *Current Biography Yearbook 1990*. New York: H.W. Wilson.
Wattleton, Faye. 1996. *Life on the Line*. New York: Ballantine Books.

JSB

Weeks Shaw, Clara Shaw (1857–1940)
Nurse

Clara Weeks Shaw was the first American nurse to write a textbook on nursing. She was born in Sanbornton, New Hampshire, on February 28, 1857, to Dr. Alpheus and Anna Coe Weeks. Weeks Shaw's early education was at a school that her mother opened in Kingston, Rhode Island and at the state's East Greenwich Seminary. At age 17, she graduated from the Rhode Island State Normal School and then got a job teaching at a public school in Newport. She hated teaching and turned to nursing as an alternative.

In a letter to the superintendent of the New York Hospital Training School for Nurses, she wrote, "I can hardly tell whether I have an especial vocation for the work [of nursing], for I have had absolutely no experience in sickness, but it has a strong attraction for me as offering a wider field for usefulness, and a better opportunity for actual *work*, than any other. The prospect of constant and absorbing employment invites rather than deters me" (Shaw). She was accepted at New York Hospital and graduated in 1880, following 18 months of training.

Weeks Shaw then organized the nursing school at Paterson General Hospital in Paterson, New Jersey, where she was superintendent for five years (1883–1888). During this time, she wrote *A Text-Book of Nursing for the Use of Training Schools, Families, and Private Students* (1885). It covered all aspects of nursing, with chapters on such topics as nurses and nursing, beds and bed making, the observation of symptoms, surgical nursing, and surgical and medical emergencies. The book was extremely popular; by 1946 it had gone through three editions and 58 printings and had sold more than 100,000 copies.

Clara S. Weeks married Cyrus W. Shaw in 1888 and retired from nursing. She died on January 14, 1940, in Mountainville, New York.

References

"Mrs. Clara S. Weeks Shaw." 1940. *American Journal of Nursing* 40 (3):356.

Shaw, Clara S. Weeks. Student Records (Graduates), Class of 1880, Cornell University-New York Hospital School of Nursing. New York Weill Cornell Medical Center Archives, New York.

Weeks-Shaw, Clara. 1932. *A Text-Book of Nursing for the Use of Training Schools, Families, and Private Students.* 3rd, rev., and enl. ed. New York: D. Appleton.

LS

Welsh, Lilian (1858–1938)
Physician

Lilian Welsh spent most of her career as a physician pioneering in what is now known as preventive medicine in Baltimore. She was born on March 6, 1858, in Columbia, Pennsylvania, the fourth of six children of Thomas and Annie Eunice (Young) Welsh. She graduated from Columbia High School in 1873 and from the State Normal School at Millersville, Pennsylvania in 1875. She later taught at both schools and was principal of Columbia High School (1881–1886).

An interest in chemistry led Welsh to study at the Woman's Medical College of Pennsylvania in Philadelphia (now MCP Hahnemann University). She later wrote in her autobiography, *Reminiscences of Thirty Years in Baltimore* (1925), that she was not convinced that she wanted to practice medicine; rather, she was drawn to medicine by an interest in science. One year before finishing her medical degree she considered transferring to the Massachusetts Institute of Technology to further her studies in chemistry. Rachel Bodley, dean and chemist at Woman's Medical, pointed out the limited opportunities available to women in chemistry and urged her to finish her degree. Consequently, Welsh remained at the college and graduated in 1889.

After graduation, Welsh went to the University of Zurich for a year and a half to study physiological chemistry, histology, and bacteriology. Her goal was a career teaching physiological chemistry and doing medical research. At the time, research positions for women physicians were difficult to obtain, and she was unable to secure such a job. Instead, she took a position as resident physician at the State Hospital for the Insane at Norristown, Pennsylvania, in 1890. The Norristown hospital, under medical superintendent Dr. Alice Bennett, was one of the first mental hospitals in the United States where women patients were entirely under the care of women physicians.

In February 1892, Welsh moved to Baltimore to open a private practice with Dr. Mary Sherwood, whom she had met in Zurich. Their practice floundered at first, because of prejudice against women doctors. In 1893, Welsh and Sherwood became codirectors of Baltimore's Evening Dispensary for Working Women and Girls (founded in part by physician Kate Campbell Hurd-Mead two years earlier) and worked there until its close in 1910. Women physicians of the dispensary emphasized prenatal and postnatal care, lectured on hygiene, developed a visiting nurse service, and distributed sterile milk. They also conducted several studies, including an investigation of the practice of midwives in Baltimore, a study of the conditions of birth registration there, and a study of the prevalence of tuberculosis deaths in Baltimore from 1890 to 1910. By the time of its close, 52 women had served on the dispensary's staff, and 22,000 women and children were provided medical care.

In 1894, Welsh was appointed professor of physiology and physical training at Woman's College (later, Goucher College) in Baltimore. At Goucher, she required physical examinations of every student and assigned students to levels of physical education class based on that exam. She believed that studying the performance of the women in these classes could be used to dispel the widely held belief that a woman's reproductive organs and menstrual cycle limited her physical abilities. In addition to her physical education program, she taught a freshman hygiene course at Goucher. In that class, she taught students basic physiology and bacteriology and the importance of public as well as personal hygiene. She continued her work at Goucher for the next 30 years, retiring in 1924.

In addition to practicing medicine and teaching, Welsh was active in the National American Woman Suffrage Association, and she and Mary Sherwood participated in suffrage marches. When Sherwood died in 1935, Welsh returned to her hometown of Columbia, Pennsylvania. She died there three years later of encephalitis lethargica on February 23, 1938.

See also Bennett, Alice; Hurd-Mead, Kate Campbell; Sherwood, Mary

References

Miller, Genevieve. 1971. "Welsh, Lilian." In *Notable American Women, 1607–1950: A Biographical Dictionary*, edited by E.T. James, J.W. James, and P.S. Boyer. Cambridge: Belknap Press of Harvard University Press.

Rishworth, Susan Knoke. 1999. "Welsh, Lilian." In *American National Biography*, edited by J.A. Garraty and M.C. Carnes. New York: Oxford University Press.

Welsh, Lilian. "A Tribute to Lilian Welsh." Deceased Alumnae Files, Special Collections on Women in Medicine, Archives and Special Collections, MCP Hahnemann University, Philadelphia.

Welsh, Lilian. 1925. *Reminiscences of Thirty Years in Baltimore*. Baltimore: Norman Remington.

LS

Willeford, Mary Bristow (1900–1941)
Nurse-midwife

Mary Willeford was one of the first nurse-midwives employed by the famed Frontier Nursing Service, a health care and midwifery service in rural Leslie County, Kentucky. She was born to William and Ellen (Bristow) Willeford on February 4, 1900, in Flatonia, Texas. Her education included a bachelor's degree from the University of Texas at Austin (1920), a diploma from the Army School of Nursing, Walter Reed Hospital, Washington, D.C. (1925), and an M.A. in public health from Teachers College, Columbia University (1927).

In 1926, Willeford took a midwifery course at York Lying-In Hospital in London, England and received a certificate from that country's midwifery board. In August of that year, she began work as a district nurse-midwife at the Frontier Nursing Service (FNS), founded by Mary Breckinridge in 1925. Willeford was one of 16 charter members of the Kentucky State Association of Midwives (1928), which later became the American Association of Nurse-Midwives. In 1929, she returned to England and received a certificate to teach midwifery. From 1930 to 1938, she was the assistant director of the FNS. In addition to her duties as a nurse-midwife and assistant director, she conducted research studies of infant and maternal mortality rates in rural areas of the country. She was also one of the first nurses in the United States to earn a doctorate (Columbia University, 1932). Her dissertation, "Income and Health in Remote Rural Areas," was based on data collected in Leslie County.

In 1938, Willeford was named a maternal and child health consultant for the California State Board of Health, and in 1940, she became a public health nursing consultant for the federal Children's Bureau in Washington, D.C. In that position she helped to establish the school of midwifery at the Tuskegee Institute in Alabama, consulted with schools of midwifery, and consulted with states and counties where nurse-midwives were practicing and supervising lay midwives.

Willeford died on December 24, 1941, in New York City.

See also Breckinridge, Mary

References

Degree information provided by Diploma Services, Office of the Registrar, University of Texas at Austin, and Office of the Registrar, Teachers College, Columbia University, New York City.

Friedman, Alice Howell. 1988. "Willeford, Mary B." In *Dictionary of American Nursing Biography*, edited by M. Kaufman. New York: Greenwood Press.

"Mary B. Willeford." 1942. *American Journal of Nursing* (February):231.

National Society of the Daughters of the American Revolution. *Daughters of the American Revolution Lineage Books.* Online. http://www.ancestry.com. 22 January 2001.

LS

Willits, Mary (1855–1902)
Physician

In June 1888, Mary Willits became the first woman physician admitted to the prestigious Philadelphia County Medical Society. She was born to Thomas and Susan (Parvin) Willits on October 16, 1855, in Maidencreek Township, Pennsylvania. She attended Swarthmore College's Preparatory Department in Swarthmore, Pennsylvania (1870–1872), and then entered Swarthmore College itself. She graduated in 1876 with an A.B., then returned home for two years.

In 1878, Willits entered the Woman's Medical College of Pennsylvania in Philadelphia and chose the college's more difficult and innovative three-year course of study. Her graduation thesis on diphtheria reflected an understanding of the traditional views of the cause of the disease as well as knowledge of the emerging germ theory of disease transmission. She graduated "distinguished" from the college in 1881 and then served a yearlong internship at a hospital on Staten Island, New York.

In 1882, Willits established a private practice, and in 1886 she was made part-time instructor at the Woman's Medical College.

Also in 1886, she was recording secretary for the Philadelphia Clinical Society, an organization made up of medical women and progressive medical men. In 1887, she became an assistant to a neurologist at the Philadelphia Polyclinic School of Medicine.

While Willits was working part-time at Woman's Medical College and at the Polyclinic, she was chosen by women from the Woman's Medical College and the Philadelphia Clinical Society as a candidate for admission to the Philadelphia County Medical Society. The society had a history of animosity toward women physicians. In 1858, it had forbidden members to consult with women practitioners and male physicians teaching at Woman's Medical. Since that time, sympathetic society members had regularly submitted the names of renowned, qualified women for admission—to no avail. In 1888, Willits' name was submitted. She differed from previous women nominees in that she was not very well known. That year, her supporters vigorously lobbied members of the society to support her. Finally, on June 20, 1888, the society voted to admit her, and another barrier to women's acceptance as physicians was broken.

After the election, Willits continued to live her quiet life. In 1892, she began working at the State Hospital for the Insane at Norristown, Pennsylvania, the first mental hospital in the United States where women patients were entirely under the care of women physicians. At Norristown, she was a staff physician under Dr. Alice Bennett, and her duties included obtaining detailed histories of new admissions and the medical care of 900 women patients. Her career as a physician was cut short by cancer; she died from the disease on December 16, 1902.

See also Bennett, Alice

References

Peitzman, Steven J. 1979. "The Quiet Life of a Philadelphia Medical Woman: Mary Willits (1855–1902)." *Journal of the American Medical Women's Association* 34 (12):443–460.
Peitzman, Steven J. 1982. "The Society's First Woman Member: Mary Willits, M.D." *Philadelphia Medicine* 78 (January):22–24.

LS

Withington, Alfreda Bosworth (1860–1951)
Physician

Alfreda Withington described her life as a notable early American woman physician in her autobiography, *Mine Eyes Have Seen: A Woman Doctor's Saga* (1941). She was born in Germantown, Pennsylvania, on August 15, 1860, to James Harvey and Alfreda (Bosworth) Withington. She received her early education at the Hicksite Quaker School and from her father and brother, George. In 1881, she earned a B.A. degree from Cornell University in New York. Her interest in medicine was sparked by the death of family members from tuberculosis. When her brother, George, died from the same disease in 1881, she wrote: "If I had known more of illness, and the means of combating it, I might have been able to do more for [George]. Out of these emotions came a decision which set the course of my life. I would become a doctor" (1945, p. 21).

Despite family opposition, Withington entered the Woman's Medical College of the New York Infirmary in 1883, founded by Dr. Elizabeth Blackwell 15 years earlier. Withington graduated in 1887 and then completed an internship at the infirmary. Afterward, she furthered her education at European hospitals and clinics. She arrived in Vienna in September 1888, where she was the first woman admitted to the K.K. Allgemeines Kranken-

haus teaching hospital. She studied obstetrics, gynecology, and surgery and was also the first woman to perform an autopsy at the hospital. In 1889, she moved on to Prague and became the first woman resident physician at the Czech National Obstetrical Hospital. The following year, she attempted to earn a post in a Dresden hospital but was refused because she was female.

When Withington returned to the United States in 1891, she opened a medical and surgical practice in Pittsfield, Massachusetts, and joined the staff of Berkshire County's House of Mercy Hospital. She was also elected by the Berkshire County Medical Society as delegate to the state society, the first woman so honored. She later served as the first woman president of the County Medical Society (1906–1907).

During the summer of 1907, Withington volunteered for the Labrador Medical Mission, formed to meet the health needs of fishermen in that area. At the end of the summer, she returned to Pittsfield and was instrumental in the formation of a Tuberculosis Society, which in turn established a tuberculosis hospital. She was also involved in forming the Berkshire chapter of the American National Red Cross. In 1917, she went abroad with the Red Cross as the chief physician at the Franco-American Dispensary in Dreux, France, despite objections by male physicians to a woman chief physician. When her tenure came to a close, she was sent to Paris as a consultant and examiner at the Refugee Clinic. However, she returned to Dreux shortly after leaving, as many of the same doctors who opposed her appointment urged her to return.

Soon after returning to Pittsfield in 1921, Withington responded to an announcement in the *Journal of the American Medical Association* seeking a woman physician to serve in the remote Kentucky mountains. She was accepted and left for Kentucky in the spring of 1924. In *Mine Eyes Have Seen*, she describes her life as a mountain doctor: "To patients who could pay I charged a small fee to preserve their self-respect. I kept no regular surgery hours, for those seeking medical attention came when they could. Most of the time between was spent calling on patients, climbing up and down the steep trails on [my horse]" (1945, p. 217). She also established a public health program, provided physical examinations and inoculations, educated her patients on preventive medicine, and introduced pre- and postnatal care to the area.

Withington is also notable for her work as a biographer of other women physicians. In *Mine Eyes Have Seen*, she paid tribute to the women pioneers who came before her by weaving their story within the context of her own. Additionally, she wrote biographies of women for *A Cyclopedia of American Medical Biography* (1912) and for the *Dictionary of American Medical Biography* (1928). She died in Pittsfield General Hospital on October 1, 1951.

See also Blackwell, Elizabeth

References

Leonard, John William, ed. 1914. *Woman's Who's Who of America*. New York: American Commonwealth.

"Obituary." 1951. *New York Times* (October 2): 27.

Withington, Alfreda. 1932. "Mountain Doctor." Series in *Atlantic Monthly* 150 (3, 4, 6):257–267, 469–476, 768–774.

Withington, Alfreda. 1945. *Mine Eyes Have Seen: A Woman Doctor's Saga*. Reprint ed. London: Robert Hale.

JSB

Y

Yarros, Rachelle Slobodinsky (1869–1946)
Physician

Rachelle Yarros was an obstetrician and gynecologist during her early career. She later expanded her work to include activism in social causes that affected the health and welfare of women. She was born on May 18, 1869, in Berdechev, Russia, to Joachim and Bernice Slobodinsky. She emigrated to the United States as a teenager, forced to leave Russia for her involvement in subversive political activities.

In 1890, Yarros entered the College of Physicians and Surgeons in Boston as its first woman student. After one year, she matriculated at the Woman's Medical College of Pennsylvania in Philadelphia. She earned an M.D. in 1893, interned for one year at New England Hospital for Women and Children, and then completed postdoctoral work in pediatrics at the New York Infirmary for Women and Children. In 1894, she married Victor Yarros, and the couple moved to Chicago, where they adopted a daughter, Elise Donaldson. Yarros completed postdoctoral studies and a medical residency at the Michael Reese Hospital and opened a private obstetrical and gynecological practice (1895).

In 1897 Yarros was appointed instructor of obstetrics at the College of Physicians and Surgeons of Chicago (later, the University of Illinois medical school). At that time, she was one of only two women in the United States teaching medicine in coeducational classes. From 1902 to 1926, she was associate professor of obstetrics, the first woman to achieve that rank at a coeducational institution. Her most notable work as a teacher was the establishment of an obstetrical dispensary in a Near West Side Chicago neighborhood in 1897, where students from the College of Physicians and Surgeons received hands-on obstetrical training. During this 12-year teaching effort, she brought the most advanced obstetric care to poor families and elevated standards for obstetric teaching and practice. In addition to her teaching duties, she was associate director of Chicago Lying-In Hospital.

From 1907 to 1927, Yarros and her husband lived at Hull House, a settlement house in Chicago, where she became active in several social reform movements directly concerned with the health of women. She began a birth control education campaign to help poor women avoid the financial and health difficulties associated with consecutive childbirths. She established the Birth Control Committee of the Chicago Woman's Club

(1915), which eventually became the Illinois Birth Control League, and was director of the organization. In 1923, she was urged by Margaret Sanger to establish Chicago's first birth control clinic. The clinic was opened in a poor Chicago neighborhood, and by 1930, she had established eight clinics in other impoverished Chicago neighborhoods.

As a prominent member of the social hygiene movement Yarros was instrumental in founding the American Social Hygiene Association (1914). The association's purpose was to reduce venereal disease by dealing with prostitution as a health problem rather than as a moral issue. A year later, she became vice president of the Illinois Social Hygiene League. In addition, she led social hygiene programs for the Illinois Board of Health and the Chicago Health Department and served as consultant on venereal diseases to the U.S. Public Health Service. In 1925, she traveled to Paris, Berlin, and London to study venereal disease and its relation to prostitution. During the 1920s, she delivered lectures on sex education to groups of young people. For her efforts in this field, the University of Illinois School of Medicine created a professorship for her in the newly formed Social Hygiene Department in 1926.

As an extension of her work in sex education and social hygiene, Yarros opened a nursery and a premarital counseling clinic. In 1933, she published *Modern Woman and Sex*, in which she supported equality in marriage, liberalization of divorce laws, sex education for youth and adults, birth control, and marital counseling. True to her concerns for the working class, she reissued a less expensive version of *Modern Woman and Sex*, as *Sex Problems in Modern Society* (1938). Her thoughts on social causes and medicine were summarized in her unpublished autobiography: "The enlightened, socially-minded doctor will sympathize with labor,

with victims of exploitation and industrial autocracy, with the . . . delinquents who are the products of slums and blighted, ugly depressing districts. He will work and fight for ripe and genuine reforms" (*Journal of Social Hygiene* [1946]: 332).

In 1939, Yarros suffered a heart attack and moved to Florida and then to California. She died in San Diego in 1946 of congestive heart failure and heart disease.

See also Sanger, Margaret Louise Higgins

Selected Additional Achievements

"Birth Control and Democracy," *World Democracy* (September 1925); "Birth Control and Its Relation to Health and Welfare," *Medical Woman's Journal* (October 1925); "Women Physicians and the Problems of Women," *Medical Woman's Journal* (January 1943); "Training and Guidance in Recreation," *Journal of Social Hygiene* (February 1929); "Social Hygiene Observations in Soviet Russia," *Journal of Social Hygiene* (November 1930). Honorary life membership, American Social Hygiene Association; fellow, American College of Surgeons; president, West Side Branch of the Chicago Medical Society.

References

"In Memoriam: Tributes to Social Hygiene Pioneers." 1946. *Journal of Social Hygiene* 32:329–332.

Lasch, Christopher. 1971. "Yarros, Rachelle Slobodinsky." In *Notable American Women, 1607–1950: A Biographical Dictionary*, edited by E.T. James, J.W. James, and P.S. Boyer. Cambridge: Belknap Press of Harvard University Press.

The National Cyclopaedia of American Biography. 1949. Vol. 35. New York: James T. White.

Van Hoosen, Bertha. 1931. "Dr. Rachel Yarros: Physician, Scientist, Humanitarian." *Medical Woman's Journal* 38 (1): 10–24.

Yarros, Rachelle S. 1933. *Modern Woman and Sex: A Feminist Physician Speaks.* New York: Vanguard Press.

JSB

Yeomans, Amelia Le Sueur (1842–1913)
Physician

Amelia Le Sueur Yeomans was a pioneer Canadian physician, suffragist, and social reformer. She was born in Quebec in 1842 to Peter and Barbara (Dawson) Le Sueur and was educated in private schools in Montreal, Quebec, and Toronto, Ontario.

In 1860, she married American army surgeon Augustus A. Yeomans. The couple settled in Winnipeg and had three daughters. Sometime after her husband's death, Yeomans decided to become a physician. She enrolled in the Department of Medicine at the University of Michigan in Ann Arbor in 1880, where her daughter, Lilian, had already been studying for one year. Lilian graduated in 1882 and returned to Winnipeg to establish a practice specializing in midwifery and diseases of women and children. Although credit is given to Lilian for being the first woman to practice medicine in Winnipeg, she is not as well known as her mother.

Yeomans graduated in 1883 and joined her daughter in Winnipeg, becoming the second female doctor in the city. In the 1880s Winnipeg was rapidly becoming one of the largest cities in Canada. Along with this growth came the amplification of social problems, and Yeomans found herself compelled to provide health care for the poor and disadvantaged in the community. Her role soon extended beyond that of physician as she campaigned for improved housing, increased wages, and better working conditions for laborers, especially those who were female.

Yeomans crusaded against prostitution and drunkenness, which she considered to be the basis of the moral decay of society. She was an active member in, and served as the president of, the Dominion Women's Christian Temperance Union. In public addresses she used graphic detail, unusual during the Victorian era, to describe the devastating effects of venereal disease on the lives of her young female patients. She also publicly appealed to the male citizenry's sense of social responsibility by charging them to protect young women from a life of prostitution and its unhealthy consequences, rather than condemning their behavior.

Tightly linked with Yeomans' crusades against drunkenness and prostitution was her commitment to the suffragist movement. She believed that women could gain equality only when men were sober and did not partake in licentious activities, so she helped establish the Equal Franchise Association in 1894. The association generated a large amount of public support and forced the Winnipeg police to stop ignoring public drunkenness and prostitution and to begin to imposing fines and making arrests.

Yeomans died in 1913, three years before legislation for both prohibition and suffrage was enacted in Manitoba.

References

Hacker, Carlotta. 1974. *The Indomitable Lady Doctors.* Toronto: Clarke, Irwin.
Time Links: Dr. Amelia Yeomans. Online. http://timelinks.merlin.mb.ca/referenc/db0014.htm. 10 September 1998.

CMB

Z

Zabriskie, Louise (1887–1957)
Nurse

Triumphing over a severe handicap that greatly limited her physical abilities, Louise Zabriskie became a prominent maternity educator. She devoted her life to improving the care of mothers and their babies. She was born in Preston City, Connecticut, in 1887. After a career in teaching was cut short by illness, she underwent an operation in a New York hospital. She was so impressed by a nurse who cared for her that she decided to apply for nursing school.

Zabriskie graduated from New York Hospital School of Nursing in 1913 and did graduate work in New York City at Teachers College, Columbia University and at New York University. Following graduation from nursing school, she worked as a night supervisor at New York Lying-In Hospital and as a public health nurse in Nashville, Tennessee. In 1919, she became a staff nurse for the Maternity Center Association (MCA) in New York City. Recognizing the connection between maternal health and the mortality rate of newborns, she worked to improve the prenatal care of mothers through her position at the MCA. She was soon promoted to assistant field director to teach other nurses the basics of prenatal care.

In 1922, Zabriskie was seriously injured in an automobile accident and suffered a broken neck. She was severely handicapped for the remainder of her life but was determined not to let the disability impede her work. After returning to work, she was promoted to field director of the MCA in 1923. In 1929, her book *Nurses Handbook of Obstetrics* was published, followed by *Baby Care in Pictures* in 1935. She conducted seminars and consultations for parents as well as other maternity care providers and was a frequent contributor to professional journals.

Zabriskie continued her work after founding the Maternity Consultation Service in New York City in 1939 and served as director of the service from its creation until 1957. The Maternity Consultation Service offered free classes to prospective mothers and was the first in the country to offer courses for prospective fathers as well. In 1946, Zabriskie began writing a regular column for *My Baby Magazine*. In addition, she served as a lecturer at New York University School of Education in 1952.

Zabriskie died on December 12, 1957, in New York City of pernicious anemia.

Selected Additional Achievements

Board member, National Council on Family Relations, National Nursing Council, Frontier Nursing Service; member, Nursing Committee, Planned Parenthood Federation of America.

References

DeVincenzo, Doris K. 1988. "Louise Zabriskie." In *American Nursing: A Biographical Dictionary*, edited by V.L. Bullough, O.M. Church, and A.P. Stein. New York: Garland.

Hawkins, Joellen Watson. 1988. "Zabriskie, Lou-ise." In *Dictionary of American Nursing Biography*, edited by M. Kaufman. New York: Greenwood Press.

"Louise Zabriskie." 1958. *American Journal of Nursing* 58 (June):802–803.

Taves, Isabella. 1945. *Successful Women: And How They Attained Success.* New York: E.P. Dutton.

DTW

Zakrzewska, Marie Elizabeth (1829–1902)
Physician

Marie Zakrzewska (pronounced Zak-*shef-ska*) was a pioneering American woman physician. She founded New England Hospital for Women and Children, the second all-female hospital in the country. The hospital was dedicated to the clinical training of women physicians and nurses and to the medical care of women.

Zakrzewska was born on September 6, 1829, in Berlin, Germany, the eldest of seven children of Ludwig Martin Zakrzewska and Frederika C. W. (Urban) Zakrzewska. In 1840, Frederika entered the school for mid-

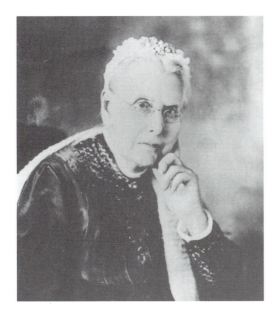

Marie Elizabeth Zakrzewska. Archives & Special Collections on Women in Medicine, MCP Hahnemann University.

wives at the Royal Hospital Charité in Berlin. In the midst of her mother's residency, the 10-year-old Zakrzewska contracted an eye infection, leaving her temporarily blinded. The frightened girl went to live with her mother at the hospital and was treated by Dr. Johannes Müller. Dr. Müller was so impressed with his "little blind doctor" that he allowed Zakrzewska to accompany him on rounds and lent her books on surgery and midwifery (Zakrzewska, p. 17).

At 13 years of age, Zakrzewska left school and spent her time reading medical works. She also accompanied her mother on midwifery calls, further developing her interest in medicine. At 18, she applied to the Royal Hospital Charité for formal training but was rejected twice for being too young. She was finally admitted at the age of 20 after she befriended Dr. Joseph Herman Schmidt, professor and director of the school for midwifery.

Schmidt was impressed with Zakrzewska's talents and made her his teaching assistant during her second year. The doctor was ill and planned to have Zakrzewska take over his position and to install her as chief midwife of the hospital upon her graduation. His plans stirred a heated debate in the medical community, and many of the male physicians at the hospital opposed her appointment. Dr. Schmidt, using political favors owed to him, was successful in his endeavor. She graduated in 1851 and on May 15, 1852, began her new duties; however, Schmidt died the next day. Without his support, opposition to her placement grew, and the "position soon be-came very disagreeable," forcing her to re-sign after only six months (Zakrzewska, p. 56).

In the meantime, Zakrzewska had heard positive reports of the Female (later, Woman's) Medical College of Pennsylvania. She left Germany in 1853, hoping to con-tinue her medical career freely in the United States. She arrived in New York and opened a private practice but was unable to find even one patient. She soon discovered that "fe-male physicians in this country were of the lowest rank and that they did not even hold the position of a good nurse" (Zakrzewska, p. 84).

In 1854, Zakrzewska met Elizabeth Black-well, the first woman to earn a medical de-gree in the United States. Blackwell tutored Zakrzewska in English and helped her apply to medical colleges. While waiting to be ad-mitted, Zakrzewska worked in Blackwell's women's hospital. In the fall of 1854, she was accepted to Western Reserve University in Cleveland, where Blackwell's sister, Emily, had earned her medical degree.

Zakrzewska was one of four women in a class of 200 (one of these four was Cordelia Greene, who would later head the Castile Sanitarium in New York). Zakrzewska de-scribed her experiences in her autobiography, *A Woman's Quest* (1924). She wrote that "[the] young men did not like our presence; some of the professors acted as if we did not exist" (p. 126). The male students circulated a petition asking that the women leave at the end of the term. The faculty's response was a promise to accept no more women.

Zakrzewska graduated in 1856 and re-turned to New York to join Elizabeth and Emily Blackwell in their endeavor to open the New York Infirmary for Women and Children. Zakrzewska traveled to Boston and Philadelphia to secure financial support for the infirmary. The infirmary was the first hos-pital in the United States to be staffed en-tirely by women and provided women opportunities for the clinical experience that they could not get elsewhere. Zakrzewska

served as a resident physician and as general manager for two years.

In 1859, Zakrzewska accepted an invita-tion to serve as professor of obstetrics and diseases of women and children and as resi-dent physician at the New England Female Medical College in Boston. However, she was disappointed at the inadequate educa-tional standards of the hospital. The school's founder, Samuel Gregory, was not a medical doctor and did not share Zakrzewska's pas-sion for providing a superior medical educa-tion for women. She was convinced that the women students were unfit to serve as phy-sicians, and she refused to sign the degrees for the first graduating class. Increasingly dis-satisfied, she resigned in 1862.

With the help of several board members and trustees of the Female Medical College, Zakrzewska founded New England Hospital for Women and Children in July 1862. The hospital was the first of its kind in New Eng-land and the second of its kind in the country (after Blackwell's). Although she supported coeducation, she limited staff to women be-cause few hospitals would admit women phy-sicians for clinical training. The hospital trained many women physicians, including Lucy Sewall, who served as resident physi-cian. In 1881, Zakrzewska began requiring that all women entering her hospital for clin-ical training have a medical degree. She served the hospital in many capacities for a period of 40 years.

Zakrzewska's adherence to high standards in her training courses helped contribute to the eventual acceptance of women as physi-cians. She never married or had children, de-voting her life to her cause. She wrote in *A Woman's Quest* that "[we] stood no longer alone as the bearers of an idea—hundreds of young women had joined us. The path had been broken; and the profession had been obliged to yield, and to acknowledge the ca-pacity of women as physicians" (pp. 358–359). She retired in 1899, suffering from ar-teriosclerosis and heart disease. She died from a stroke on May 12, 1902, at her home in Jamaica Plain, Massachusetts.

See also Blackwell, Elizabeth; Blackwell,

Emily; Greene, Cordelia Agnes; Sewall, Lucy Ellen

Selected Additional Achievements

Zakrzewska, Marie E., *A Practical Illustration of "Woman's Right to Labor,"* edited by Caroline H. Dall. Boston: Walker, Wise, 1860.

References

Blake, John B. 1971. "Zakrzewska, Marie Elizabeth." In *Notable American Women, 1607–1950: A Biographical Dictionary*, edited by E.T. James, J.W. James, and P.S. Boyer. Cambridge: Belknap Press of Harvard University Press.

Drachman, Virginia G. 1985. "Zakrzewska, Marie Elizabeth." In *American Reformers: An H.W. Wilson Biographical Dictionary*, edited by A. Whitman. New York: H.W. Wilson.

Kelly, Howard A., and Walter L. Burrage, eds. 1928. *Dictionary of American Medical Biography: Lives of Eminent Physicians of the United States and Canada, from the Earliest Times*. New York: D. Appleton.

Kingston, Maureen A. 1994. "Marie E. Zakrzewska." In *Women Educators in the United States, 1820–1993: A Bio-bibliographical Sourcebook*, edited by M.S. Seller. Westport, Conn.: Greenwood Press.

Viets, Henry R. 1936. "Zakrzewska, Marie Elizabeth." In *The Dictionary of American Biography*, edited by D. Malone. New York: Charles Scribner's Sons.

Zakrzewska, Marie E. 1972. *A Woman's Quest: The Life of Marie E. Zakrzewska, M.D.* Edited by A.C. Vietor. New York: Arno Press. Original ed., New York: D. Appleton, 1924.

JSB

Appendix I: List of Women by Occupation

MIDWIVES

Aragon, Jesusita

Armstrong, Penny Bradbury

Ballard, Martha Moore

Beeman, Ruth Coates

Berryhill, Elizabeth

Breckinridge, Mary

Browne, Helen Edith

Burton, Pearlie

Callen, Maude Evelyn

Erickson, Hilda Anderson

Ernst, Eunice Katherine MacDonald [Kitty]

Führer, Charlotte Heise

Gaskin, Ina May

Goggans, Lalla Mary

Goldman, Emma

Hale, Mamie Odessa

Hamilton, Elizabeth Jane Soley

Hogan, Aileen I.

Hutchinson, Anne Marbury

James, Susan Gail

Lang, Raven

Leonard, Carol L.

Logan, Onnie Lee

Lubic, Ruth Watson

Mageras, Georgia Lathouris

Mason, Biddy [Bridget]

McDougall, Adelaide

McNaught, Rose Madeline

Milton, Gladys

Murdaugh, Mary Angela

Nichols, [Margaret Carrie] Etta Grigsby

Pelletier, Henriette Blier

Peterson, Mary

Porn, Hanna

Reinders, Agnes Shoemaker [Sister M. Theophane]

Richardson, Luba Lyons

Ross, Marie-Henriette LeJeune

Sessions, Patty Bartlett

Sharpless, Amy Mildred

Smith, Margaret Charles

Van Blarcom, Carolyn Conant

Ventre, Fran

Willeford, Mary Bristow

NURSES

Aikens, Charlotte Albina

Arnstein, Margaret Gene

Barton, Clarissa Harlowe [Clara]

Batterham, Mary Rose

Beard, Mary

Bickerdyke, Mary Ann Ball

Birtles, Mary Ellen

Blanchfield, Florence Aby

Butler, Ida de Fatio

Clayton, S. Lillian

Corbin, Hazel

Crandall, Ella Phillips

Davis, Frances Elliott

Davis, Mary E.P.

Delano, Jane Arminda

Deming, Dorothy

Dix, Dorothea Lynde

Dock, Lavinia Lloyd

Dyke, Eunice Henrietta

Fagin, Claire Mintzer

Foley, Edna Lois

Franklin, Martha Minerva

Freeman, Ruth Benson

Gardner, Mary Sewall

Gault, Alma Elizabeth

Geister, Janet Marie Louise Sophie

Goodrich, Annie Warburton

Gunn, Jean Isabel

Hall, Lydia Eloise

Hegan, Eliza Parks

Henderson, Virginia Avenel

Jean, Sally Lucas

Johns, Ethel Mary Incledon

Jumper, Betty Mae Tiger

Kinney, Dita Hopkins

Leete, Harriet L.

Leone, Lucile Petry

Livingston, Nora G.E. [Gertrude Elizabeth]

Logan, Laura Rebekah

Loveridge, Emily Lemoine

Lytle, Nancy A.

Macleod, Charlotte

Mahoney, Mary Eliza

Mance, Jeanne

Maxwell, Anna Caroline

McMaster, Elizabeth Jennet

Minnigerode, Lucy

Mundinger, Mary O'Neil

Noyes, Clara Dutton

Nutting, [Mary] Adelaide

Ohlson, Agnes K.

Osborne, Geneva Estelle Massey Riddle

Osborne, Mary D.

Palmer, Sophia French

Peplau, Hildegard E.

Phillips, Harriet Newton

Porter, Elizabeth Kerr

Reiter, Frances Ursula

Richards, Linda Ann Judson

Robb, Isabel Adams Hampton

Roberts, Mary May

Rogers, Martha Elizabeth

Sanger, Margaret Louise Higgins

Schlotfeldt, Rozella May

Seton, Elizabeth Ann Bayley

Shaw, Flora Madeline

Sheahan, Marion Winifred

Smellie, Elizabeth Lawrie

Snively, Mary Agnes

Staupers, Mabel Keaton

Stewart, Isabel Maitland

Stimson, Julia Catherine

Sutliffe, Irene H.

Taylor, Euphemia Jane [Effie]

Thoms, Adah Belle Samuels

Titus, Shirley Carew

Tompkins, Sally Louisa

Wald, Florence Schorske

Wald, Lillian D.

Wattleton, [Alyce] Faye

Weeks Shaw, Clara Shaw

Zabriskie, Louise

PHYSICIANS

Abbott, Maude Elizabeth Seymour

Alexander, Virginia M.

Angwin, Maria L.

Apgar, Virginia

Bagshaw, Elizabeth

Baker, S. [Sara] Josephine

Barringer, Emily Dunning

Barry, James Miranda Stuart

Bass, [Mary] Elizabeth

Bates, Mary Elizabeth

Bennett, Alice

Black, Elinor Frances Elizabeth

Blackwell, Elizabeth

Blackwell, Emily

Broomall, Anna Elizabeth

Brown, Charlotte Amanda Blake

Brown, Dorothy Lavinia

Buckel, C. [Cloe] Annette

Calderone, Mary Steichen

Chinn, May Edward

Clark, Nancy Talbot

Cleaves, Margaret Abigail

Cleveland, Emeline Horton

Cole, Rebecca J.

Comfort, Anna Amelia Manning

Craighill, Margaret

Crumpler, Rebecca Davis Lee

Cushier, Elizabeth

Daniel, Annie Sturges

Darrow, Anna Albertina Lindstedt

Dickey, Nancy Wilson

Dimock, Susan

Dixon Jones, Mary Amanda

Dodge, Eva Francette

Dolley, Sarah Read Adamson

Duckering, Florence West

Eliot, Martha May

Follansbee, Elizabeth A.

Fowler, Lydia Folger

Gannt, Love Rosa Hirschmann

Gleason, Rachel Brooks

Greene, Cordelia Agnes

Guion, Connie Myers

Gullen, Augusta Stowe

Hamilton, Alice

Hastings, Caroline Eliza

Howell, Mary Catherine Raugust

Hunt, Harriot Kezia

Hurd-Mead, Kate Campbell

Hurdon, Elizabeth

Huson, Florence

Jackson, Mary Percy

Jacobi, Mary Corinna Putnam

Johnson, Halle Tanner Dillon

La Roe, Else Kienle

L'Esperance Elise Depew Strang

Lockrey, Sarah Hunt

Longshore, Hannah E. Myers

Love, Susan M.

Lovejoy, Esther Pohl

Lozier, Clemence Sophia Harned

MacMurchy, Helen

Magee, Joni Lahr

Marshall, Clara

Matheson, Elizabeth Beckett Scott

Mayo, Sara Tew

McGee, Anita Newcomb

McKane, Alice Woodby

McKinney Steward, Susan Maria Smith

McLean, Mary Hancock

Mendenhall, Dorothy Reed

Mergler, Marie Josepha

Merrick, Myra King

Minoka-Hill, Lillie Rosa

Morani, Alma Dea

Morton, Rosalie Slaughter

Mosher, Clelia Duel

Mosher, Eliza Maria

Nichols, Mary Sargeant Neal Gove

Novello, Antonia Coello

Owens-Adair, Bethenia Angelina

Parker, Valeria Hopkins

Picotte, Susan La Flesche

Preston, Ann

Putnam, Helen Cordelia

Robertson, Jennie Smillie

Ross, Charlotte Whitehead

Roys-Gavitt, Elmina M.

Rutherford, Frances Armstrong

Sabin, Florence Rena

Safford, Mary Jane

Sewall, Lucy Ellen

Sherwood, Mary

Shipp, Ellis Reynolds

Shortt, Elizabeth Smith

Sirridge, Marjorie

Stevenson, Sarah Ann Hackett

Stone, Hannah Mayer

Stowe, Emily Jennings

Sturgis, Katharine Rosenbaum Boucot

Taussig, Helen Brooke

Thomas, Mary Frame Myers

Thompson, Mary Harris

Trout, Jenny Kidd

Van Hoosen, Bertha

Walker, Mary Edwards

Warner, Estella Ford

Welsh, Lilian

Willits, Mary

Withington, Alfreda Bosworth

Yarros, Rachelle Slobodinsky

Yeomans, Amelia Le Sueur

Zakrzewska, Marie Elizabeth

Appendix II: Notable Events Related to Women Healers

1607	Jamestown, Virginia founded.
1608	Quebec founded.
Ca. 1634–1643	**Anne Marbury Hutchinson** (ca. 1591–1643) practices midwifery in the Massachusetts Bay Colony. In colonial and early American times, childbirth was regarded as a natural, woman-centered event, with the midwife as primary attendant and caregiver.
1642	Ville Marie (Montreal) established. There, **Jeanne Mance** (1606–1673) founds the Hôtel-Dieu, one of the first hospitals in North America. Mance is considered the first lay nurse in Canada.
1763	France cedes Canada to Britain.
1776	The Declaration of Independence is signed.
1785–1812	**Martha Moore Ballard** (1735–1812) keeps a diary of her midwifery practice in Maine. By this time, male physicians are replacing female midwives in the birthing rooms of urban women.
1835	**Harriot Kezia Hunt** (1805–1875) begins practicing medicine in the United States; she is considered to be the first American woman to practice medicine.
1838	In Boston, water cure physician **Mary Sargeant Neal Gove Nichols** (1810–1884) gives a course of lectures on anatomy and physiology, the first such lectures given by a woman.
1848	The first women's rights convention in the United States is held in Seneca Falls, New York. Participants produce a Declaration of Sentiments, listing the grievances of American women.
1848	Samuel Gregory establishes a school of midwifery in Boston, the New England Female Medical College. (In the 1850s, it becomes a training school for women physicians.)
1849	**Elizabeth Blackwell** (1821–1910), graduates from Geneva Medical College in western New York, becoming the first woman to earn an M.D.
1849	The first co-educational medical school in the United States, Central Medical College, in Syracuse, New York, opens.

1850	The first women's medical school, Female (later, Woman's) Medical College of Pennsylvania is established in Philadelphia. The school becomes the primary training ground for women physicians and continues long after other women's medical colleges close. (It becomes co-educational in the 1970s and continues today as MCP Hahnemann University.)
1857	**James Miranda Stuart Barry** (ca. 1795–1865), is assigned by the British army to the post of inspector general of hospitals in Montreal, becoming the first female physician to practice medicine in Canada. (This fact is not known until after her death; Barry, who earned a medical degree in Scotland in 1812, led her life disguised as a man.)
1857	The New York Infirmary for Women and Children, the first American hospital administered entirely by women, is established by physicians **Elizabeth Blackwell** (1821–1910), **Emily Blackwell** (1826–1910), and **Marie Elizabeth Zakrzewska** (1829–1902).
1861	The American Civil War begins. Thousands of women like **Mary Ann Ball Bickerdyke** (1817–1901), **Clarissa [Clara] Harlowe Barton** (1821–1912), and **Sally Louisa Tompkins** (1833–1916) volunteer as nurses.
1861	**Dorothea Lynde Dix** (1802–1887) is appointed Superintendent of Women Nurses for the Union Army.
1862	Physician **Marie Elizabeth Zakrzewska** (1829–1902) founds the New England Hospital for Women and Children in Boston.
1864	**Rebecca Davis Lee Crumpler** (1831–1895) graduates from New England Female Medical College in Boston, becoming the first African American woman to earn a medical degree in the United States.
1866	**Mary Edwards Walker** (1832–1919), a volunteer surgeon during the Civil War, becomes the first and only woman to earn the Congressional Medal of Honor. (The award is rescinded in 1917, but reinstated in 1977.)
1867	The Dominion of Canada is established with the passage of the British North America Act.
1867	**Emily Jennings Stowe** (1831–1903), the first Canadian-born woman to practice medicine in Canada, graduates from the New York Medical College and Hospital for Women (Homeopathic).
1868	Physicians **Elizabeth Blackwell** (1821–1910) and **Emily Blackwell** (1826–1910) found the Woman's Medical College of the New York Infirmary for Women and Children. (The school lasts until 1899, when Cornell University Medical College begins accepting women students.)
1873	The first hospital-based nurse training schools patterned on famed English nurse Florence Nightingale's model are established in New York City; New Haven, Connecticut; and Boston.
1873	**Linda Ann Judson Richards** (1841–1930) earns a diploma from the nurse training school at New England Hospital for Women and Children. (Often considered America's first trained nurse, Richards actually graduated several years after lesser-known nurse **Harriet Newton Phillips** (1819–1901) was trained at Woman's Hospital in Philadelphia.)
1873	The Comstock Act (U.S.) passes. The law severely hinders efforts to distribute information on birth control, as it defines such information as obscene.

1875   Nurse **Elizabeth Jennet McMaster** (1847–1903) founds Canada's first children's hospital, the Toronto Hospital for Sick Children.

1876   Physician **Mary Corinna Putnam Jacobi** (1842–1906) becomes the first woman to win Harvard's Boylston Prize; her essay is entitled "The Question of Rest for Women during Menstruation."

1876   Physician **Sarah Ann Hackett Stevenson** (1841–1909) becomes the first female member of the American Medical Association.

1879   **Mary Eliza Mahoney** (1845–1926), the first African American woman to earn a degree in nursing graduates from the nursing school at New England Hospital for Women and Children.

1881   Nurse **Clarissa [Clara] Harlowe Barton**, (1821–1912) founds the American Red Cross.

1883   Through the efforts of physicians **Jenny Kidd Trout** (1841–1921) and **Emily Jennings Stowe** (1831–1903), Women's Medical College in Kingston, Ontario and Woman's Medical College in Toronto open.

1885   **Clara Shaw Weeks Shaw** (1857–1940), the first American nurse to write a textbook on nursing, publishes *A Text-Book of Nursing for the Use of Training Schools, Families, and Private Students.*

1889   **Susan La Flesche Picotte** (1865–1915), the first Native American woman to earn a medical degree, graduates from Woman's Medical College of Pennsylvania.

1892   Physician **Clelia Duel Mosher** (1863–1940) begins a thirty-year survey on women's sexuality, which refutes the Victorian notion of the passionless woman. (The survey remains unpublished until 1980.)

1893   In New York, **Lillian D. Wald** (1867–1940) founds the Nurses' Settlement, later called the Henry Street Settlement. Wald's work with this visiting nurse service helps to define the field of public health nursing.

1893   Johns Hopkins Medical School opens, with a $500,000 gift from the women's community and the stipulation that it accept women students on an equal basis.

1893   The first national nursing organization in the United States, the American Society of Superintendents of Training Schools for Nurses of the United States and Canada, is founded. (It continues today as the National League for Nursing.)

1893   Physician **Elmina M. Roys-Gavitt** (1828–1898) founds and is first editor of *Woman's Medical Journal*. (Later entitled the *Medical Woman's Journal*, the journal is published until 1952.)

1896   The first general membership organization for nurses, the Nurses' Associated Alumnae of the United States and Canada, is founded. (It is renamed the American Nurses Association in 1911, and continues today.)

1897   The first visiting nurse service in Canada, the Victorian Order of Nurses, is established.

1900   The first nurse-owned and operated publication, the *American Journal of Nursing*, is established, with nurse **Sophia French Palmer** (1839–1920) as its first editor in chief.

1901   The Army Nurse Corps is established, largely through the efforts of physician **Anita Newcomb McGee** (1864–1940). Nurse **Dita Hopkins Kinney** (1854–1921) becomes the corps' first superintendent.

1902   North Carolina becomes the first state to require the registration of nurses.

1907   **[Mary] Adelaide Nutting** (1858–1948) becomes the first nurse to hold a professorship, with her appointment to the faculty of Teachers College, Columbia University.

1908   **Mary Agnes Snively** (1847–1933) helps found the Canadian National Association of Trained Nurses (it becomes the Canadian Nurses Association in 1924).

1908   **Martha Minerva Franklin** (1870–1968), **Adah Belle Samuels Thoms** (ca. 1863–1943), and other African American nurses found the National Association of Colored Graduate Nurses.

1910   The Flexner Report, which recommends more rigorous requirements for medical schools, is published. As a result of the report, many medical schools close and the number of women admitted to medical school begins to decline. (In this year, 9,000 women are practicing medicine in the United States.)

1910–1920   Between 1910 and 1920, physician opposition to midwives heightens, resulting in the decline of midwifery. Midwives deliver approximately 50 percent of all babies in the United States in 1910.

1913   The American College of Surgeons is founded and accepts women, including **Florence West Duckering** (1869–1951) and **Elizabeth Hurdon** (1868–1941).

1915   Physician **Bertha Van Hoosen** (1863–1952) founds the American Medical Women's Association.

1914–1918   World War I.

1916   Nurse **Margaret Louise Higgins Sanger** (1879–1966) and her sister open the first birth control clinic in the U.S. in Brooklyn, New York.

1916   **Mary Sewall Gardner** (1871–1961) publishes *Public Health Nursing*, the first textbook on the subject.

1917   McGill University in Montreal begins accepting women medical students.

1918   Women in Canada are granted the right to vote.

1918   A worldwide influenza epidemic strikes.

1918   The Maternity Center Association is established in New York City to combat high maternal and infant death rates.

1920   In the United States, the Nineteenth Amendment is ratified and women are granted the right to vote.

1921   The Sheppard-Tower Act passes. The legislation funds maternity, infant, and child hygiene programs, including midwife training programs. (It is repealed in 1929, with pressure from the American Medical Association.)

1921   Nurse **Margaret Louise Higgins Sanger** (1879–1966) founds the American Birth Control League, precursor to the Planned Parenthood Federation of America.

1923   The first extensive study of nursing education and practice, *Nursing and Nursing Education in the United States*, is published. The report advocates high standards in nursing education and leads to the establishment of a university school of nursing at Yale.

1924   The Federation of Medical Women of Canada is founded.

1925   Nurse-midwife **Mary Breckinridge** (1881–1965) establishes the Frontier Nursing Service (originally named the Kentucky Committee for Mothers and Babies), bringing the profession of nurse-midwifery to the United States.

1929   The U.S. stock market collapses, triggering a worldwide economic depression.

1932   Canada's first birth control clinic, the Birth Control Society, opens in Hamilton, Ontario. Physician **Elizabeth Bagshaw** (1881–1982) becomes the organization's first medical director.

1936   Comstock Act (U.S.) overturned; birth control information ruled not to be obscene.

1937   The Kate Depew Strang Cancer Prevention Clinic, the first clinic established to prevent cancer in women through early diagnosis (and the first cancer detection facility in the world), is founded by physician **Elise Depew Strang L'Esperance** (ca. 1878–1959).

1939–1945   World War II. Nursing comes to be a profession practiced chiefly in hospitals. (Before this, nurses were mostly self-employed and worked largely in private homes.)

1948   The American Nurses Association begins admitting African Americans; the National Association of Colored Graduate Nurses disbands three years later.

1952   Physician **Virginia Apgar** (1909–1974) introduces a method of evaluating the condition of newborn babies within one minute of birth. This method is still in use today.

1955   The American College of Nurse-Midwifery, the first national organization devoted solely to the professional needs and concerns of nurse-midwives is founded. (The name is changed to the American College of Nurse-Midwives in 1969, and the organization continues today.)

1963   The Loeb Center for Nursing and Rehabilitation in Bronx, New York, the first nurse-administered, in-patient institution is established with the help of **Lydia Eloise Hall** (1906–1969). (The center becomes a nursing home in 1984.)

1965   The United States Supreme Court declares the ban on birth control unconstitutional.

1969   Canada legalizes advertising for contraceptives and legalizes abortion in cases where a woman's life or health is jeopardized.

1971   *Our Bodies, Ourselves*, an outgrowth of the women's health movement, is published by the Boston Women's Health Book Collective. Women become interested in returning to natural childbirth, and lay midwives like **Raven Lang** (1942–   ) begin to practice.

1973   The U.S. Supreme Court rules in *Roe v. Wade* that a woman has a constitutional right to abortion.

1978   Nurse **[Alyce] Faye Wattleton** (1943–   ) becomes the first woman since **Margaret Louise Higgins Sanger** (1879–1966) and the first African American to head the Planned Parenthood Federation of America.

1982   The Midwives' Alliance of North America is founded by midwives, including **Carol L. Leonard** (1950–   ), **Ina May Gaskin** (1940–   ), and **Fran Ventre** (1941–   ).

1990   **Antonia Coello Novello** (1944–   ) becomes the first female U.S. Surgeon General.

1994   For the first time, more women than men enter training programs in the speciality of obstetrics and gynecology.

1998–1999   **Nancy Wilson Dickey** (1950–   ) serves as the first female president of the American Medical Association. At this point in time, 23 percent of all practicing physicians in the United States are women.

Selected Bibliography

Abram, Ruth J. 1985. *Send Us a Lady Physician: Women Doctors in America, 1835–1920*. New York: Norton.

Alsop, Gulielma Fell. 1950. *History of the Woman's Medical College, Philadelphia, Pennsylvania 1850–1950*. Philadelphia: J.B. Lippincott.

Apple, Rima D., ed. 1990. *Women, Health, and Medicine in America: A Historical Handbook*. New Brunswick, N.J.: Rutgers University Press.

Arms, Suzanne. 1975. *Immaculate Deception: A New Look at Women and Childbirth in America*. Boston: Houghton Mifflin.

Benoit, Cecilia. 1991. *Midwives in Passage: The Modernisation of Maternity Care*. St. John's, Nfld.: Institute of Social and Economic Research, Memorial University of Newfoundland.

Biggs, C. Lesley. 1983. "The Case of the Missing Midwives: A History of Midwifery in Ontario from 1795–1900." *Ontario History* 75 (1):21–35.

Boston Women's Health Book Collective. 1998. *Our Bodies, Ourselves for the New Century: A Book by and for Women*. Newly rev. and updated ed. New York: Simon and Schuster.

Bullough, Bonnie, Vern L. Bullough, and Barrett Elcano. 1981. *Nursing: A Historical Bibliography*. New York: Garland.

Bullough, Vern L., and Bonnie Bullough. 1978. *The Care of the Sick: The Emergence of Modern Nursing*. New York: Prodist.

Bullough, Vern L., Olga M. Church, and Alice P. Stein, eds. 1988. *American Nursing: A Biographical Dictionary*. Vol. 1. New York: Garland.

Bullough, Vern L., and Lilli Sentz, eds. 2000. *American Nursing: A Biographical Dictionary*. Vol. 3. New York: Springer.

Bullough, Vern L., Lilli Sentz, and Alice P. Stein, eds. 1992. *American Nursing: A Biographical Dictionary*. Vol. 2. New York: Garland.

Chaff, Sandra L. 1977. *Women in Medicine: A Bibliography of the Literature on Women Physicians*. Metuchen, N.J.: Scarecrow Press.

Chester, Penfield. 1997. *Sisters on a Journey: Portraits of American Midwives*. New Brunswick, N.J.: Rutgers University Press.

Cutter, Irving S., and Henry R. Viets. 1964. *A Short History of Midwifery*. Philadelphia: W.B. Saunders.

Dodd, Dianne, and Deborah Gorham, eds. 1994. *Caring and Curing: Historical Perspectives on Women and Healing in Canada, Social Sciences, Canadian Society*. Ottawa: University of Ottawa Press.

Donahue, M. Patricia. 1996. *Nursing, the Finest Art: An Illustrated History*. 2nd ed. St. Louis: Mosby.

Donegan, Jane B. 1978. *Women and Men Midwives: Medicine, Morality, and Misogyny in Early America.* Westport, Conn.: Greenwood Press.

Drachman, Virginia G. 1984. *Hospital with a Heart: Women Doctors and the Paradox of Separatism at the New England Hospital, 1862–1969.* Ithaca, N.Y.: Cornell University Press.

Edwards, Margot, and Mary Waldorf. 1984. *Reclaiming Birth: History and Heroines of American Childbirth Reform.* Trumansburg, N.Y.: Crossing Press.

Ehrenreich, Barbara, and Deirdre English. 1973. *Witches, Midwives, and Nurses: A History of Women Healers.* New York: Feminist Press at City University of New York.

Friedman, Emily, ed. 1994. *An Unfinished Revolution: Women and Health Care in America.* New York: United Hospital Fund.

Gevitz, Norman. 1987. "Sectarian Medicine." *JAMA* 257 (12):1636–1640.

Gibbon, John Murray, and Mary S. Mathewson. 1947. *Three Centuries of Canadian Nursing.* Toronto: Macmillan.

Hackett, Lise L. 1998. *Midwifery in Canada, 1980–1997: A Brief History and Selective Annotated Bibliography of Publications in English.* Halifax, Nova Scotia: School of Library and Information Studies, Dalhousie University.

Henderson, Virginia, ed. 1984. *Nursing Studies Index.* Reprint ed. Vols. 1–4. New York: Garland.

Herman, Kali. 1984. *Women in Particular: An Index to American Women.* Phoenix, Ariz.: Oryx Press.

Hurd-Mead, Kate Campbell. 1933. *Medical Women of America: A Short History of the Pioneer Medical Women of America and of a Few of Their Colleagues in England.* New York: Froben Press.

James, Edward T., Janet Wilson James, and Paul S. Boyer, eds. 1971. *Notable American Women, 1607–1950: A Biographical Dictionary.* Cambridge: Belknap Press of Harvard University Press.

Kaufman, Martin, ed. 1988. *Dictionary of American Nursing Biography.* New York: Greenwood Press.

Kaufman, Martin, Stuart Galishoff, and Todd L. Savitt, eds. 1984. *Dictionary of American Medical Biography.* Westport, Conn.: Greenwood Press.

Kelly, Howard A., and Walter L. Burrage, eds. 1928. *Dictionary of American Medical Biography: Lives of Eminent Physicians of the United States and Canada, from the Earliest Times.* New York: D. Appleton.

Lang, Raven. 1972. *Birth Book.* Palo Alto, Calif.: Genesis Press.

Leavitt, Judith Walzer, ed. 1984. *Women and Health in America: Historical Readings.* Madison: University of Wisconsin Press.

Leavitt, Judith Walzer. 1986. *Brought to Bed: Childbearing in America—1750–1950.* New York: Oxford University Press.

Leavitt, Judith Walzer. 1990. "Medicine in Context: A Review Essay of the History of Medicine." *American Historical Review* 95 (5):1471–1484.

Leavitt, Judith Walzer, ed. 1999. *Women and Health in America: Historical Readings.* 2nd ed. Madison: University of Wisconsin Press.

Litoff, Judy Barrett. 1978. *American Midwives: 1860 to the Present.* Westport, Conn.: Greenwood Press.

Lovejoy, Esther Pohl. 1957. *Women Doctors of the World.* New York: Macmillan.

Marshall, Clara. 1897. *The Woman's Medical College of Pennsylvania: An Historical Outline.* Philadelphia: P. Blakiston, Son.

Mason, Jutta. 1987. "A History of Midwifery in Canada." In *Report of the Task Force on the Implementation of Midwifery in Ontario.* Toronto, Ont.: Task Force.

McPherson, Kathryn M. 1996. *Bedside Matters: The Transformation of Canadian Nursing, 1900–1970.* Toronto: Oxford University Press.

Melosh, Barbara. 1982. *"The Physician's Hand": Work Culture and Conflict in American Nursing.* Philadelphia: Temple University Press.

Morantz-Sanchez, Regina Markell. 1985. *Sympathy and Science: Women Physicians in American Medicine.* New York: Oxford University Press.

Nutting, M. Adelaide, and Lavinia Lloyd Dock. 1907–1912. *A History of Nursing.* 4 vols. New York: G.P. Putnam's Sons.

Peitzman, Steven J. 2000. *A New and Untried Course: Woman's Medical College and Medical College of Pennsylvania, 1850–1998.* New Brunswick, N.J.: Rutgers University Press.

Pennock, Meta Rutter, ed. 1940. *Makers of Nursing History: Portraits and Pen Sketches of One-hundred and Nine Prominent Women.* New York: Lakeside.

Reid, Margaret. 1989. "Sisterhood and Professionalization: A Case Study of the American Lay Midwife." In *Women as Healers: Cross-Cultural Perspectives*, edited by C.S. McClain. New Brunswick, N.J.: Rutgers University Press.

Reverby, Susan. 1987. *Ordered to Care: The Dilemma of American Nursing, 1850–1945.* Cambridge: Cambridge University Press.

Rich, Adrienne. 1986. *Of Woman Born: Motherhood as Experience and Institution.* 10th anniversary ed. New York: W.W. Norton.

Roberts, Mary M. 1954. *American Nursing: History and Interpretation.* New York: Macmillan.

Ruzek, Sheryl Burt. 1978. *The Women's Health Movement: Feminist Alternatives to Medical Control.* New York: Praeger.

Scholten, Catherine M. 1977. " 'On the Importance of the Obstetrick Art': Changing Customs of Childbirth in America, 1760 to 1825." *William and Mary Quarterly* 34 (3):426–445.

Shoemaker, M. Theophane. 1984. *History of Nurse-Midwifery in the United States.* Reprint ed. New York: Garland.

Shryock, Richard Harrison. 1966. "Women in American Medicine." In *Medicine in America: Historical Essays*, edited by R.H. Shryock. Baltimore: Johns Hopkins University Press.

Sicherman, Barbara, and Carol Hurd Green, eds. 1980. *Notable American Women: The Modern Period: A Biographical Dictionary.* Cambridge: Belknap Press of Harvard University Press.

Snodgrass, Mary Ellen. 1999. *Historical Encyclopedia of Nursing.* Santa Barbara, Calif.: ABC-Clio.

Strong-Boag, Veronica. 1979. "Canada's Women Doctors: Feminism Constrained." In *A Not Unreasonable Claim: Women and Reform in Canada, 1880s–1920s*, edited by L. Kealey. Toronto: University of Toronto Press.

Strong-Boag, Veronica. 1991. "Making a Difference: The History of Canada's Nurses." *Canadian Bulletin of Medical History* 8 (2):231–248.

Tom, Sally Austen. 1978. "With Loving Hands: The Life Stories of Four Nurse-Midwives." Master's thesis, College of Nursing, University of Utah.

Tom, Sally Austen. 1982. "The Evolution of Nurse-Midwifery: 1900–1960." *Journal of Nurse-Midwifery* 27 (4):4–13.

Walsh, Mary Roth. 1977. *"Doctors Wanted, No Women Need Apply": Sexual Barriers in the Medical Profession, 1835–1975.* New Haven, Conn.: Yale University Press.

Wear, Delese, ed. 1996. *Women in Medical Education: An Anthology of Experience.* New York: State University of New York Press.

Wertz, Richard W., and Dorothy C. Wertz. 1977. *Lying In: A History of Childbirth in America.* New Haven, Conn.: Yale University Press.

Index

The page numbers set in **boldface** indicate the location of a main entry.

About the Authors and Contributors

LAURIE SCRIVENER is an assistant professor of bibliography and social sciences reference librarian at the University of Oklahoma Libraries. She earned a B.A. and an M.L.I.S. from the University of Oklahoma. Ms. Scrivener was a co-editor of the International Biographical Directory of National Archivists, Documentalists, and Librarians, second edition, and has been published in the *Journal of Government Information*.

J. SUZANNE BARNES currently works for Ebsco Subscription Services, Inc. in Los Angeles, California. She received both a B.A. and an M.L.I.S. from the University of Oklahoma. Ms. Barnes has worked for the University of Oklahoma Libraries, the Tulsa City-County Library System, the Santa Monica Public Library, and the Gemological Institute of America Library.

CECELIA M. BROWN is an assistant professor in the School of Library and Information Studies at the University of Oklahoma. She received her M.S. and Ph.D. in Nutritional Sciences from the University of Illinois at Urbana-Champaign, her M.L.I.S. at the University of Oklahoma, and her B.A.Sc. in Applied Human Nutrition from the University of Guelph. Dr. Brown's research on the information seeking behaviors of scientists, information literacy of science students, and scientific databases has been published in the *Journal of Nutrition*, the *Bulletin of the Medical Library Association*, *College & Research Libraries*, and the *Journal of the American Society for Information Science and Technology*.

DANA TULEY-WILLIAMS is a circulation/reference librarian at Oklahoma City Community College and is a former cataloging instructor at East Central University in Ada, Oklahoma. She earned a B.A. and an M.L.I.S. from the University of Oklahoma.